Contents

CONTENTS

Contributors

Patrick F D'Arcy OBE BPharm PhD DSc FRPharmS Cchem FRCS FPSNI, Formerly Emeritus Professor of Pharmacy, Queen's University of Belfast, Northern Ireland

Jane R Griffin BA(Hons) MSc, Boehringer Ingelheim Ltd, Bracknell, Berkshire, UK

John P Griffin BSc PhD MBBS FRCP MRCS FRCPath FFPM, John Griffin Associates Ltd, Welwyn, Hertfordshire, UK

Dean WG Harron BSc PhD FRPharmS MPSNI, Professor, School of Pharmacy, Queen's University of Belfast, Northern Ireland

Janice Hirshorn BSc (Hons) PhD FAICD, Consultant, Rose Bay NSW, Australia

Christopher JS Hodges MA (Oxon), CMS Cameron McKenna, London, UK; Honorary Research Associate, New College, Oxford, UK

Peter Barton Hutt, Partner in the law firm of Covington and Burling, Washington DC, USA; Lecturer in Food and Drug Law, Harvard Law School; former Chief Counsel to the US FDA

Judith K Jones MD PhD, President, The Degge Group; President, The Pharmaceutical Education and Research Institute; Adjunct Professor of Pharmacology, Georgetown University, Washington DC, USA

Yuichi Kubo, Daiichi Pharmaceutical Co. Ltd, Tokyo, Japan

Louis Lasagna MD, Dean, Sackler School of Graduate Biomedical Sciences, Tufts University School of Medicine, Boston MA, USA

Deborah Monk BPharm Dip Hosp Pharm BA, Director Scientific and Technical Affairs, Medicines Australia, Deakin ACT, Australia

John O'Grady MD FRCP FFPM FBIRA MRCPath, European Medical Director, Daiichi Pharmaceutical Co. Ltd, London, UK

Rashmi R Shah BSc MB MD FRCP FFPM, Senior Medical Officer, Medicines Control Agency, London, UK

Richard N Spivey Pharm D PhD, Vice President, Medical and Regulatory Affairs, MedPointe Inc, Somerset NJ, USA

William Wardell MD PhD, President, Wardell Associates International, Princeton NJ, USA

Amanda Wearing MA(Oxon), Solicitor, Arnold & Porter, London, UK

Preface

The Regulation of Medical Products has been expanded from *The Textbook of Pharmaceutical Medicine* (Griffin and O'Grady) – the syllabus course book for the Diploma in Pharmaceutical Medicine – and introduces new material into some of the existing chapters, including new chapters and appendices.

In early 2002, the British Government agreed to recognise pharmaceutical medicine as an accredited medical specialty. This has necessitated the formalisation of Higher Medical Training (HMT), which leads to the Certificate of Completion of Specialist Training (CCST) with the General Medical Council (GMC). The road to a CCST in pharmaceutical medicine will mean a minimum of two years' general medical training after full registration by the GMC. Such experience requires clinical care of general medical patients, and two years spent in, for example, histopathology alone would not suffice. This will be followed by at least four years' experience, during which an *ad personum* period of specialist training in pharmaceutical medicine would be taken. An integral part of this schedule will be the need to pass the Diploma in Pharmaceutical Medicine after a minimum of two years' experience in pharmaceutical medicine. This diploma is a knowledge based examination, and as stated previously, *The Textbook of Pharmaceutical Medicine* has been specifically written to cover the diploma syllabus.

Successful completion of the diploma examination allows a candidate to apply for Membership of the Faculty of Pharmaceutical Medicine. Candidates pursuing their CCST will have an *ad personum* course drawn up for them. All candidates must complete six modules of HMT. Two modules may be taken as some of their "on the job" experience (in whole or in part), and four modules are taught again in whole or in part. The breakdown will depend on the breadth of work experience each person can expect to receive. Exemption from a module may be claimed in some circumstances. For example, a person with a CCST in clinical pharmacology may be exempt from that module, or a person with an MSc in medical statistics may not have to take the statistics module. However, the six modules for HMT will be geared to assess competence as well as knowledge.

It is hoped that this book will be a convenient format for use in the module of Medicines Regulation.

The book will also be of value to those working in regulatory affairs, prescribing doctors, and pharmacists.

JP Griffin
J O'Grady

vii

Acknowledgements

The editors would like to thank the contributors for the prompt manner in which they produced their manuscripts and processed their proofs. We would also like to thank the staff of BMJ Books for their courteous efficiency in dealing with the production of this and our other books; our particular thanks are extended to Mary Banks, who has the ability to keep things moving and to schedule with great charm.

We would also like to thank Greenwich Medical Ltd for permission to publish a revised version of Christopher Hodges' chapter on the regulation of medical devices in this book, which draws upon his earlier chapter in *Medicines, medical devices and the law*, edited by John O'Grady, I Dodds Smith, N Walsh and M Spencer.

JP Griffin
J O'Grady

The editors

Professor John P Griffin BSc PhD MBBS FRCP MRCS FRCPath FFPM qualified in medicine at the Royal London Hospital, where he was also in clinical practice. He was a lecturer in Physiology at King's College, London and held the post of Head of Clinical Research at Riker Laboratories from 1967 to 1971. Professor Griffin joined the then Medicines Division of the Department of Health, now Medicines Control Agency (MCA) London, as a Senior Medical Officer, in 1971, and was subsequently appointed Medical Assessor to the Committee on Safety of Medicines. From 1977 to 1984, Professor Griffin was Senior Principal Medical Officer and Professional Head of Medicines Division as well as being Medical Assessor to the Medicines Commission. As Professional Head of Medicines Division he also attended the Scientific Sub-Committee of the Veterinary Products Committee of the Ministry of Agriculture, Food and Fisheries. During this time he was a member of the EC committee on Proprietary Medicinal Products and Chairman of the CPMP's Working Party on Safety Requirements.

From 1976 to 1984 John Griffin served on the Joint Formulary Committee of the British National Formulary, during which period the first eight issues of the current format were produced.

John Griffin was the Director of the Association of the British Pharmaceutial Industry from 1984 to 1994. During this time he was a member of the Executive Board of the European Federation of Pharmaceutical Industries' Associations and a council member of the International Federation of Pharmaceutical Industry Associations IFPMA.

John Griffin chaired the ICH Safety Expert Working Group from 1988 to 1994 and presented papers at ICH1 and ICH2 in the plenary sessions.

Since June 1994 John Griffin has run his own independent consultancy company, which has provided independent and impartial advice to governments on the development of a pharmaceutical policy, to national trade associations and individual companies. John Griffin is Visiting Professor in Pharmaceutical Medicine at the University of Surrey, and is also Honorary Consultant Clinical Pharmacologist at the Lister Hospital in Hertfordshire, UK.

Professor Griffin is on the Board of the Faculty of Pharmaceutical Medicine and Chairman of the Board of Examiners of the Faculty of Pharmaceutical Medicine of the Royal Colleges of Physicians, and serves on the Task Force on Specialist Medical Training in Pharmaceutical Medicine. He served on a number of Royal College of Physicians London Working Parties including that on the "Development of Clinical Pharmacology and Therapeutics in a Changing World".

Professor Griffin is the author and co-author of over 250 publications on adverse drug reactions and iatrogenic disease, aspects of neurophysiology and clinical pharmacology and toxicology and drug regulation. Among his publications are the four following standard texts:

Iatrogenic Diseases Oxford University Press, 1st ed. 1972, 3rd ed. 1986; jointly with Professor PF D'Arcy

A Manual of Adverse Drug Interactions John Wright Bristol, 1st ed. 1975; Elsevier Press Amsterdam, 5th ed. 1997; jointly with Professor PF D'Arcy

The Textbook of Pharmaceutical Medicine The Queen's University of Belfast Press, 1st ed. 1993, 2nd ed. 1994, 3rd ed. 1998, 4th ed. BMJ Books 2002 jointly with Professor J O'Grady.

Medicines, Research, Regulation and Risk The Queen's University of Belfast Press, 1st ed. 1989, 2nd ed. 1992.

Since 1991 he has been Editor in Chief of *Adverse Drug Reactions and Toxicological Reviews*, a peer-reviewed journal produced quarterly by Oxford University Press, which publishes in-depth assessments relating to drug and chemical safety issues.

Professor John O'Grady MD FRCP FFPM FBIRA MRCPath, after graduating in medicine, trained in general medicine and also in clinical pharmacology and therapeutics to achieve specialist registrations. He held medical appointments at the Radcliffe Infirmary in Oxford, Royal Postgraduate Medical School, Hammersmith Hospital, Hospital for Nervous Diseases Queen's Square, London and St Bartholomew's Hospital, London.

Formerly Head of Clinical Pharmacology at Wellcome Research Laboratories, he was then made Medical Director at Rhone-Poulenc and Visiting Professor at the University of Cape Town, South Africa.

Currently, he is a Medical Director for Europe, Daiichi Pharmaceuticals UK Ltd, a director of Imperial Cancer Research Technology Ltd, Visiting Professor of Clinical Pharmacology and Therapeutics at the University of Vienna, Austria, and Visiting Professor of Clinical Pharmacology, University of London.

Professor O'Grady is Examiner to the Royal College of Physicians, Faculty of Pharmaceutical Medicine. He is a Fellow of the Royal Statistical Society and a member of the British Pharmacopoeia Commission.

He has published widely in the field of medicine, in clinical pharmacology and therapeutics and in pharmaceutical medicine. He is editor of several books dealing with drug effects in man and with medicines and the law, including *The Textbook of Pharmaceutical Medicine* jointly with JP Griffin.

1: History of drug regulation in the UK

JOHN P GRIFFIN, RASHMI R SHAH

1.1 Introduction

Our concepts on how medicines should be tested and regulated have evolved very gradually over time, perhaps dating back to 120 BC. This chapter is a brief account of some of the major events that have guided drug regulation to what it is today in the UK.

Mithridates VI, 120 BC, King of Pontus, concocted a compound preparation called "Mithridatium" which was held as a panacea for almost every illness until the 1780s. Having investigated the powers of a number of single ingredients, which he found to be antidotes to various venoms and poisons individually, he evaluated them experimentally. The required "clinical trials" were conducted on condemned criminals! Once an ingredient was found to be effective, Mithridates proceeded to incorporate it into his compound preparation, which included 41 individual components when fully formulated. Another formulation of Mithridatium, known as "Galene", which included 55 components, was also available from the days of Andromachus (c.50 AD). "Galene" means "tranquility" and also became known as a "theriac". The concoction took some 40 days to prepare, after which the process of maturation began. Twelve years was considered by Galen the proper period to keep it before use. The quality of Mithridatium and Galene was important since, as late as 1540, failure of their efficacy was attributed to the use of poor quality ingredients.

Mithridatium and Galene had also found their way into England, where, after the founding of the Royal College of Physicians in 1518, their manufacture was made subject to supervision under the Apothecary Wares, Drugs and Stuffs Act of 1540. This Act was one of the earliest British statutes on the control of drugs and it empowered the Physicians to appoint four inspectors of "Apothecary Wares, Drugs and Stuffs".

Standards for the manufacture of Mithridatium and Galene were laid down in *The London Pharmacopoeia* in 1618 (see Figure 1.1). The

1

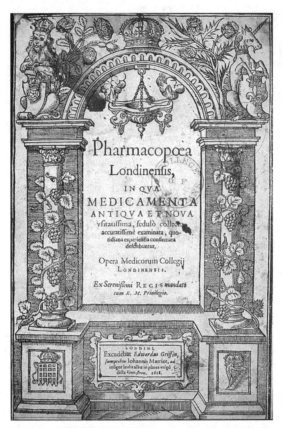

Figure 1.1 Frontpiece of *The London Pharmacopoeia*, 1618. (Reproduced with kind permission from The Hunterian Libraries, The Royal College of Physicians, London.)

manufacture of these theriacs took place in public with much pomp and ceremony (Figure 1.2). It was commonly thought by those in authority that if Mithridatium did not produce the desired cure, this was due to incorrect preparation (perhaps with adulterated or poor quality materials) or to incorrect storage after use. However, Galen records that Marcus Aurelius consumed the preparation within two months of its being compounded without ill effect.

In 1665, during the Great Plague of London, Charles II turned to the Royal College of Physicians for advice. This advice recommended, among other measures, that the victims of the plague who developed buboes were to be treated with a plaster of either Mithridatium or Galene applied hot thrice daily.

Many physicians in the early eighteenth century had doubts as to whether Mithridatium was the universal panacea of all illness as claimed. The ultimate mortal attack on the remedy came from Dr William Heberden (1710–1801), better known clinically for his description of the "Heberden's nodes" in osteoarthritis (see Figure 1.3). Consequently, the

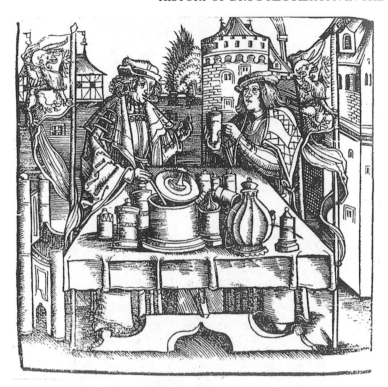

Figure 1.2   Manufacture of Mithridatium.

1746 edition of *The London Pharmacopoeia* was the last in which references to Mithridatium appear. With its disappearance, the long-used complex remedy attributable to an experimental toxicologist from the first century BC came to an end. Perhaps in the final analysis the contribution of Mithridatium to modern medicine was that concerns about quality stimulated the earliest concepts of medicines regulation.

Concerns on the safety of medicines began to emerge when the laws on vaccination against smallpox were tightened in 1853 and later in 1871 when a House of Commons Select Committee, set up to investigate the efficacy of the compulsory system, was concerned by a report by Dr Jonathan Hutchinson who gave an account of the transmission of syphilis in two patients by arm-to-arm inoculation.

Following the discovery and clinical use of chloroform in 1847, The Royal Medical and Chirurgical Society (later to become The Royal Society of Medicine) had already set up in 1864 a committee to enquire "into the uses and the physiological, therapeutical and toxicological effects of chloroform". There had been 109 fatalities following administration of chloroform. A critical relationship had been demonstrated between the

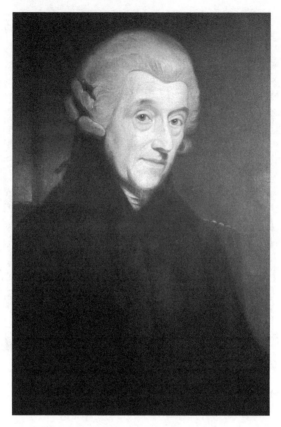

Figure 1.3 Dr William Heberden (1710–1801). (Reproduced with kind permission from The Hunterian Libraries, The Royal College of Physicians, London.)

dose and effect of this anaesthetic. The committee commented on the need for animal experiments to compare chloroform with ether and also on the relative cardiac safety of ether.

At the British Medical Association meeting in Manchester in 1877, Spencer Wells strongly advocated urgent investigations into how anaesthesia, effective as it was, might be rendered safe for the future. The British Medical Association too set up its own working party in 1877 to investigate sudden deaths following chloroform anaesthesia and had suggested setting up an independent body to assess its safety. This BMA working party published its report in 1880 but this had little impact on generating public or political concern to set up a regulatory authority. The safety of chloroform was to resurface as late as 1978 (see later).

The stimulus ultimately came following the publications of two BMA papers entitled "Secret Remedies" in 1909 and "More Secret Remedies" in 1912. These prompted a Parliamentary Select Committee on Patent Medicines to be set up. This Select Committee reported in 1914, but the outbreak of war resulted in the shelving of all proposed legislation.

Following the discovery of arsphenamine (Salvarsan) in Germany in 1907, it was imported into the UK until the beginning of World War I, when the Board of Trade issued licences to certain British manufacturers to produce it. Each batch had to be submitted to the Medical Research Council (MRC) for approval before marketing.

The forerunner to monitoring of adverse reactions can be traced to a recommendation in 1922 by the MRC Salvarsan Committee. This Committee, set up to investigate epidemics of jaundice and hepatic necrosis following the use of Salvarsan, encouraged reporting "to the Ministry of Health of details concerning such accidents, for it is only in the light of such information that investigation and measures with regard to their prevention can be successfully undertaken".

Following concerns on impurities and standardisation, the Therapeutic Substances Act was passed in 1925 with the aim of regulating the manufacture of biological substances, providing the standards to which they must conform and regulating their labelling. This Act recognised the significance of the manufacturing process and factory inspection and in-process controls played a large part in supervision by the Ministry of Health. This Therapeutic Substances Act was later consolidated and strengthened in 1956 when Part II was added, which dealt with control of sale and supply. Records of sale had to be kept and the container had to identify both the manufacturer and the batch. The first schedule to the 1956 Act included the substances commonly known as vaccines, sera, toxins, antitoxins, and antigens.

The Venereal Disease Act of 1917 and The Cancer Act of 1939 had already prevented public advertisement and promotion of drugs for these conditions to protect sufferers from inadequate or unsuitable treatment and fraudulent claims (of efficacy).

Clearly, by the 1950s, fragments of legislation controlling the quality, sale, and promotion of drugs had existed in the UK for many years but these had in general been disease orientated and had little relevance to the therapeutic revolution that was taking place at the time. There seemed to be no major concerns of deficiencies in Europe with the way the drugs were manufactured, placed on the market, and, in a broad sense, controlled.

In France, 102 people had died and 100 more were affected by paraplegia in 1957 as a result of the administration of Stalinon capsules for the treatment of boils. The Stalinon episode had resulted from a formulation error – Stalinon capsules for marketing contained 15 mg diiodoethyltin and 100 mg isolinoleic acid esters. Clinical trials were carried out with capsules containing only 3 mg of diiodoethyltin (one-fifth of the marketed dose)! Subsequent studies in animals and in humans confirmed the neurotoxicity of diiodoethyltin, which was characterised by intramyelinic vacuolation and

5

astrocyte swelling with no evidence of neuronal degeneration. This tragedy, however, was a foretaste of an even much greater disaster – that due to thalidomide.

The thalidomide disaster in 1961 was to blow apart the complacency on regulation of drugs. The confidence in the therapeutic revolution promised by the pharmaceutical industry was shattered and there was considerable public outcry.

1.2 The thalidomide disaster and its immediate aftermath

Thalidomide was a sedative and a hypnotic that first went on sale in 1956 in West Germany. Between 1958 and 1960 it was introduced in 46 countries under 51 different trade names. It was first introduced on the UK market in April 1958 under the name Distaval. It enjoyed good sales because of its prompt action, lack of hangover and addiction observed with barbiturates, and apparent safety.

Following anecdotal reports of benefit in the treatment of vomiting in early pregnancy, it was heavily promoted for this purpose. This use in early pregnancy was soon followed by an epidemic of a previously unknown congenital malformation of the limbs, termed "phocomelia" due to its resemblance to the flippers of a seal, and other associated internal malformations. The first cases were reported from Germany beginning in 1959 but the malformation also began to make an appearance in other countries where the drug was on sale. Curiously, among the West European countries the drug was not marketed in France, which was spared the tragedy.

Of considerable concern was the scale of the disaster resulting from its protracted marketing, the manufacturer continuing to deny all evidence of a causal relationship between these congenital abnormalities and the drug. Worldwide, there were an estimated 10 000 babies with phocomelia and other allied deformities, including more than 500 in England. The frequency of the malformations in Germany followed the absolute sales of the drug with a time lag of a little less than one year. The drug was withdrawn from the market in Germany in November 1961, in the UK in December 1961 and, over the next 10 months thereafter, from most countries of the world. Eight to nine months after the withdrawal of the drug from the market, the wave of the unique malformations disappeared as suddenly as it had appeared after the same time lag that had followed the introduction of the drug. The drug was soon confirmed as a potent teratogen in a number of animal studies.

Governments throughout the Western world were now galvanised into introducing effective drug regulation. Even in the USA, despite the strength of the prevailing legislation on safety, news reports on the role of Dr Frances Kelsey, a medical officer at the Food and Drug Administration

(FDA), in keeping the drug off the US market, aroused much public support for even stronger drug regulation.

For their part, the UK Government set up in August 1962 the Joint Sub-Committee of the English and Scottish Standing Medical Advisory Committees, under the Chairmanship of The Lord Cohen of Birkenhead, with the following terms of reference:

To advise the Minister of Health and the Secretary of State for Scotland on what measures are needed:

* to secure adequate pharmacological and safety testing and clinical trials of new drugs before their release for general use
* to secure early detection of adverse effects arising after their release for general use and
* to keep doctors informed of the experiences of such drugs in clinical practice.

1.3 Voluntary controls in the UK (1963–1971)

In its interim advice delivered on 2 November 1962, the Joint Sub-Committee of the English and Scottish Standing Medical Advisory Committees, set up in the aftermath of the thalidomide disaster, made three main recommendations:

* that the responsibility for the experimental laboratory testing of new drugs before they are used in clinical trials should remain with the individual pharmaceutical manufacturer
* that it was neither desirable nor practical that at this stage of their evaluation the responsibility for testing drugs should be transferred to a central authority
* that there should be an expert body to review the evidence and offer advice on the toxicity of new drugs, whether manufactured in Great Britain or abroad, before they were used in clinical trials. (The Sub-Committee proposed in the light of further consideration and consultations, to formulate detailed advice on the composition and terms of this advisory body.)

On 6 November 1962, the Minister of Health announced that the Government had accepted the first two recommendations and would await the advice on the third.

In the period intervening between its interim advice and its final report, the Joint Sub-Committee received memoranda from, and met representatives of, the Association of the British Pharmaceutical Industry (ABPI), the British Medical Association (BMA), the Pharmaceutical Society of Great Britain, and the College of General Practitioners.

Despite reservations expressed by a number of these bodies, the Joint Sub-Committee took the view that public opinion was unlikely to be content with anything short of Ministerial responsibility for verifying that adequate precautions had been taken to secure the safety of drugs, the more so because of the number and nature of new drugs.

The Joint Sub-Committee issued its Final Report on "Safety of Drugs" in March 1963, which states in paragraph 10:

We think that a Committee on Safety of Drugs should be established with sub-committees to advise it on each of the three aspects, namely:

(i) toxicity
(ii) clinical trials and therapeutic efficacy and
(iii) adverse reactions.

1.3.1 Committee on Safety of Drugs (CSD)

The three Health Ministers of the United Kingdom, in consultation with the medical and pharmaceutical professions and the ABPI, set up the Committee on Safety of Drugs (CSD) in June 1963. The three Health Ministers were the Secretary of State for Scotland, the Minister of Health, and the Minister of Health and Social Services, Northern Ireland.

The Committee had the following terms of reference:

(i) To invite from the manufacturer or other person developing or proposing to market a drug in the United Kingdom any reports they may think fit on the toxicity tests carried out on it; to consider whether any further tests should be made and whether the drug should be submitted to clinical trials; and to convey their advice to those who submitted reports.
(ii) To obtain reports of clinical trials of drugs submitted thereto.
(iii) Taking into account the safety and efficacy of each drug, and the purposes for which it is to be used, to consider whether it may be released for marketing, with or without precautions or restrictions on its use; and to convey their advice to those who submitted reports.
(iv) To give to manufacturers and others concerned any general advice they may think fit.
(v) To assemble and assess reports about adverse effects of drugs in use and prepare information thereon which may be brought to the notice of doctors and other concerned.
(vi) To advise the appointing Ministers on any of the above matters.

The Committee consisted of a panel of independent experts from various fields of pharmacy, medicine, and pathology among others, with Sir Derrick Dunlop as its first Chairman. In tribute to his personal charm, considerable skills, and foresight, it soon became popularly known as the "Dunlop Committee".

Table 1.1 Membership of the Committee on Safety of Drugs and its Sub-Committees (1963)

Committee on Safety of Drugs	Sub-Committee on Adverse Reactions	Sub-Committee on Toxicity	Sub-Committee on Clinical Trials and Therapeutic Efficacy
(All committee papers to be printed on white paper)	*(All sub-committee papers to be printed on yellow paper)*	*(All sub-committee papers to be printed on green paper)*	*(All sub-committee papers to be printed on pink paper)*
Sir Derrick Dunlop *(Chairman)*	Prof LJ Witts *(Chairman)*	Prof AC Frazer *(Chairman)*	Prof RB Hunter *(Chairman)*
Prof AC Frazer *(Deputy Chairman)*	Prof OL Wade *(Deputy Chairman)*	Prof EF Scowen *(Deputy Chairman)*	Prof GM Wilson *(Deputy Chairman)*
Prof LJ Witts	Dr EV Kuenssberg	Dr F Hartley	Dr W Linford-Rees
Prof EF Scowen	Prof DJ Finney	Dr LG Goodwin	Sir Austin Bradford Hill
Prof GM Wilson	Dr KR Capper	Prof GJ Cunningham	Prof TNA Jeffcoate
Prof OL Wade	Prof WW Mushin	Dr PN Magee	Prof DR Laurence
Prof WW Mushin		Mr TC Denston	
Dr EY Kuenssberg			
Dr F Hartley			
Mr TC Denston			
Sir Austin Bradford Hill			
Prof RB Hunter			

The Committee had no legal powers but worked with the voluntary agreement of the ABPI and the Proprietary Association of Great Britain (PAGB). These associations promised that none of their members would put on clinical trial or release for marketing a new drug against the advice of the Committee and whose advice they would always seek. In an attempt to make sure that the manufacturers adhered to this, the Health Ministers undertook, in a circular sent to all dentists and doctors in the UK, to inform the prescribers of any cases of drugs being marketed or put to clinical trials without the Committee's approval.

A number of sub-committees were also established to assist the main Committee. These were the Sub-Committee on Toxicity and the Sub-Committee on Clinical Trials and Therapeutic Efficacy. Against the background of the thalidomide tragedy, an important sub-committee established was the Sub-Committee on Adverse Reactions. The memberships of the main Committee and its three Sub-Committees when first established in 1963 are shown in Table 1.1.

The Committee spent the first six months of its existence (the latter half of 1963) in completing its preparatory work. By 1 January 1964, the Committee was in a position to invite submissions (this is what they were called, and not "applications") on drugs intended for clinical trials or about to be released for the market.

In 1967, the Sub-Committee on Toxicity and the Sub-Committee on Clinical Trials and Therapeutic Efficacy were merged since the interests of the two were shown by experience to overlap considerably. The new sub-committee, the Sub-Committee on Toxicity, Clinical Trials and Therapeutic Efficacy, was chaired by Professor AC Frazer with Professor EF Scowen (later Sir Eric Scowen) as the Deputy Chairman.

1.3.2 CSD secretariat

The Committee on Safety of Drugs was serviced by a professional secretariat of pharmacists and medical officers who undertook the assessment of the submissions and presented these to the Committee and its various sub-committees. The secretariat initially included three doctors and two pharmacists. In 1965, the number of professional staff had been increased to six doctors and three pharmacists. Among the six doctors was Dr Denis Cahal, who headed the secretariat. Others were Drs J Broadbent, M Hollyhock, WH Inman, D Mansel-Jones, and C Ruttle. Dr Cahal was one of the founder members of the Medicines Division in 1964. The close collaboration between Dr Cahal and Sir Derrick Dunlop was pivotal in guiding the Medicines Act through Parliament and setting the foundation of a system that became a model to the rest of the world for fairness and efficiency.

The secretariat was originally based at Queen Anne's Mansions, Queen Anne's Gate, London SW1, where the Committee and the sub-committees also held their meetings. The secretariat was moved on 1 April 1971 to new accommodation at Finsbury Square House, 33/37a Finsbury Square, London EC2A 1PP. Still later in March 1980, it moved to its current imposing location, overlooking the River Thames, at Market Towers, 1 Nine Elms Lane, Vauxhall, London SW8 5NQ.

Each manufacturer was given a four-digit company number for identification and this number was to be used for all their product-related documents – a system that prevails even today. For example, Geigy (UK) Ltd was 0001, Glaxo Group Ltd was 0004, John Wyeth & Brother Ltd was 0011, Astra-Hewlett Ltd was 0017, Parke Davis & Co. was 0018, AB Kabi was 0022, ER Squibb & Sons Ltd was 0034, Abbott Laboratories Ltd was 0037, and for those who are given to reminisce and remember it, Beecham Research Laboratories was 0038. The order of the allocation of these numbers was determined by the order in which the submissions were received by the new regulatory body from the companies. Thus, Geigy (UK) Ltd was the first company ever to make a submission to CSD. A second four-digit set of numbers followed the company number (that is, 0000/0000) and related to the individual products licensed for sale to that company, again in a numerical order by which the submissions for marketing authorisations were received.

1.3.3   The legacy of the Committee on Safety of Drugs

Even in these embryonic days, the Committee was to set down many important principles that still dominate drug regulation today.

The Committee had required as a minimum teratogenicity testing in two species, one of which should preferably be a non-rodent, for one generation only. They also recognised the limitations of teratogenicity tests in animals but emphasised that only in the most exceptional circumstances would they release any drug for clinical trial in women of child-bearing age until the appropriate tests on animals had been carried out satisfactorily.

The Committee also required a wider interpretation of the term "new drugs" to include "*new formulations of existing drugs, drugs to be presented for a new purpose, and existing substances not previously used as drugs, covering virtually all new products introduced*". The Committee had clearly appreciated that new formulations ought to be subject to scrutiny since reformulation did occasionally introduce additional hazards.

Perhaps one of the most important years in drug regulation in the UK was 1965. That year, the manufacturers began to challenge the right of the Committee to require under its terms of reference evidence of efficacy of a drug. The Committee took the view that for serious diseases failure of efficacy constituted an unacceptable risk, while for trivial diseases where efficacy may be irrelevant, even a trivial safety hazard is not acceptable – the concept of modern day "risk/benefit". The Committee also emphasised that it was not concerned with efficacy and its clearance of a drug for the market did not necessarily imply its approval of it as a valuable remedy. The Committee also noted "*Medicines are not sacrosanct however simply because they have been in use for a long time*".

During the year there were a number of reports in the press of deaths associated with phenacetin. The Committee emphasised that the hazard was associated with the abuse of the drug (excessive doses taken over a long term) and reiterated that, consequently, no special action was necessary. Furthermore, because a drug (including phenacetin) could be marketed under different proprietary names, it could confuse a doctor. Therefore, the Committee decided that they would not consider an application by a manufacturer to market a new substance unless the applicant gave an assurance that an Approved Name had been obtained or applied for.

When considering new drug submissions, the Committee also paid attention to the claims and indications that the promoter intended to include on the label of a drug or in promotional literature. Another significant step taken by the Committee related to labelling of the prescribed medicines by pharmacists. The practice of labelling the container as "The Tablets" was no longer considered acceptable (unless the prescribing doctor specified otherwise). After canvassing the opinions of many professional bodies, including all Royal Colleges, the BMA and the Pharmaceutical Society of Great Britain had agreed by 1971 to the proposal of marking of prescriptions "Nomen Proprium".

The period 1966–7 was one of consolidation. The Committee had received considerable support for and re-emphasised all their previous recommendations. Between 1964 and 1967 the Committee received representatives from the World Health Organisation (WHO) and many European and Far and Middle Eastern countries, as well as from Canada and the USA, to study its methods.

In 1966 the Committee made observations on a hazard that increasingly plagues many drugs even today – the problems of drug–drug interactions. The Committee noted

> It is now well known that the administration of one drug may considerably modify the actions of another being given at the same time. Both the toxicity and the metabolism of each drug may be affected by the other. This applies to combinations of drugs in one preparation as well as to those separately administered. However, it is still too readily assumed by some manufacturers that no additional hazard is incurred by combining two or more drugs in one preparation.

The first drug–drug interaction alert issued by the Committee in 1966 concerned the risks from interactions between preparations containing adrenaline or noradrenaline and monoamine oxidase inhibitors (MAO) used for the treatment of depression.

In its final report, in 1969–70, the Committee expressed safety concerns arising from the names of products that differ, for example, only by a suffixed letter, and expressed a desire to see the naming of products put on a more rational basis.

It is interesting that for entirely new chemical entities, submissions in these early days of drug regulation were "often voluminous: a submission containing over 1000 pages of reports, drafts and tables was not unusual". Rejection of drugs outright was a comparatively minor part of the Committee's operations; by far the more important actions involved persuading manufacturers to make changes in their intentions (formulation, indication, etc.).

In 1965, a great majority of submissions had concerned reformulation of established drugs. The number of submissions for reformulated preparations of established drugs was even higher in 1966, a matter that concerned the Committee in respect of "the extent to which the drug houses have tended to flood the market with so many similar preparations". As a result, Mr CA Johnson (a pharmacist) and Dr DFJ Mason (a toxicologist) were also then appointed to the Sub-Committee on Toxicity. The work of the Committee during their tenure from January 1964 to 31 August 1971 in terms of submissions received and determined is shown in Table 1.2.

Table 1.2 Submissions to the Committee on Safety of Drugs (1964–1971)

	1964	1965	1966	1967	1968	1969	1970	1971
Clinical trial submissions	66 (11·0%)	168 (19·2%)	203 (22·4%)	202 (26·4%)	239 (30·2%)	218 (25·7%)	178 (24·9%)	122 (22·0%)
Marketing submissions	534	706	705	563	552	630	536	432
Total (inc. NCEs)	600 (55)	874 (69)	908 (66)	765 (56)	791 (56)	848 (66)	714 (69)	554 (??)
Approved	386	807	771	698	669	694	499	411
Rejected	15 (2·5%)	19 (1·8%)	24 (2·4%)	36 (4·1%)	36 (4·1%)	33 (3·5%)	53 (6·3%)	38 (5·0%)
Withdrawn by applicant	32 (5·3%)	119 (11·4%)	86 (8·6%)	70 (7·9%)	83 (9·5%)	86 (9·2%)	79 (9·4%)	66 (8·7%)
Further information requested	99 (16·5%)	49 (4·7%)	39 (3·9%)	43 (4·8%)	34 (3·9%)	47 (5·0%)	68 (8·1%)	74 (9·7%)
Pending further consideration	68	47	84	41	53	75	137	170
Total	600	1041	1004	888	875	935	836	759

NCEs, new clinical entities.

From time to time, the Committee received submissions relating to vaccines or immunological products. When considering these, the Committee felt the need to seek advice of experts in that special field. Therefore, in November 1969 it was decided to set up a Vaccine Advisory Group. This initiative ultimately culminated in the establishment of the Sub-Committee on Biological Substances, and the Biological Standards Act received the Royal Assent in February 1975. This Act provided for the establishment of a National Biological Standards Board to manage the activities carried out at the National Institute for Biological Standards and Control. The Institute undertook the control of testing of biological substances used for therapeutic, prophylactic, and diagnostic purposes (for example, vaccines, sera, antibiotics) to discharge their obligations under the Therapeutic Substances Act 1956 and the Medicines Act 1968.

In 1969, it came to the attention of the Committee that unidentified tablets of a drug purporting to be nitrazepam were being distributed in the United Kingdom. The Ministers issued a press statement warning those concerned not to use any other but the branded product that the Committee had cleared. Likewise, in early 1970 it came to public (!) notice that one manufacturer was proposing to market L-dopa, a drug which at

Table 1.3   Membership of Committee on Safety of Drugs and its Sub-Committees (December 1970)

Committee on Safety of Drugs	Sub-Committee on Adverse Reactions	Sub-Committee on Toxicity, Clinical Trials and Therapeutic Efficacy
Prof EF Scowen (*Chairman*)	Prof WRS Doll (*Chairman*)	Prof GM Wilson (*Chairman*)
Prof WI Cranston	CW Barrett	Prof CT Dollery
Prof T Crawford	Prof WI Cranston	Sir Austin Bradford Hill
Prof CT Dollery	Prof J Crooks	Prof PJ Huntingford
Sir Austin Bradford Hill	Dr DM Davies	Prof DR Laurence
Dr DC Garratt	Prof DJ Finney	Prof PN Magee
Prof PJ Huntingford★	Dr MJ Linnett	Dr DFJ Mason
Dr EV Kuenssberg	Prof GR Lowe	Prof DVW Parke
Prof DR Laurence	Prof WW Mushin	Prof W Linford-Rees
Prof PN Magee	Prof DA Price Evans	
Prof WW Mushin	Dr DW Vere	
Prof DVW Parke	Prof RD Weir	
Prof W Linford-Rees		
Prof JB Stenlake		
Prof GM Wilson		
Prof JS Scott★		

★Appointed to a new post abroad. Therefore Prof PJ Huntingford resigned and he was replaced by Prof JS Scott in September 1971.

the time was still under clinical trial for the treatment of Parkinsonism, without first making a submission to the Committee. The Department of Health responded by issuing a statement advising strongly against the use of this drug from any source that had not been approved by the Committee. By the end of 1969, the Committee was able to "fast track" the only two submissions for approval of clinical trials with L-dopa for its use in Parkinsonism. These manufacturers were encouraged by the Committee to submit the data early and it was possible to release some L-dopa preparations for marketing during the earlier part of 1970.

The membership of the Committee on Safety of Drugs and its sub-committees changed further following the resignation of Sir Derrick Dunlop in May 1969 as a result of his appointment as the first Chairman of the Medicines Commission (MC), established under the Medicines Act 1968.

Professor AC Frazer was appointed to succeed Sir Derrick but unfortunately died shortly thereafter. During 1969, therefore, Professor EF Scowen succeeded Professor Frazer as the Chairman of the Committee. In June 1970 the membership of the Committee was revised to correspond with that of the then newly established (under section 4 of the Medicines Act) Committee on Safety of Medicines (CSM). The full membership of the Committee on Safety of Drugs as at 31 December 1970 is shown in Table 1.3.

1.3.4 Voluntary adverse reactions reporting system: the "Yellow Card Scheme"

The Committee on Safety of Drugs had also started studies of adverse reactions to drugs (ADRs) by the beginning of 1964. On 15 June 1964, Sir Derrick Dunlop wrote to all the doctors and dentists, inviting them "to report to us promptly details of any untoward condition in a patient which might be the result of drug treatment". They were assured that "all the reports or replies that the Committee receive from them will be treated with complete professional confidence by the Committee and their staff. The Health Ministers have given an undertaking that the information supplied will never be used for disciplinary purposes or for enquiries about prescribing costs".

This spontaneous adverse reaction reporting system was the brainchild of Professor Leslie Witts and was, and still is, based upon the submission of ADR reports by doctors and dentists by means of reply-paid yellow cards, and hence it is popularly known as the "Yellow Card Scheme".

In the first year up to 100 yellow card reports were received each week. In the case of "serious suspected adverse reactions which might call for action it is necessary, therefore, to have more information about the reported incident and a number of doctors have been appointed throughout the country who will help the Committee on a part-time basis by following up reports". At the end of 1965, there were 35 such part-time doctors helping with the follow up of serious reports. During the first five years the number of reports received averaged about 60 per week, but the problem of determining number of prescriptions was soon recognised. The Committee needed to relate the number of reports with exposure. It concluded, "it is possible to determine the ratio of adverse reactions only by asking a number of doctors who have prescribed a drug about their experience of it with special reference to the adverse reactions which, from reports, appear to be associated with its use".

The Committee, as early as 1964, seemed to have anticipated Prescription Event Monitoring as well as the need for compiling large databases. It thought of a scheme which "involves taking a sample of prescriptions written by doctors for the drugs being investigated. In the United Kingdom the assembly of National Health Service prescriptions for pricing purposes offers a unique opportunity for this sort of analysis which is not available anywhere else in the world and the pricing bureaux have kindly offered their help." Regarding large databases, it went on "prescription scripts are not at present filed in a way which allows easy identification of particular drugs but with the co-operation of the pricing bureaux, the Committee are developing a satisfactory procedure".

Since new drugs are often at first used in hospitals and "it is at this stage that serious adverse reactions are likely to be noticed", a pilot scheme was set up with a number of hospitals for recording prescriptions and the Committee devised a "list of specially monitored drugs" which at "any time will contain all the new substances introduced during the previous two years and a number of older drugs which still need special observation". This clearly was the forerunner to the present "Black Triangle" Scheme that operates today to identify drugs requiring intensive monitoring for at least two years.

When a safety problem was suspected, the promotion of information on safety of drugs was an important remit of the Committee and this they discharged by issuing a series of leaflets to all the doctors and dentists in the UK. The first alert leaflet in this series entitled *"Adverse Reactions Series"* was issued by the Committee on Safety of Drugs in February 1964. It dealt with reports of liver damage and blood pressure changes following the use of monoamine oxidase inhibitor drugs. Nine such alert leaflets were issued over the next five years to December 1969. The contents of these alerts are summarised in an earlier account.[1]

In 1967, computer facilities were installed for handling the yellow card reports and, after consultation, a method of confidential feedback to the profession was designed. A doctor reporting an adverse reaction to a drug was automatically sent a summary of all the reports received by the Committee on the drug and on similar drugs. Where possible, an estimate of the extent to which the drug was prescribed was also given.

By 1965, the value of the Yellow Card Scheme was clearly established and two other countries had introduced a similar scheme. By the beginning of 1967, the Committee was also cooperating in the WHO's Pilot Study on the Monitoring of Adverse Reactions to Drugs at an international level. By the end of 1968, a total of ten countries were participating in this Pilot Study. This study matured into the international WHO ADR Monitoring Centre with a membership which now stands at 67 with six others enjoying associate status.

The Yellow Card Scheme was now beginning to pay dividends. In early 1966, the Yellow Card Scheme had identified methyldopa as a cause of haemolytic anaemia and an appropriate advice was issued. Another success was the detection of a faulty batch of a particular product, which the manufacturer immediately withdrew, underlining the value of an efficient procedure for tracing a batch. During June 1967 the Committee distributed a leaflet on the use of aerosols in asthma. This was prompted by the death rate amongst asthmatic patients aged 5 to 34 years that had risen some 300% above the level in 1959–60 when such preparations were introduced. By September 1968, the rate had dropped to only 50% above that seen in 1959–60 despite sales having dropped only 20%.

Among the first three "old" drugs to be withdrawn from the market during the tenure of the Committee on Safety of Drugs were benziodarone, a vasodilator launched in 1962 and withdrawn in 1964 due to reports of jaundice, pronethalol, a β-blocker introduced in 1963 and withdrawn in 1965 due to animal carcinogenicity, and phenoxypropazine, an antidepressant introduced in 1961 and withdrawn in 1966 due to its hepatotoxicity.

The first major new drug to be approved and withdrawn from the market by the CSD was ibufenac, the first of the non-steroidal anti-inflammatory drugs (NSAID) to be marketed. Ibufenac was a precursor of ibuprofen and its use in the UK was associated with serious and frequent hepatotoxicity. Two other drug withdrawals (also approved during their tenure by CSD) were chlormadinone and fenclozic acid.

During 1969–1970, the nephropathic hazards of phenacetin again attracted much attention and the Committee made a seminal observation that has profoundly influenced our regulatory philosophy even today: "*It is the safety of drugs in normal usage that is the Committee's concern, and because all drugs have their hazards when abused, particularly by over-dosage, the Committee has not considered that it should take special action in connection with phenacetin*".

The "demise" of the CSD was marked by a reception at Lancaster House in December 1971. It was attended by the Secretary of State together with the Health Ministers of Scotland, Wales and Northern Ireland as well as by the current and previous members of CSD, its first Chairman, Sir Derrick Dunlop, the Presidents of the Royal Colleges, and representatives of the medical and pharmaceutical professions and pharmaceutical industry.

The Committee on Safety of Drugs had already set the pattern for effective drug controls in the future.

1.4   The Medicines Act 1968

The Joint Sub-Committee of the English and Scottish Standing Medical Advisory Committee, chaired by The Lord Cohen of Birkenhead, had included as its members seven distinguished clinicians and pharmacists of the day.[2] They were:

Prof S Alstead, CBE, MD, FRCP, FRFPS
AB Davies, BSc, MD, ChB, MRCS, LRCP
Prof Sir Charles Dodds, MVO, MD, DSc, FRCP, FRS
JB Grosset, MPS, DBA
Sir Hugh Linstead, OBE, LLD, FPS, MP
Prof EJ Wayne, MD, FRCP, FRFPS
Prof GM Wilson, MD, FRCP

The Joint Sub-Committee had concluded that testing was the responsibility of the manufacturers and they appeared to favour a voluntary scheme of control.

Para 25: Sanctions under a Voluntary Scheme

While a voluntary scheme could have no formal legal sanctions, we think that the following measures might help, nevertheless, to ensure that new drugs were subject to adequate toxicity testing and clinical trials ...

However, the two eminent pharmacists, John Grosset and Hugh Linstead, appended to the report a lengthy note of dissent that was forceful and stated with uncompromising clarity:

Voluntary or Statutory Control of Toxicity Testing and Clinical Trials?
Our main disagreement with our colleagues lies in the answer to this question. They favour a voluntary system until time can be found for legislation. We believe that any voluntary system must have so many loopholes that it can offer no real additional safeguards to the public. In consequence, we consider that there is no satisfactory alternative to early legislation.

In their note, they also commented extensively on the deficiencies of a voluntary system. Grosset and Linstead concluded their note with a plea "to set on foot, with or without further enquiry, the preparation of a comprehensive statute dealing with drugs and medicines which will bring the whole field, including the supervision of toxicity testing and clinical trials, under the responsibility of the Health Ministers advised by a central body of experts".

Full voluntary cooperation was clearly not as assured as might have been anticipated. During 1965, the Committee on Safety of Drugs itself seemed to articulate in its Annual Report a carefully concealed aspiration for the introduction of statutory controls on drug regulation. After a period of review and consultation, a White Paper "Forthcoming Legislation on the Safety, Quality and Description of Drugs and Medicines" was published in September 1967 and the Medicines Act based on these proposals received the Royal Assent on 25 October 1968. The Committee on Safety of Drugs "welcomes the statutory provisions which provide a firm basis for the continued evaluation of drug safety in the future".

The Medicines Act 1968 is a comprehensive set of measures replacing most of the previous legislation on the control of medicines for human use and for veterinary use in the UK. It is a consolidation into a single Act of the most desirable features of all previous rules, regulations and Acts in the UK and also includes controls on promotion and sale of drugs. The Act has 136 sections divided into eight Parts (Parts I to VIII) and has a further eight schedules appended to it. Among the important sections for licensing and monitoring purposes are:

- sections 18–24 regarding applications for, and grant and renewal of, licences with section 19 requiring evidence for safety, efficacy and quality when determining an application
- sections 28–30 in respect of suspension, revocation and variation of licences
- sections 31–39 on clinical trials
- sections 51–59 on sale and supply
- sections 85–88 on labelling and leaflets

- sections 92–97 on promotion and advertising
- sections 104–128 on enforcement.

Under section 118 of the Act, all data submitted by a company in support of an application to conduct clinical trials or market a medicinal product are confidential; indeed even the existence of such an application is confidential. Breach of confidentiality attracts penalties and "any person guilty of an offence under this section shall be liable (a) on summary conviction, to a fine not exceeding £400; (b) on conviction on indictment, to a fine or to imprisonment for a term not exceeding two years or to both".

Given the remarkable degree of similarity between the requirements under the Medicines Act 1968 and the legislations prevailing at the time in the USA and the European Economic Community (EEC), the existence of four major legislations, together with their amendments and consequential secondary legislations, is worth bearing in mind.

One was the Federal Pure Food and Drugs Act (also known as the "Wiley Act") that was introduced in the USA in 1906. This law was enacted in response to revelations of worthless, impure and dangerous patent medicines that were claimed to cure almost anything. Another was the Federal Food, Drug and Cosmetic Act 1938 that had been passed following the Elixir Sulfanilamide disaster in the USA during 1937 in which 107 people (mostly children) had died from renal failure associated with its therapeutic use. As the drug was called "elixir", implying that the preparation contained alcohol, the FDA could only make seizure of the product for misbranding. In reaction to this calamity, the US Congress passed the 1938 Act, which, for the first time, required proof of safety before release of a new drug. However, no proof of efficacy was required. Following the thalidomide tragedy in Western Europe, a subsequent New Drug Amendment (the Kefauver–Harris Amendment) was introduced in 1962 that required the FDA to monitor all stages of drug development. As a result of the Kefauver–Harris Amendment, even investigational drugs then required comprehensive animal testing before extensive human trials could be started. Proof of efficacy and safety was mandatory and the time constraints for disposition of new drugs, previously deemed approved by default if the FDA had failed to consider the new drug application by 60 days, were removed.

The EEC had already in place the Council Directive 65/65/EEC on the approximation of provisions laid down by law, regulation or administrative action relating to medicinal products. Many of the requirements of Council Directive 65/65/EEC had already formed part of the Medicines Act. When Directives 75/318/EEC and 75/319/EEC were adopted by the Council of Ministers on 20 May 1975, they only supplemented and amended the original Directive 65/65/EEC. Therefore, the provisions of these two new Directives did not substantially affect the licensing system that operated in the UK under the Medicines Act, although certain relatively minor amendments were necessary.

19

The first provisions laid down in the Medicines Act regarding licensing of medicinal products and other aspects of control came into effect on 1 September 1971 – the "duly appointed day". The Act was administered by the Health and Agriculture Ministers of the United Kingdom acting together as the Licensing Authority or in some cases separately as the health ministers or the agriculture ministers in respect of human and veterinary medicines respectively. The Act allows for Orders and Regulations to be made implementing its provisions and 98 Statutory Instruments had been made by the end of 1977. The first four were made in 1970 (SI 1970/746, 1257, 1304, and 1256), establishing respectively the Medicines Commission, Committee on Safety of Medicines, Veterinary Products Committee, and the British Pharmacopoeia Commission. A full list of these is contained in the Annual Reports for 1976 and 1977 of the Medicines Commission and the section 4 Committees.

1.4.1 The Licensing Authority

Under section 6 of the Medicines Act 1968, the Licensing Authority (LA) is the authority responsible for the grant, renewal, variation, suspension and revocation of licences and certificates. In 1971, the LA was constituted of a body of Ministers consisting of the Secretary of State for Social Services, the Secretary of State for Scotland, the Secretary of State for Wales, the Minister of Health and Social Services for Northern Ireland, the Minister of Agriculture, Fisheries and Food, and the Minister of Agriculture in Northern Ireland.

1.4.2 Medicines Division (DHSS)

The day-to-day administration of the Act for human medicines was delegated to the Medicines Division of the Department of Health and Social Security (DHSS) and was managed jointly by an Under Secretary and the Professional Head of the Division. These Professional Heads of the Medicines Division held the rank of Senior Principal Medical Officer.

Over the period, the successive Professional Heads of the Medicines Division have been Dr DA Cahal (1964–70), Dr D Mansel-Jones (1970–74), Dr EL Harris (1974–77), Dr JP Griffin (1977–84) and Dr G Jones (1984–89). In 1989, when the Medicines Division was reorganised into the Medicines Control Agency (MCA), Dr KH Jones was appointed the first Director of the new Agency.

Before the UK joined the EU, the Medicines Division had developed close links with other authorities both within and outside the EU. Notable among these were the "Tripartite Meetings" held biannually with the US FDA and the Canadian Health Protection Branch. These meetings, lasting a few days, discussed all areas of drug regulation generally and problems with specific drugs. Having first started in 1971, these meetings continued, while the EU system was evolving during the UK membership, until 1991 (apart from a very brief lull during the mid-1980s). By 1991, the

International Conference on Harmonisation (ICH) initiative (see later) had fully matured into the first ICH meeting, to be held in Brussels in November 1991.

1.5 Statutory Controls in the UK (1971 and thereafter)

1.5.1 Medicines Commission

The Medicines Commission, provided for in section 2 of the Act, was established by the Ministers to give them advice generally relating to the execution of the Act (SI 1970/746), with Sir Derrick Dunlop as its first Chairman.

The scope of the functions of the Commission is very wide, but as defined in 1975 may be summarised as follows:

- to advise the LA on matters relating to the execution of the Medicines Act
- to recommend to the Ministers the number and functions of committees to be established under section 4 of the Act and to recommend such persons as they consider well qualified to serve as members of such committees
- to advise the LA in cases where it consults the Commission, including cases where the LA arranges for the applicant for the grant of a licence to have an opportunity of appearing before, and being heard by, the Commission.

Sir Derrick Dunlop's tenure of office ended on 31 December 1971. The Medicines Commission has since then been successively chaired by Lord Rosenheim (from January 1972 to 2 December 1972 when he died suddenly), Professor A Wilson (Acting Chairman December 1972 to the middle of 1973), Sir Ronald Bodley Scott (middle of 1973 to December 1975), Professor WJH Butterfield (later Sir John Butterfield and later still Lord Butterfield, January 1976 to December 1981), Professor Rosalinde Hurley (later Dame Rosalinde Hurley, January 1982 to December 1993), Professor DH Lawson (January 1994 to December 2001), and Professor Parveen Kumar (January 2002 to present).

The establishment of the Medicines Commission in May 1969 was followed by the establishment of a number of expert committees with specific advisory functions, appointed by Ministers after considering the recommendations of the Commission as proposed in section 4 of the Medicines Act. These expert committees, whose members are appointed by Ministers on the advice of the Medicines Commission, advise the Licensing Authority and consist of independent experts such as hospital clinicians, general practitioners, pharmacists, and clinical pharmacologists, and not the staff of the DHSS.

The relevant advisory committees with a remit for medicines for human use established under the Medicines Act 1968 were the Committee on Safety of Medicines (CSM), set up in June 1970 (SI 1970/1257) under the Chairmanship of Professor EF Scowen and the British Pharmacopoeia Commission (BPC), also set up in June 1970 (SI 1970/1256) under the Chairmanship of Dr F Hartley (later Sir Frank Hartley). The Veterinary Products Committee (VPC), chaired by Professor CSG Grunsell (with a remit for medicines for veterinary use and administered through the Ministry of Agriculture Food and Fisheries), was also established in June 1970 (SI 1970/1304). Other important bodies set up were the Joint Sub-Committee on the Use of Antibiotics and Related Substances and Standing Joint Sub-Committee on the Classification of Proprietary Preparations, both of which reported directly to the Medicines Commission.

The products already on the market on 1 September 1971, the date for implementation of the Medicines Act, were given the Product Licences of Right (PLR) that were subject to a review process at a later date. This proposal for review of PLRs is reminiscent of the FDA contract with the National Academy of Sciences/National Research Council (NAS/NRC) in 1966 to evaluate the effectiveness of some 4000 different drug formulations approved on the basis of safety alone between 1938 and 1962 – the year of the Kefauver–Harris Amendment.

In 1977, the Medicines Commission reached a significant milestone when the work on classification of medicines was completed. New arrangements provided for three categories of medicines according to their safety factor – those available on prescription only (POM), those sufficiently safe to be on general sale to the public through any retail outlet (GSL), and an intermediate category of those which should only be sold at pharmacies (P). Under section 59 of the Medicines Act, all new medicinal products, not previously on the market, are prescription only for the first five years. A conscious decision is made for reclassification of each before the five-year period expires. This requires updating the Prescription Only Medicines (POM) Order or the General Sales List (GSL) Order.

Rule 13(1) of the Poisons Rules (1972) allowed a pharmacist to supply a POM medicine without a prescription when, by reason of some emergency, a doctor was unable to furnish a prescription immediately.

Section 96 of the Act provided that after the duly appointed day (1 September 1971), no advertisement relating to medicinal products may be sent to a practitioner unless a data sheet had been sent some time in the previous 15 months. Final regulations on long term arrangements for data sheets appeared in 1972.

The issue of chloroform had surfaced again in 1978. In June 1977, a consultation letter was issued by the Licensing Authority (MLX 90) introducing a proposal to make an Order under section 62 of the Act prohibiting the sale, supply, and importation of any medicinal products containing chloroform (with certain exceptions such as its use as a preservative in pharmaceuticals). Many organisations, including the Joint UK Working Party on Chloroform, made representations and the Commission considered the safety of chloroform in the context of its alleged carcinogenicity in animals and safety in humans. It was concluded that chloroform was not mutagenic and hence did not present a carcinogenic risk to humans. It was also concluded that the upper permitted level of chloroform in medicinal products should be that of the saturated aqueous solution, which is 0·5% volume in volume. The exceptions to the prohibition included the use of chloroform as an anaesthetic agent, its use in dental surgery, and the right of doctors and dentists to exercise clinical judgement to have prepared for their patients products containing a higher concentration.

1.5.2 Committee on Safety of Medicines (CSM)

The Committee on Safety of Medicines, first chaired by Professor EF Scowen, replaced the previous Committee on Safety of Drugs and first met on 25 June 1970. Its functions may be summarised as follows:

- giving advice with respect to safety, quality, and efficacy, in relation to human use, of any substance or article (not being an instrument, apparatus or appliance) to which any provision of the Act is applicable; and
- promoting the collection and investigation of information relating to adverse reactions, for the purpose of enabling such advice to be given.

A number of sub-committees assisted the main Committee. Originally, these were the Sub-Committee on Toxicity, Clinical Trials, and Therapeutic Efficacy, the Sub-Committee on Chemistry, Pharmacy, and Standards, the Sub-Committee on Adverse Reactions, and the Sub-Committee on Biologicals.

In order to permit a smooth transition, the two committees (that on Safety of Drugs and that on Safety of Medicines) met simultaneously from June 1970 onwards, the CSD continuing to appraise products for clinical trials and marketing while the CSM had been concerned with preparation for the implementation of the Medicines Act. On 1 September 1971, the "duly appointed day", the CSM took over the work formerly done by the CSD and the applicants, responsible for submissions still awaiting consideration by the CSD on 1 September 1971, were invited to convert those submissions into applications for Clinical Trial Certificates or for Product Licences. The CSD, however, continued to meet several times after 1 September 1971 to deal with some residual matters arising directly from its own decisions.

Consistent with the emphasis on drug safety, the terms of reference of the Sub-Committee on Adverse Reactions were reviewed in 1971 and revised as follows:

- to promote and assemble reports about possible adverse effects of medicinal products administered to man
- to assess the meaning of such reports
- to recommend to the Committee any special or extended investigations which it considered desirable
- to keep under review the methods by which adverse reactions are monitored
- to make recommendations to the Committee based on its assessment of any action which it considers should be taken, and
- to advise the Committee on communications with the professions relating to the work of the Sub-Committee.

The Licensing Authority was already empowered by the Medicines Act to suspend, revoke or vary licences under section 28 and to control clinical trials in patients under section 36. At the outset in 1971, the Committee recognised the need to adhere to the policy stated by the CSD in respect of considering efficacy but took a much firmer line in 1972, bearing in mind section 19 of the Act. The Committee stated explicitly that, in future, it would require applications to be supported by some evidence of efficacy before advising that a product licence should be granted.

Since its establishment, the CSM has been chaired successively by Professors EF Scowen (June 1970 to March 1976), GM Wilson (April 1976 to December 1976), EF Scowen (January 1977 to June 1980), A Goldberg (later Sir Abraham Goldberg, July 1980 to December 1986), AW Asscher (later Sir William Asscher, January 1987 to December 1992), MD Rawlins (later Sir Michael Rawlins, January 1993 to December 1998), and AM Breckenridge (January 1999 to date).

1.5.3 Committee on the Review of Medicines (CRM) and Committee on Dental and Surgical Materials (CDSM)

The proposed review of Product Licences of Right (PLRs) was already considered desirable by the UK but became a requirement when the UK joined the EU. It was to correspond to the requirements under Directives 65/65/EEC and 75/318/EEC of the European Community which required that, throughout the Community, proprietary medicinal products granted licences before 22 November 1976 should be reviewed by 20 May 1990. All Member States of the European Community were similarly required to review the quality, safety, and efficacy data of products on their market.

In 1974 the Health Ministers consulted the UK Medicines Commission on a proposal to set up a committee under section 4 to advise the Licensing Authority on applications for product licences for dental and other surgical materials. Therefore, under the Act, the Committee on the Review of Medicines (CRM) was also established in 1975 (SI 1975/1006), under the Chairmanship of Professor EF Scowen with Professor OL Wade as the Deputy Chairman, to review all PLRs.

This Committee first met in October 1975. Initially, the review was organised in approximately 30 therapeutic categories such as analgesics, NSAIDs, psychotropics, etc. The priority was antirheumatics first, followed by analgesics and psychotropics, the priority being determined by the fact that adverse reactions related to these drugs were reported frequently. Therefore, a number of sub-committees, such as the Sub-Committee on Anti-Rheumatic Agents, Sub-Committee on Analgesics and Sub-Committee on Psychotropic Agents, were established. This approach proved slow and it was modified to a review of products of all companies, each company in two five-yearly cycles. The Herbal Standards Sub-Committee of the CSM also contributed to the review of PLRs.

The Committee on Dental and Surgical Materials (CDSM) was also established (SI 1975/1473) in 1975 under the Chairmanship of Professor RA Cawson to advise on dental and ophthalmic products and surgical materials. It dealt with PLRs within its area of expertise and held its first meeting in October 1976.

These two main review Committees had their own dedicated professional secretariat with a remit to review the evidence of safety, quality, and efficacy of all 39 035 PLRs. Of these some 6000 PLRs related to homeopathic or blood products, vaccines, toxins, sera, and radiopharmaceuticals which were excluded from review requirements since these were excluded from Directives EEC/65/65, 75/318 and 75/319 as they stood in 1976. Subsequently, however, the Extension Directive brought even these products within the scope of review.

The number of PLRs that were allowed to lapse by the manufacturers or were revoked or suspended in the UK between 1971 and 1982 was 22 376, and by 1988 this number had increased to 27 938. By 1982, the number of PLRs that were converted into full Product Licences was only 598. At the completion of the review in 1990, the number of applications received for full Product Licences was 6272 and of these just under 5300 were converted into full licences, most after changes had been agreed to the terms of the licences.[3] Of the 6272 applications, only 706 required referral to CRM or CDSM for advice. The CRM was deemed to have completed its work in 1991 and was disestablished on 31 March 1992 (SI 1992/606) while similarly, the CDSM was disestablished on 31 December 1994 (SI 1994/15).

During their existence, the CRM and the CDSM had four chairmen each – Professors EF Scowen (October 1975–December 1978), OL Wade (January 1979–December 1984), W Asscher (January 1985–December 1986) and DH Lawson (January 1987–March 1992) chairing the CRM, while Professors RA Cawson (October 1976–December 1979), R Hurley (January 1980–December 1981), CL Berry (later Sir Colin Berry, January 1982–December 1992), and D Poswillo (January 1993–December 1994) chaired the CDSM.

1.5.4 Earlier controls on conduct of clinical trials in the UK

The Medicines Act 1968 includes the definitions of a clinical trial and of a medicinal product. Clinical studies involving healthy volunteers do not meet this definition of a clinical trial and, as a result, do not come under the remit of regulatory controls. Such studies were subject to self-regulation by the pharmaceutical industry. Consequently, only the clinical trials in patients had to be covered by a clinical trial certificate (CTC).

The Licensing Authority did not lay down rigid requirements concerning the data that must be provided before authorisation can be given for a certificate for the clinical trial of a new drug. It did, however, issue guidelines for applicants.

In view of the regulatory delay that was caused by the need to apply for a CTC, a Statutory Order (SI 1974/498) was made during 1974 to provide an exemption from the need to hold a CTC in such cases, subject to certain conditions (this order applied to trials conducted by doctors and dentists on their own responsibility (DDX)). The basis of the clinical trial exemption (CTX) scheme introduced in 1981 included studies initiated by the pharmaceutical industry, is that together with a detailed clinical trial protocol and summaries of chemical, pharmaceutical, pharmacological, pharmacokinetic, toxicological, and human volunteer studies, a clinical trial in patients may proceed without the need of the additional details normally required for a Clinical Trial Certificate or Product Licence application. This exemption scheme is based on the requirement that:

- a doctor must certify the accuracy of the data
- the applicant undertakes to inform the Licensing Authority of any refusal to permit the trial by an ethical committee, and
- the applicant also undertakes to inform the Licensing Authority of any data or reports concerning the safety of the product.

The Licensing Authority has 35 days to respond to the notification but can in exceptional circumstances require a further 28 days to consider the notification. If the CTX is refused, the applicant can apply for a CTC, in which case complete data has to be filed. If the CTC application is refused the statutory appeal procedures come into play if the applicant company wishes to avail itself of this provision. These appeal procedures are identical with those applying to marketing applications. The CTX scheme proved highly successful in encouraging inward investment into research in the UK (see also p. 51). In a sample of 42 companies, an increase in research investment of 10% or more was attributed to the scheme by 23 of them.[4,5]

This introduction of the CTX scheme is widely cited as an example of the benefits of deregulation. Australian drug regulatory authorities subsequently also introduced a similar scheme.

1.5.5 The CSM and monitoring adverse reactions

One of the most important aspects of the United Kingdom regulatory system is the scheme that provides for the voluntary reporting of adverse reactions to a marketed drug. Since most serious adverse drug reactions (ADRs) are rare events, they are unlikely to be detected in early clinical trials.

In order to stimulate a decreasing rate of reporting, the CSM in 1971 adopted a new version of the yellow card that was simple to complete but provided for more information to be included. The trial proved successful. In addition, to promote reporting of adverse drug reactions from general practitioners, the Sub-Committee on Adverse Reactions convened a conference at the Royal College of General Practitioners in September 1973. In order to explore the ways of improving the dissemination of information about adverse drug reactions, a conference was also organised at the Royal College of Physicians in October 1975. Sustaining the efforts of the CSD, the CSM continued close cooperation with the WHO and with other regulatory authorities, in particular on matters relating to adverse reactions to medicinal products.

The first two safety letters from CSM to the doctors were sent out in 1973. One in May dealt with a range of issues, including the reports of subacute myelo-optic neuropathy (SMON) in association with clioquinol (some 10 000 cases in Japan but in the UK none of SMON and only a few cases of reversible neurotoxicity following prolonged exposure) and vaginal adenocarcinoma in daughters of mothers who had taken stilboesterol during pregnancy (80 cases in the USA but none in the UK). The other dated 3 January 1974 reported on 130 cases (66 fatal) of halothane-induced jaundice, 94 of which were associated with repeated exposures to this anaesthetic.

During 1974, the Committee discussed the introduction of a special mark to identify recently introduced products. This resulted in the introduction in January 1976 of the "Black Triangle" Scheme to identify drugs requiring intensive monitoring. This involves the Product Name to be followed immediately by an inverted black triangle (▼) as a superscript next to it in all product literature. Products requiring this symbol would include new drugs, established products having significantly new indications or new routes of administration, and entirely novel combinations of potent medicinal substances. In 1977, the Committee also produced detailed guidelines for the improved post-marketing surveillance of drugs. Following consultations in 1978, final guidelines were agreed with the ABPI and BMA.

The Yellow Card Scheme, at first restricted to receive reports from doctors, dentists and coroners, has been gradually expanded to receive reports from other sources. From October 1996 the scheme was extended to include reporting of suspected adverse reactions to unlicensed herbal remedies. In April 1997, the Yellow Card Scheme was further extended to include hospital pharmacists as recognised reporters of suspected adverse drug reactions. In addition, there are specially targeted extensions of the scheme such as adverse reactions to HIV medicines and adverse reactions in children.

In compliance with Data Protection legislation and the General Medical Council guidelines on confidentiality, the Yellow Card was updated in September 2000 to ask for an *identification number* for the patient; for instance, a practice or hospital number. The CSM no longer asked for personal patient identifiers on Yellow Cards; all that is now required is the patient's initials and age instead of their name and date of birth. The inclusion of the identification number enables the patient to be identifiable to the reporter but not to the CSM, thus allowing the reporter to know to whom the report refers for any potential future correspondence.

Apart from these changes necessary to keep pace with the changing times, the system has continued unchanged from when it was first set up, and the number of reports and fatal reactions each year of the scheme's operation to 2000 is shown in Table 1.4. By then, the CSM had received well over 400 000 reports since 1964. Despite relatively low reporting rates (a common feature of all spontaneous reporting systems worldwide), the UK Yellow Card Scheme has enjoyed a remarkable success and international recognition and has been responsible in uncovering many important drug safety hazards.

Communication with the profession was at first maintained by continuing (until January 1985) the *Adverse Reaction Series* leaflets started by CSD, and later by a regularly published bulletin on "Current Problems". The first issue of *Current Problems* in September 1975 led with the adverse oculo-cutaneous effects and sclerosing peritonitis associated with β-adrenergic receptor blocking agents and also included items on loss of consciousness associated with prazosin and on the risks of anti-inflammatory agents and asthma.

Major drugs withdrawn between 1971 and 1982 for safety reasons included polidexide (introduced 1974 and withdrawn 1975), oral formulation of practolol (1970 and 1976), alclofenac (1972 and 1979), tienilic acid (1979 and 1980), clomacron (1977 and 1982) and indoprofen (1982 and 1982).

Practolol illustrated well not only the value of a spontaneous reporting system but also the depth to which the Committee would investigate a signal of a serious ADR. Practolol-induced eye damage first came to light as a result of a publication by an ophthalmologist. Prior to this, the Committee had received only one report over a period of nearly three years. Subsequent to the publication, more than 200 cases of eye damage were reported retrospectively. In January 1975, a warning leaflet in the *Adverse Reaction Series* was issued and the Committee continued to receive additional reports. Later that year, the manufacturer proposed restrictions in the use of practolol. Ultimately, the oral formulation was withdrawn from the market.

The full might of the statutory control on regulation of drugs and their safety became evident in 1982 with the suspension of benoxaprofen, the first drug to be suspended from the UK market.[6] Benoxaprofen, also an NSAID, was approved in 1980 and marketed by Eli Lilly under the name

Table 1.4   Annual number of total and fatal Adverse Reaction Reports to the CSD and CSM

Year	Total ADR reports	Total fatal reports	Fatal reports (% of total)
1964	1415	86	6·1
1965	3987	169	4·2
1966	2386	152	6·4
1967	3503	198	5·7
1968	3486	213	6·1
1969	4306	271	6·3
1970	3563	196	5·5
1971	2851	203	7·1
1972	3638	211	5·8
1973	3619	224	6·2
1974	4815	275	5·7
1975	5052	250	4·9
1976	6490	236	2·6
1977	11 255	352	3·1
1978	11 873	396	3·3
1979	10 881	286	2·6
1980	10 179	287	2·9
1981	13 032	303	2·3
1982	10 922	340	3·1
1983	12 689	409	3·2
1984	12 163	340	2·8
1985	12 652	348	2·8
1986	15 527	403	2·6
1987	16 431	390	2·4
1988	19 022	410	2·2
1989	19 246	475	2·5
1990	18 084	377	2·1
1991	20 272	541	2·7
1992	20 161	478	2·4
1993	18 078	480	2·7
1994	17 556	412	2·3
1995	17 748	467	2·6
1996	17 109	393	2·3
1997	16 637	455	2·7
1998	18 062	529	2·9
1999	18 505	560	3·0
2000	33 094	610	1·8

Opren. It was launched amidst massive publicity and its marketing was "explosive". However, reports of serious adverse drug reactions and associated fatalities began to appear at an alarming rate. The first reports of deaths associated with benoxaprofen appeared in April and May 1982, when there were reported a total of eight cases of elderly women who developed jaundice while taking benoxaprofen; six of them died. Many other reports soon followed and the incidence of hepatotoxicity was

29

estimated to be 2–4%. Before long, there were 61 fatalities associated with benoxaprofen and the drug was immediately suspended from the market on 3 August 1982.

The experience with benoxaprofen and later with other drugs given to elderly patients was ultimately to result in a clinical guideline, adopted by the CPMP in September 1993, requiring the "Investigation of Medicinal Products in Geriatrics" focusing on pharmacokinetics, pharmacodynamics, and drug interactions as well as on the influence of renal or hepatic diseases on drug disposition. This also illustrates how guidelines have evolved with experience.

At the time the Yellow Card System celebrated its Silver Jubilee in 1989 at the Royal College of Physicians in London, the number of ADR reports in the CSM register was well in excess of 210 000 and the UK was a major contributor to the reports held by the WHO ADR Monitoring Centre in Uppsala. In relation to the size of the population, this represented a reporting rate in Britain that was among the highest in the world. In 1991, the existing computer system was completely replaced by inauguration and introduction of ADROIT (Adverse Drug Reactions On-line Information Tracking), which was developed by the Medicines Control Agency (MCA). This system makes use of state-of-the-art information technology and highly interrelational databases including a medical dictionary designed by the Agency staff. All major regulatory authorities now use this dictionary, MedDRA, for the purposes of monitoring and communicating information on adverse drug reactions. Data held on the previous system were transferred to ADROIT, which allowed assessors to set up complex enquiries of the database and respond rapidly to emerging safety issues.

1.6   General safety measures

The Commission and the CSM also made recommendations on the introduction of many other broad safety measures. These included the phenacetin prohibition order (SI 1974/1082), presentation of medicines in relation to child safety (SI 1975/2000), and declaration of alcohol in medicinal products on the package as active ingredient where this is likely to be pharmacologically active. Other labelling issues culminated in an Order (SI 1976/1726) which set out the standard particulars that must be shown on the containers and packaging of medicinal products. Consultations on other generally applicable warnings on the labels of certain medicines to protect children and to ensure that more general advice and information is provided resulted in SI 1977/996.

In the USA, the FDA had first required patient information leaflets in 1970. Following consultations with the Pharmaceutical Society, the ABPI, BMA, Health Council and other bodies, regulations on leaflets (SI 1977/1055) were introduced to make sure that the public had greater information on the medicines they were prescribed.

Concerns on promotion of drugs were beginning to emerge and regulations were introduced under section 95 of the Act to control advertising to practitioners (SI 1975/298 and 1326). The former dealt with the advertising of products covered by PLRs while the latter dealt with specifying the information that must appear in all advertisement, including succinct statements on contraindications, warnings, and adverse effects relevant to the indications. In addition, the generic name and the NHS cost were also required to appear. Further regulations (SI 1978/41) were also introduced on 1 February 1978 in respect of advertising direct to the public. Part of this made it an offence to advertise any product for certain serious diseases. In 1977, agreement was also reached with the ABPI for voluntary control and monitoring of advertisements by the industry and the ABPI instituted a Code of Practice and a Committee to supervise its implementation.

In 1975, the Medicines Division set up the Advertising Action Group to monitor advertising. The group included doctors, pharmacists, lawyers, and administrators. Although a number of small companies had been prosecuted for breaching the regulations on advertising, these cases attracted little attention or interest within the industry at large. However, in 1984, monitoring of advertisements reached its climax with the successful prosecution of a major pharmaceutical company in respect of its advertisement for its drug Surgam (tiaprofenic acid).[7] The outcome of this prosecution has greatly influenced the behaviour of, and within, the industry and strengthened the case for the professional independence and responsibilities of physicians working in the industry.

1.7 Medicines Control Agency

Because of the rising future demands and delays in licensing, the Minister of Health announced on 11 March 1987 that he had commissioned a study of the control of medicines in the UK. The terms of reference were:

> To examine the issues for DHSS arising from continued increase in licence applications and other work under the Medicines Act and to recommend ways of dealing expeditiously with this work, while maintaining adequate standards for the safety, efficacy, and quality of human medicines in the UK.

The study was undertaken by Dr John Evans, a previous Deputy Chief Medical Officer at the DHSS, and Mr Peter Cunliffe, Chairman of the Pharmaceutical Division of ICI. In 1988 the DHSS was split into two Departments, the Department of Health (DoH) and the Department of Social Security (DSS). Following the Cunliffe/Evans report, the Medicines Division of the DoH was reorganised in April 1989 to become the Medicines Control Agency (MCA) under a Director and Dr Keith Jones was appointed the first Director of the Agency. The Agency was expected to be self-funding from fees commensurate with the services provided. In July 1991, the Agency became an Executive Agency of the DoH under the Government's "Next Steps" initiative. Dr Jones, now the Chief Executive, was thereafter accountable to the Secretary of State for Health.

The Agency is the competent national authority responsible for human medicinal products in the UK and continues to discharge the functions of its predecessor, the Medicines Division, in implementing the Medicines Act and all European legislation. As at January 2001, the total staff had increased to 530 of whom 153 were working in the Licensing Division and 152 in the Post-licensing Division. These 305 included 49 medical, 53 pharmaceutical, and 85 preclinical or scientific staff.

The Agency continued to thrive and play a key role in Europe and also in all the regulatory and scientific activities of the European Committee for Proprietary Medicinal Products (see section 1.9 below) and all its Working Parties. Dr Susan Wood represented the UK at CPMP and until her death in 1998 was the first Chairperson of its Pharmacovigilance Working Party. Dr PC Waller who succeeded her as the UK representative at CPMP also chaired this important Working Party. Mr AC Cartwright, another officer from the UK, chaired the Quality Working Party. Over the period, the UK has remained among the leading regulatory authorities in the EU in terms of rapporteurship for the applications going through the Centralised Procedure, acting as a Reference Member State for the applications intended to go through the Mutual Recognition Procedure and as a coordinator of scientific advice from the CPMP.

At a European level, the UK has continued to contribute extensively to the many subsequent EU Directives and Regulations that control drugs in the European Union. All these, once adopted, have been incorporated into UK national legislation. In the UK now, for example, Council Directive 92/27/EEC of 31 March 1992 regulates labelling and leaflets while Council Directive 92/28/EEC of 31 March 1992 regulates advertising of medicinal products for human use.

1.8   The Medicines and Healthcare Products Regulatory Agency (MHRA)

On the 12 September 2002 the Health Minister, Lord Philip Hunt announced that the MCA and the Medical Devices Agency (MDA) would merge with effect from April 2003. The merged agencies would be known as the Medicines and Healthcare Products Regulatory Agency (MHRA).

1.9   European dimensions

The UK joined the European Community in January 1973 but the data requirements for granting marketing authorisations have, since the implementation of the Medicines Act 1968, been in accordance with European Community Directive 65/65/EEC and the subsequent Directive 75/318 as amended, which elaborated on the requirements for preclinical testing, pharmaceutical quality, and manufacture. It was vital that during 1973, following the UK entry into the Community, they also had the opportunity to consider and comment extensively on the two draft directives (later to become 75/318/EEC and 75/319/EEC). Directive 75/318/EEC has largely introduced the common dossier that has harmonised the standards and requirements across the EU while Directive 75/319/EEC established the Committee for Proprietary Medicinal Products, introduced the Mutual Recognition Procedure and brought in the requirements for expert reports.

The European Union's advisory Committee for Proprietary Medicinal Products (CPMP) was set up in 1975 under Directive 75/319. The first meeting was held on 26 November 1976 and Mr Leon Robert from Luxembourg was appointed its first Chairman. The Professional Head of the then UK Medicines Division, Dr EL Harris, who was also the UK Representative to CPMP, was elected a Deputy Chairman. Dr JP Griffin, his alternate, was appointed Chairman of the CPMP Working Party on Toxicity. Dr NMG Dukes from the Dutch regulatory authority was appointed Chairman of the Efficacy Working Party at the same time. He was later succeeded by Professor JM Alexandre (from the French regulatory authority) who then proceeded to become the Chairman of the CPMP (1995 to 2000).

The proposed review of Product Licences of Right in the UK, already considered desirable even earlier, was to correspond to the requirements under these Directives. These Directives required that throughout the Community proprietary medicinal products granted licences before 22 November 1976 should be reviewed by 20 May 1990. Indeed, the UK was among the first to complete this review on time. This review eliminated from the market all medicinal products that were released for clinical use previously without scrutiny and which were ineffective, unsafe or which had an unacceptable benefit to risk ratio.

Much later, Directive 83/570 required the applicants to produce a draft Summary of Product Characteristics (SPC) as an integral part of the documentation. In September 1995 an order was made (SI 1995/2321) to the effect that, in the UK, data sheets were no longer required where a product had an approved SPC and also that data sheets no longer had to be sent to all doctors and dentists prior to advertising.

In the UK, healthy volunteer studies were subject to self-regulation by the pharmaceutical industry and consequently only the clinical trials in patients had to be covered by a clinical trial certificate (CTC). However, with a view to harmonising the controls on clinical trials, a draft Directive concerning the conduct of clinical trials in the European Union was finally agreed on 14 December 2000 and formally adopted in May 2001 with a three year transition period for its implementation.

The EU Clinical Trials Directive contains specific provisions regarding the conduct of clinical trials, including multicentre trials, on human subjects. It defines "clinical trial" as any investigation in human subjects intended to discover or verify the clinical, pharmacological and/or other pharmacodynamic effects of one or more investigational medicinal product(s), and/or to identify any adverse reactions to one or more investigational medicinal product(s) and/or to study absorption, distribution, metabolism, and excretion of one or more investigational medicinal product(s) with the object of ascertaining its (their) safety and/or efficacy and defines "subject" as an individual who participates in a clinical trial as either a recipient of the investigational medicinal product or a control. Thus, healthy volunteer studies are included.

Further stringent requirements have evolved over time in respect of investigations to be carried out during the clinical development of drugs, the data required before they are approved for marketing, and subsequently the requirements for safety monitoring during the post-marketing period (pharmacovigilance).

The raft of rules, regulations, guidelines, and procedures (both EU and ICH) governing the human medicinal products in the EU can be found in the following five volumes published by the European Commission:

Volume 1 Pharmaceutical Legislation
Volume 2 Notice to Applicants

> 2A: Procedures for Marketing Authorisation
> 2B: Presentation and Content of the Dossier
> 2C: Regulatory Guidelines

Volume 3 Guidelines

> 3A: Quality and Biotechnology
> 3B: Safety, Environment, and Information
> 3C: Efficacy

Volume 4 Good Manufacturing Practice
Volume 9 Pharmacovigilance
(Volumes 5–8 relate to veterinary medicinal products)

Many of the Directives originally adopted have been frequently amended over the period. In the interests of clarity and rationality, a whole range of the latest versions of these Directives was codified by assembling them in a single text, that is Directive 2001/83/EC of 6 November 2001. Therefore, the reader should also cross-refer to this Directive, which codifies the following:

Council Directive 65/65/EEC of 26 January 1965 on the approximation of provisions laid down by law, regulation or administrative action relating to medicinal products

Council Directive 75/318/EEC of 20 May 1975 on the approximation of the laws of Member States relating to analytical, pharmacotoxicological and clinical standards and protocols in respect of the testing of proprietary medicinal products

Council Directive 75/319/EEC of 20 May 1975 on the approximation of provisions laid down by law, regulation or administrative action relating to proprietary medicinal products

Council Directive 89/342/EEC of 3 May 1989 on immunologicals (vaccines, toxins or serums and allergens)

Council Directive 89/343/EEC of 3 May 1989 on radiopharmaceuticals

Council Directive 89/381/EEC of 14 June 1989 on products derived from human blood or human plasma

Council Directive 92/25/EEC of 31 March 1992 on the wholesale distribution

Council Directive 92/26/EEC of 31 March 1992 on classification for the supply

Council Directive 92/27/EEC of 31 March 1992 on labelling and package leaflets

Council Directive 92/28/EEC of 31 March 1992 on advertising

Council Directive 92/73/EEC of 22 September 1992 on homeopathic medicinal products.

The EU legislation and procedures are likely to undergo further profound changes following the Review 2001 as anticipated in Article 71 of Regulation EEC/2309/93 which required that: "Within six years of the entry into force of this Regulation, the Commission shall publish a general report on the experience of the procedures laid down in this Regulation, in Chapter III of Directive 75/319/EEC and in Chapter IV of Directive 81/851/EEC". This Review has been completed and all interested parties, such as the national authorities, the European Commission, and the EFPIA, have considered its findings and offered their solutions. These have been actively debated and discussed and the EC has now proposed comprehensive reform of the EU pharmaceutical legislation.

During its first reading of the proposed changes to the pharmaceutical legislation, the European Parliament has already approved 144 of the 167 amendments to Regulation EEC/2309/93 and 160 of the 202 amendments to Directive 2001/83/EC.

1.10 International dimensions

In June 1984 the Commission decided that a meeting with the Japanese authorities, attended by Mr F Sauer and the Chairman and Vice-Chairman of the Safety Working Party, Dr JP Griffin and Professor R Bass respectively, and the Chairman of the Efficacy Working Group, Professor JM Alexandre, should take place in Tokyo. The efforts following this initial meeting were ultimately to culminate in the International Conference on Harmonisation (ICH). The main players at ICH are now the European

Commission/EMEA, European Federation of Pharmaceutical Industry Associations (EFPIA), Japanese Ministry of Health and Welfare (JMHW), Japanese Pharmaceutical Manufacturers Association (JPMA), US FDA, and Pharmaceutical Research and Manufacturers of America (PhRMA). The WHO, Canadian Health Protection Branch, and the European Free Trade Area (EFTA) countries enjoy an observer status at ICH meetings.

The ICH Steering Committee established expert working groups to discuss areas where harmonisation was possible and to produce universally acceptable guidelines. Thus under the auspices of the ICH a large number of guidelines have been issued in the areas of quality, safety, and efficacy, with the objective of achieving harmonisation of requirements for registration between regulatory authorities and thereby reducing the need to duplicate studies. It must be made clear that these documents should be regarded as guidelines and not requirements.

These guidelines may not be at the cutting edge of science but they represent acceptable compromises based on sound science. As at May 2001, there were at least 12 safety, 11 efficacy, 14 quality, and a number of pharmacovigilance guidelines accepted since the first meeting of ICH in Brussels in November 1991. Once adopted by the CPMP and published, the guidelines resulting from the ICH process are incorporated and applied as EU Community guidelines.

Regarding pharmacovigilance, there are a number of ICH/CPMP guidelines and a Joint Pharmacovigilance Plan (CPMP/PhVWP/2058/99 Revision 1) for the Implementation of the ICH guidelines E2B, M1, and M2. Two major advances were the acceptance of MedDRA (ICH topic M1) and the acceptance of Periodic Safety Update Reports (PSUR) (ICH topic E2C) for new drugs approved in the EU. The ICH guidelines adopted by the CPMP include ICH/135/95 (Good Clinical Practice), ICH/285/95 (Guidance on Recommendations on Electronic Transmission of Individual Case Safety Reports Message Specification (M2)), ICH/287/95 (Guidance on Clinical Safety Data Management: Data Elements for Transmission of Individual Case Safety Reports (E2B)), ICH/288/95 (Guidance on Clinical Safety Data Management: Periodic Safety Update Reports for Marketed Drugs (E2C)), and ICH/377/95 (Clinical Safety Data Management: Definitions and Standards for Expedited Reporting (E2A)). If harmonisation could be achieved, as it has been, across a broad range of areas in quality, safety, and efficacy, there seemed no logical reason why a Common Technical Document or dossier could not be prepared that would be acceptable to all drug regulatory authorities. At the last meeting of ICH in November 2000 in San Diego (USA), agreement was reached on a Common Technical Document (CTD) that represented a common format for the submission of dossiers to the three regions of the USA, the EU, and Japan. Many other non-ICH regulatory authorities have expressed their desire to accept the dossier in CTD format.

In order to expedite and optimise drug development, clinical trials are now conducted in different parts of the world. Recognising that drug development is a global process and in order that the data from one ethnic group can be confidently extrapolated to another, an ICH guideline (CPMP/ICH/289/95) has been agreed taking into account the genetic and non-genetic influences on drug responses. Application of this and all other national, regional, and international guidelines relevant to quality, toxicity testing, and demonstrating efficacy in clinical trials has ensured that public safety is not compromised while still ensuring that safe and effective medicines are made available to the UK public without the need for repeating lengthy clinical trials.

1.11 Conclusions

This chapter has provided, hopefully, a brief but interesting account of the events that have been responsible for the evolution of the present drug controls in the UK. Importantly, it highlights how the broad pattern of drug regulation was already set during the early period that led to the implementation of the Medicines Act in 1971 and how this pattern was consolidated during the decade thereafter.

Contrary to what is generally believed, the need for an effective control was always recognised, and indeed demanded, and there was a sort of control. However, it was patchy, very limited in its scope, erratic in its implementation and of little relevance to the drugs that were beginning, and were likely in the future, to appear in the market as a result of progress in pharmacology and medicinal chemistry.

Thalidomide generated an outcry and a demand that could no longer be ignored, and spurred the Government into not only consolidating all previous legislation and extending its scope but also creating a formal regulatory structure by which to ensure that the legislation was adequately and fully implemented.

The Medicines Act, together with the associated EU legislation and EU and ICH guidelines, should ensure that the safety of drugs made to the highest quality, the acceptability of their risk/benefit ratio, and the promotion of correct information to the prescribers and consumers are the dominant features of the controls that operate today.

References

1 Shah RR. Thalidomide, drug safety and early drug regulation in the UK. *Adverse Drug React Toxicol Rev* 2001;**20**:199–255.
2 Ministry of Health, Scottish Home and Health Departments. *Safety of Drugs*. Final Report of the Joint Sub-Committee of the Standing Medical Advisory Committees. Her Majesty's Stationery Office, London, 1963.
3 Winship K, Hepburn D, Lawson DH. The review of medicines in the United Kingdom. *Br J Clin Pharmacol* 1992;**33**:583–7.
4 Speirs CJ, Griffin JP. A survey of the first year of operation of the new procedure affecting the conduct of clinical trials in the United Kingdom. *Br J Clin Pharmacol* 1983;**15**:649–55.
5 Speirs CJ, Saunders RM, Griffin JP. The United Kingdom Clinical Trial Exemption Scheme – its effects on investment in research. *Pharm Int* 1984;**5**:254–6.

6 Shah RR. Drug-induced hepatotoxicity: pharmacokinetic perspectives and strategies for risk reduction. *Adverse Drug React Toxicol Rev* 1999;**18**:181–233.
7 Collier J, Herxheimer A. Roussel convicted of misleading promotion. *Lancet* 1987;**i**:113–14.

Other sources of information

Committee on Safety of Drugs. Report of the Committee on Safety of Drugs for the year ended December 31st, 1964. Her Majesty's Stationery Office, London, 1965.

Committee on Safety of Drugs. Report for the year ended December 31st, 1965. Her Majesty's Stationery Office, London, 1966.

Committee on Safety of Drugs. Report for the year ended December 31st, 1966. Her Majesty's Stationery Office, London, 1967.

Committee on Safety of Drugs. Report for the year ended December 31st, 1967. Her Majesty's Stationery Office, London, 1968.

Committee on Safety of Drugs. Report for the year ended December 31st 1968. Her Majesty's Stationery Office, London, 1969.

Committee on Safety of Drugs. Report for 1969 and 1970. Her Majesty's Stationery Office, London, 1971.

Medicines Commission. First Annual Report to end of 1970. Her Majesty's Stationery Office, London, 1971.

Medicines Commission. Annual Report for 1971. Her Majesty's Stationery Office, London, 1972.

Committee on Safety of Medicines. Report for the year ended 31 December 1971. Her Majesty's Stationery Office, London, 1972.

Committee on Safety of Medicines. Report for the year ended 31 December 1972. Her Majesty's Stationery Office, London, 1973.

The Medicines Commission. Annual Report for 1973 (together with annual reports of standing committees appointed under section 4 of the Medicines Act 1968). Her Majesty's Stationery Office, London, 1974.

The Medicines Commission. Annual Report for 1974 (together with annual reports of standing committees appointed under section 4 of the Medicines Act 1968). Her Majesty's Stationery Office, London, 1975.

The Medicines Commission. Annual Report for 1975 (together with annual reports of standing committees appointed under section 4 of the Medicines Act 1968). Her Majesty's Stationery Office, London, 1976.

The Medicines Commission. Annual Report for 1976 (together with annual reports of standing committees appointed under section 4 of the Medicines Act 1968). Her Majesty's Stationery Office, London, 1977.

The Medicines Commission. Annual Report for 1977 (together with annual reports of standing committees appointed under section 4 of the Medicines Act 1968). Her Majesty's Stationery Office, London, 1978.

The Medicines Commission. Annual Report for 1978 (together with annual reports of standing committees appointed under section 4 of the Medicines Act 1968). Her Majesty's Stationery Office, London, 1979.

2: Regulation of human medicinal products in the European Union

RASHMI R SHAH, JOHN P GRIFFIN

2.1 Introduction

The thalidomide disaster, described in Chapter 1, resulted in an epidemic of a previously unknown malformation ("phocomelia"). The scale of the disaster reached such proportions that the drug was withdrawn from the market worldwide. The USA was essentially spared the thalidomide tragedy because of the concerns of the Food and Drug Administration (FDA) over the neurotoxicity of thalidomide. This resulted in the application being stalled in the USA. Following the thalidomide tragedy in Western Europe, a subsequent New Drug Amendment (the Kefauver Amendment) in 1962 called for the FDA to monitor all stages of drug development. As a result, even investigational drugs then required comprehensive animal testing before extensive human clinical trials could be started. Under the Kefauver Amendment, proof of efficacy and safety was mandatory and the time constraints on the FDA for disposition of new drug applications were removed.

The thalidomide disaster was to provide the impetus to the introduction, for the first time in most non-US countries (including those in Western Europe), of regulatory control for drugs to be marketed for clinical use. In the UK the result was the Medicines Act 1968 and the establishment of the Licensing Authority.

The UK joined the European Community in 1973, but the data requirements for granting marketing authorisations have, since the implementation of the Medicines Act 1968, been in accordance with European Community Directive 65/65/EEC and the subsequent Directive 75/318/EEC as amended. It is to be noted that the requirements, and also the general nature of the regulatory controls envisaged under the Medicines Act are remarkably similar to those under legislations prevailing at the time in the USA and the European Economic Community (EEC). In particular, the existence of four major pieces of legislation is worth bearing in mind:

- The US Federal Pure Food and Drugs Act (1906)
- The US Federal Food, Drug and Cosmetic Act (1938)
- US New Drug Amendment (the Kefauver–Harris Amendment) (1962)
- The EU Council Directive 65/65/EEC (1965).

Since the UK joined the EU, all EU pharmaceutical regulation and legislation is transposed into the UK national pharmaceutical regulation and legislation. The primary aim of the European Union's regulations is laid down in the preamble to the Council Directive of 26 January 1965 (65/65/EEC), which states that:

THE COUNCIL OF THE EUROPEAN ECONOMIC COMMUNITY,
Having regard to the Treaty establishing the European Economic Community and in particular Article 100 thereof ...

- Whereas the primary purpose of any rules concerning the production and distribution of medicinal products must be to safeguard public health;
- Whereas, however, this objective must be attained by means which will not hinder the development of the pharmaceutical industry or trade in medicinal products within the Community;
- Whereas trade in medicinal products within the Community is hindered by disparities between certain national provisions, in particular between provisions relating to medicinal products (excluding substances or combinations of substances which are foods, animal feedingstuffs or toilet preparations); and whereas such disparities, directly affect the establishment and functioning of the common market;
- Whereas such hindrances must accordingly be removed; and whereas this entails approximation of the relevant provisions;
- Whereas, however, such approximation can only be achieved progressively; and whereas priority must be given to eliminating the disparities liable to have the greatest effect on the functioning of the common market;

HAS ADOPTED THIS DIRECTIVE.

The scope of the regulations is defined by the breadth of its definition of a medicinal product. The regulations define a medicinal product as any substance or combination of substances presented for treating or preventing disease in human beings or animals or which may be administered in human beings or animals with a view to making a medical diagnosis or to restoring, correcting or modifying physiological functions in human beings or animals. Substance is further defined as any matter which may be of human, animal, vegetable or chemical origin.

2.2   Regulatory controls in the European Union

In order to enable the reader to appreciate better the development of regulatory controls in the European Union (EU), we have referred to various Directives by their original citation in this chapter. However, these Directives have been frequently amended subsequent to their original adoption. In the interests of clarity and rationality, a whole range of the latest versions of these Directives was codified by assembling them in a single text, namely Directive 2001/83/EC of 6 November 2001. Therefore, the reader should also cross-refer to this Directive, which codifies the following:

Council Directive 65/65/EEC of 26 January 1965 on the approximation of provisions laid down by law, regulation or administrative action relating to medicinal products

Council Directive 75/318/EEC of 20 May 1975 on the approximation of the laws of Member States relating to analytical, pharmacotoxicological and clinical standards and protocols in respect of the testing of proprietary medicinal products

Council Directive 75/319/EEC of 20 May 1975 on the approximation of provisions laid down by law, regulation or administrative action relating to proprietary medicinal products

Council Directive 89/342/EEC of 3 May 1989 on immunologicals (vaccines, toxins or serums and allergens)

Council Directive 89/343/EEC of 3 May 1989 on radiopharmaceuticals

Council Directive 89/381/EEC of 14 June 1989 on products derived from human blood or human plasma

Council Directive 92/25/EEC of 31 March 1992 on the wholesale distribution

Council Directive 92/26/EEC of 31 March 1992 on classification for the supply

Council Directive 92/27/EEC of 31 March 1992 on labelling and package leaflets

Council Directive 92/28/EEC of 31 March 1992 on advertising

Council Directive 92/73/EEC of 22 September 1992 on homeopathic medicinal products.

In the EU, a medicinal product may only be placed on the market when a marketing authorisation has been issued by the competent authority of a Member State for its own territory (national authorisation) or when an authorisation has been granted by the European Commission (EC) for the entire Community (Community authorisation).

Later, Directive 75/318/EEC introduced the requirements relating to analytical, pharmacotoxicological and clinical standards and protocols in respect of the testing of proprietary medicinal products in order to establish their quality, safety, and efficacy, while Directive 75/319/EEC established the Committee for Proprietary Medicinal Products ("old" CPMP) and introduced the multistate procedure (known now as the mutual recognition procedure). Directive 87/22/EEC introduced the concertation procedure (known now as the centralised procedure) relating to the placing on the market of high technology medicinal products, particularly those derived from biotechnology.

Since these original requirements, further stringent legislation and requirements have evolved in respect of investigations during the development of a drug, data necessary for its approval, its promotion, and monitoring of its safety during the post-marketing period (pharmacovigilance).

The CPMP is the pharmaceutical advisory committee to the EC in respect of human medicinal products. It has an elected chairman and is constituted of two members from each Member State. This "old" CPMP met for the first time on 26 November 1976. Its last meeting was on 13–14 December 1994. Article 1 of Council Regulation EEC/2309/93 of 22 July 1993 established the European Medicines Evaluation Agency (EMEA) and article 5 re-established the Committee for Proprietary Medicinal Products established by Article 8 of Directive 75/319/EEC. This "new" CPMP was to be responsible for formulating the opinion of the Agency on any question concerning the admissibility of the files submitted in accordance with the centralised procedure, the granting, variation, suspension or withdrawal of an authorisation to place a medicinal product for human use on the market arising in accordance with the provisions of this Regulation, and pharmacovigilance. The "new" CPMP met for the first time in January 1995 with Professor JM Alexandre elected as its first Chairman. It also is constituted of two members from each of the 15 Member States. On completion of his two terms in December 2000, Professor Alexandre was succeeded by the current Chairman, Dr Daniel Brasseur, from Belgium.

Legislation has also been introduced recently in respect of orphan diseases/drugs. Orphan diseases are those which are sufficiently rare that there are no commercial incentives to research these diseases and develop effective therapy. Following the success of the US orphan drug legislation passed in 1983, a number of countries introduced similar legislation (Japan in 1993 and Australia in 1998). In 1999, the EU also passed legislation relating to this important area of drug development. The applications for orphan drug designation are considered by the Committee for Orphan Medicinal Products (COMP). The relevant EU legislation establishing the COMP and the criteria for designation is the Regulation (EC) No. 141/2000 on orphan medicinal products.

In order to encourage pharmaceutical companies to invest in orphan drug development, legislation provides for a number of incentives. These include fee waiver (the extent of reduction varies with the region, and in the EU it is 50% in the year 2002), market exclusivity, and protocol assistance (100% reduction in fee applicable to providing scientific advice). The period of market exclusivity is 10 years from authorisation. In the context of market exclusivity in the EU, a Member State must not accept another application for a marketing authorisation or grant a marketing authorisation or accept an application to extend an existing marketing authorisation for the same therapeutic indication in respect of a *similar medicinal product*. However, exclusivity may be lost by the first applicant consenting to a second application from another applicant, if the first applicant is unable to meet demand, if a similar product is found to be *clinically superior*, if the criteria are no longer met or if, at the end of five years, a Member State can show that the product is profitable. Commission regulation (EC) No. 847/2000 laid down the provisions for implementation of the designation process and definitions of the concepts "similar medicinal product" and "clinical superiority".

COMP held its inaugural meeting in April 2000 and is constituted of a representative from each Member State, three nominated by the EC to liaise with CPMP and three from patient organisations, making a total of 21 representatives. COMP at present is the only advisory committee (associated with drug regulation) in the world with such direct patient representation. In addition to the 21 representatives, there is a Chairman, currently Professor Joseph Torrent-Farnell, from Spain.

The EMEA, based in London, has the executive functions of a professional secretariat and works in very close liaison with the national authorities of the Member States, the COMP, and the members of the CPMP and its various working parties. These are the Efficacy Working Party, Safety Working Party, Biotechnology Working Party, Quality Working Party, Pharmacovigilance Working Party, Blood and Plasma Working Party, and Herbal Remedies Working Party. Each Member State is represented on every working party by representatives nominated by its national authority. The working parties are responsible for regularly producing a number of Concept Papers, Points to Consider documents, and Guidelines relevant to their scientific fields. Following initial consultation with CPMP and subsequently with interested organisations, the final drafts are adopted by the CPMP for implementation. In addition, the CPMP also sets up when necessary special ad hoc groups of experts to deal with specific issues or scientific subjects of particular regulatory interest (for example, drug-induced QT internal prolongation or pharmacogenetics in drug development).

2.3 Applications for marketing authorisations in the EU

2.3.1 Legislation and guidance notes

Council Directive 65/65/EEC, referred to earlier, has been frequently amended and other Directives have extended the scope of legislation for authorising medicines and introducing new procedures.

For human medicinal products, the relevant legislation is presented in Volume 1 of *The Rules Governing Medicinal Products in the European Union*, published by the European Commission. Volume 2 comprises the *Notice to Applicants for Marketing Authorisations for Medicinal Products for Human Use in the European Union*. Procedures for marketing authorisations are described in Volume 2A, the presentation and the content of the dossier are described in Volume 2B, and various regulatory guidelines in Volume 2C. Volume 3 gives guidance notes for medicinal products for human use, Volume 4 relates to good manufacturing practice, and Volume 9 is concerned with pharmacovigilance (both for human and veterinary use). The remaining volumes (5–8) are concerned with veterinary medicinal products.

Guidance notes produced by the CPMP through its Working Parties or its membership of the International Conference on Harmonisation (ICH) are compiled in Volumes 3A (quality and biotechnology), 3B (pharmacotoxicological), and 3C (clinical). These guidelines have been prepared by experts, have undergone input from academia and the industry during consultation, and have been adopted only thereafter. None of these guidelines is legally binding and they are intended to be sufficiently flexible so as not to impede scientific progress in drug development. However, where an applicant chooses not to follow a guideline, the decision must be explained and justified in the dossier.

2.3.2 Format of the dossier

The basic requirements for the contents of the dossier of information accompanying the application for a marketing authorisation are the same whether it is submitted nationally or centrally and are laid out in detail in Directive 75/318/EEC and its subsequent amendments. Provisions are made in Directive 65/65/EEC for the omission of data in certain circumstances where information is already available to the regulatory authorities from other sources, for example, in the case of applications for line extensions to existing products or for generic drugs. Applications that do not include a full dossier of information are referred to as "abridged applications". The complex legal basis for the different types of generic or abridged applications for marketing authorisations will not be considered further in this chapter.

2.3.2.1 Current format of the dossier

Directive 75/318/EEC requires that the dossier be presented in four highly structured parts: Parts I, II, III, and IV. Directive 83/570/EEC was the amending Directive which introduced the requirements for a draft Summary of Product Characteristics (SPC) to be produced by the applicant. Volume 2B of *The Rules Governing Medicinal Products in the European Union* gives a detailed breakdown of the structure of a European regulatory dossier. This format is valid to the end of June 2003 when a new format known as the Common Technical Document (CTD) will become mandatory.

An application for a marketing authorisation must be accompanied, among other items, by specified pharmaceutical, preclinical, and clinical particulars and documents (the "dossier"). Three important summary documents in the dossier are the SPC, a Package or Patient Information Leaflet (PIL), and the sales presentation of the product (label). The SPC has a formally prescribed structure (Box 2.1), and forms the basis for *authorised* clinical prescribing of the medicinal product concerned.

Box 2.1 Contents of the summary of product characteristics

1   Trade name of the medicinal product
2   Qualitative and quantitative composition (active ingredient)
3   Pharmaceutical form
4   Clinical particulars

    4.1   Therapeutic indications
    4.2   Posology and method of administration
    4.3   Contraindications
    4.4   Special warnings and special precautions for use
    4.5   Interactions with other medicaments and other forms of interactions
    4.6   (Use during) Pregnancy and lactation
    4.7   Effects on ability to drive and to use machines
    4.8   Undesirable effects (frequency and seriousness)
    4.9   Overdose (symptoms, emergency procedures, antidotes)

5   Pharmacological properties

    5.1   Pharmacodynamic properties
    5.2   Pharmacokinetic properties
    5.3   Preclinical safety data

6   Pharmaceutical Particulars

    6.1   List of excipients
    6.2   Incompatibilities
    6.3   Shelf life (when necessary after reconstitution or opening the container for the first time)
    6.4   Special precautions for storage
    6.5   Nature and contents of container
    6.6   Instructions for use/handling

7   Marketing authorisation holder (name and address)
8   Marketing authorisation number
9   Date of first authorisation
10 Date of (partial) revision of the text

Part I is a summary of the information presented in the whole dossier and includes the application forms and administrative particulars on fees, various declarations, and the type of application as well as particulars of the marketing authorisation (IA), proposed SPC (IB1), proposals for packaging, labels, and package or patient information leaflets (IB2), and any SPCs already approved in the Member State(s) for the particular product (IB3). Also included are separate Expert Reports on chemical and pharmaceutical (IC1), toxicopharmacological (preclinical) (IC2), and clinical documentations (IC3), as required under Directive 75/319/EEC. These Expert Reports are the summaries of the dossier with a critical appraisal of the data presented by an expert on behalf of the applicant. Detailed regulatory guidance, supported by various Directives, is available on the content of each of these documents.

Part II relates to the quality of the product and gives details of its chemical, pharmaceutical, and biological testing. In cases where the active ingredient is made by a manufacturer other than the applicant or product manufacturer, some of the information required in Part II may be presented in a separate file, the Drug Master File, to maintain the confidential nature of the synthetic process. Part III describes the toxicological and pharmacological tests conducted with the drug in animals (preclinical tests). Part IV describes the clinical documentation. The details of requirements for these four parts are annexed to Directive 2001/83/EC. This Directive is a very important document since it codifies into a single document a number of previous Directives which have been amended. It can be accessed on the EMEA website at http://pharmacos.eudra.org/F2/eudralex/vol-1/home.htm.

Part II data should be provided in respect of qualitative and quantitative particulars of the constituents, description of the method of preparation, control of starting materials, control tests on intermediate products, control tests on the finished product, and stability tests. In cases where the active ingredient is made by a manufacturer other than the applicant or the product manufacturer, some of the information required in Part II may be presented in a separate file, the Drug Master File, to maintain the confidential nature of the synthetic process. Part III data should include pharmacology, safety pharmacology, pharmacokinetics, single- and repeat-dose toxicological evaluation, reproductive function, fertility, embryofetal and perinatal toxicity, mutagenic potential, and data on carcinogenicity. Part IV clinical data are divided into part IVA, which is the detailed clinical pharmacology of the medicinal product, and part IVB, which describes in detail the clinical experience. Clinical pharmacology data should provide characterisation of the pharmacodynamics and the pharmacokinetics of the drug. It is not only the primary pharmacology (responsible for the therapeutic effect of the drug) but also its secondary pharmacology (responsible for unwanted effects) that needs to be investigated. Pharmacokinetics requires full characterisation, with all the aspects that embody the term in its broadest sense, together with data on the effects of age, gender, renal or hepatic dysfunction, and food. Genetic factors are assuming greater importance and information should be provided on the effect of genetic factors on the pharmacology of a drug and the ethnic structure of the trial population.

Arising from pharmacokinetic studies there should be a detailed and well-designed programme of drug interaction studies. It is important that the dose schedule is scientifically supported by the pharmacokinetics and pharmacodynamics of the drug. Equally critical are the considerations of the time to steady state and whether the pharmacodynamic effects lag behind changes in plasma concentrations. An ideal dose-ranging studies programme should provide definitive information on the risk/benefit of a range of doses and dosage regimens.

Each study in the clinical dossier, whether clinical pharmacology or clinical experience, should be presented in a structured manner to include a summary, study objectives, detailed study design (including doses selected, duration, planned number of patients, all efficacy variables, assessment time-points and statistical methods), results, conclusion, and bibliography if necessary. The safety database (both clinical and laboratory but dealt with separately) should be presented overall and by subpopulation exposed in terms of dose, duration, age, gender, and special populations, such as those with hepatic dysfunction or renal impairment. Safety data should also include any post-marketing experience from countries (EU and non-EU) where the product is already approved and on the market. Information should be provided on the intensity and outcomes of these effects. To put these data in their perspective, data should be included on the estimated patient exposure. Every attempt should be made to obtain details of the patients withdrawn from studies, serious adverse events, and those that resulted in deaths. Expert reports are not a promotion platform for the product but an assessment of the data generated, an explanation of the results, and an interpretation. An expert report should not normally exceed 25 pages of A4. Reports should also make clear whether or not the preclinical studies submitted have been conducted according to good laboratory practice, and whether the clinical studies have been conducted according to good clinical practice principles and in accord with the Declaration of Helsinki.

2.3.2.2 Common Technical Document

Following agreement at the ICH meeting in November 2000, the format of the EU dossier described above will change to conform to the new format known as the "Common Technical Document". This new format (CTD) will be common to all the three major regions of drug regulation (EU, USA, and Japan) and most of the other major non-ICH authorities have also agreed to accept the dossier in CTD format. Information on the Common Technical Document can be accessed from the EMEA website at http://pharmacos.eudra.org/F2/pharmacos/docs.htm.

Box 2.2 Summary of the contents of the modules of the Common Technical Document

Module 1   EU-specific requirements

1.1   Module 1 Comprehensive Table of Contents (Module 1–5)
1.2   Application Form
1.3   Product Literature

  1.3.1   Summary of Product Characteristics (SPC)
  1.3.2   Labelling
  1.3.3   Package leaflet
  1.3.4   Mock-ups and specimen
  1.3.5   SPCs already approved in the Member States

1.4   Information about Experts
1.5   Specific requirements for different types of applications
    Annex: Environmental Risk Assessment

Module 2   CTD Summaries

2.1   CTD Table of Contents (Module 2–5)
2.2   CTD Introduction
2.3   Quality Overall Summary
2.4   Nonclinical Overview
2.5   Clinical Overview
2.6   Nonclinical Written and Tabulated Summary
    Pharmacology
    Pharmacokinetics
    Toxicology
2.7   Clinical Summary
    Biopharmaceutics and Associated Analytical Methods
    Clinical Pharmacology Studies
    Clinical Efficacy
    Clinical Safety
    Synopsis of Individual Studies

Module 3   Quality

3.1   Module 3 Table of Contents
3.2   Body of Data
3.3   Key Literature References

Module 4   Non-clinical Study Reports

4.1   Module 4 Table of Contents
4.2   Study Reports
4.3   Literature References

Module 5   Clinical Study Reports

5.1   Module 5 Table of Contents
5.2   Tabular Listing of All Clinical Studies
5.3   Clinical Study Reports
5.4   Literature References

CTD consists of four modules, preceded by a Module 1 which is region-specific and includes administrative and prescribing information. Module 2 comprises of CTD Summaries and Overviews of the quality, non-clinical and clinical data, Module 3 contains data on Quality, Module 4 consists of the Non-clinical Study Reports, and Module 5 comprises the Clinical Study Reports. There are guidelines on the details to be included in each module and these are summarised in Box 2.2. Before the CTD can be introduced, certain legislative changes are required in each of the three regions. The non-clinical and clinical overviews and summaries are equivalent to the present Expert Report described in Section 2.3.2.1. It is anticipated that submission of the dossier in CTD format will become mandatory by July 2003, although applicants may choose to use this format from July 2001.

The objectives behind CTD are to reduce the time and resources needed to compile applications, to facilitate electronic submissions, regulatory reviews and communications, and to facilitate exchange of information between regulatory authorities. It is not intended to indicate what studies are required – these are essentially the same as before – but to indicate merely an appropriate internationally harmonised format for the presentation of the data that have been generated.

2.4 Integrated regulatory assessment

A typical dossier for a new active substance (NAS) includes 4–6 volumes of Part I, 6–10 volumes of Part II, 20–40 volumes of Part III, and 60–100 volumes of Part IV data. During the assessment process, there is a documented interactive dialogue between each assessor and the applicant to clarify points which are complex or ambiguous or to enable the applicant to provide additional raw data, statistical appendices, and detailed protocols to facilitate the assessment process.

However, none of these four parts of the dossier is self-standing or independent of others. There are areas within each which are intricately linked to the others. In preparing a comprehensive and integrated regulatory assessment report, it is important that these areas of common interest are appropriately addressed.

2.4.1 Integration of preclinical and pharmaceutical dossier

The drug substance and finished product specification of any product allow for the presence of low levels of impurities, depending on daily dose and duration of treatment. The permitted levels are specified. It is important that the safety of these allowable impurities is confirmed. The preclinical dossier requires careful scrutiny to ensure that these impurities were present in the test product administered to animals and in quantities sufficient to provide a confident and reassuring margin of safety.

If this has not been done, then the impurities present in relatively high concentration(s) need to be isolated or synthesised and a limited programme of toxicity studies, probably consisting of acute toxicity and genotoxicity, should be conducted directly with these.

2.4.2 Integration of preclinical and clinical data

The clinical dossier has to be scrutinised to ensure that the effects observed in preclinical general toxicity studies have been looked for in the clinical studies and, if present, the level of the risk established. Typical examples would include the preclinical effect of the drug on drug metabolising enzymes or specific target organs for toxicity. Likewise, it is easier to appreciate the significance of an unexpected finding in the clinical studies if there was a corresponding finding in the animal studies.

Often, unusual preclinical findings may require specific studies in man to exclude their clinical significance. While for others, such as testicular or thyroid tumours in animals, the mechanism of their induction is sufficiently well understood that usually no additional studies are warranted.

Of course, any metabolite-related toxicity can only be relied upon if the metabolic profile of the drug in man and in the animal species concerned was similar. While some drug metabolising isoforms show polymorphism in man, the same may not apply to the animal species used in the preclinical programme. As with impurities, any unusual metabolite, if found at a significant level in man, would have to be tested preclinically in separate studies. This is more likely if the impaired metabolism of a drug in man is likely to activate alternative pathways and generate atypical metabolites. In case of drugs with chiral centre, the enantioselectivity in pharmacokinetics in man and in animals should be similar if the findings from clinical and preclinical studies are to be correlated.

The most important areas of preclinical and clinical integration are the results of the genotoxicity, oncogenicity, and reproductive studies. The findings from the latter studies are central to approving the use of the drug during pregnancy and lactation and in children.

2.4.3 Integration of pharmaceutical and clinical data

Frequently, the formulation used in clinical trials is not the one that is ultimately marketed. The pharmaceutical dossier is scrutinised for these variations and to ensure that studies have been carried out to prove the bioequivalence of the two. The same applies if more than one dose strength or dosage form is to be marketed, for example tablets for adults and liquid preparations for use in children.

Devices used for delivery of the drug (such as inhalers) are another area requiring an integrated clinical and pharmaceutical assessment for their performance, ease of use, and implications for safety and efficacy.

The content uniformity and the finished product specifications are critical for drugs with a very narrow therapeutic index. In such cases, the specifications may have to be tightened.

2.5 Procedures for clinical trials

2.5.1 Current status of clinical trials in the UK

The primary legislation regarding the clinical trials in the UK at present is the Medicines Act 1968, which includes the definition of a clinical trial and of a medicinal product. Clinical studies involving healthy volunteers do not meet this definition of a clinical trial and, as a result, do not come under the remit of the Medicines Act 1968 or Medicines Control Agency. Such studies are subject to self-regulation by the pharmaceutical industry. However, within the next three years, the legislative basis and the procedures involved in initiating clinical trials in the UK will change following the introduction of the EU Clinical Trials Directive (see Section 2.5.2) relating to the implementation of good clinical practice in the conduct of clinical trials on medicinal products for human use.

At present there are four ways of seeking approval for the commencement of clinical trials in the UK. These are by means of a Clinical Trial Certificate (CTC), a Clinical Trial Exemption (CTX), a Doctor's and Dentist's Exemption (DDX) or as a Clinical Trial on a Marketed Product (CTMP). Each requires provision of a detailed protocol of the proposed trial.

2.5.1.1 *Clinical Trial Certificate*

A Clinical Trial Certificate is granted for a period of two years and may be renewed. Variations to the Certificate are possible. The applicant for a CTC is required to provide full information on the quality and safety of the product to be used in the trial along with any early evidence of efficacy. This information is provided under the same headings as a Marketing Authorisation application and, thus, consists of data on the chemical or biological/biotechnological and pharmaceutical aspects of the drug substance and drug product (Part II), preclinical data on the pharmacodynamics, pharmacokinetics, safety pharmacology, and toxicology of the material (Part III), and any clinical data already generated (Part IV).

The full data package is submitted and assessed by assessors from each of the three disciplines. Their assessment report is then considered by the Committee on Safety of Medicines and its sub-committees. If the decision is positive then a Certificate is issued. If the decision is negative, then the applicant has the same appeal rights as those that apply to a Marketing Authorisation application (see Section 2.8.1).

The disadvantage of the CTC approach is that it can be slow. There are no statutory timelines for the process. As a result, most applicants now use the CTX scheme. A Clinical Trial Certificate is, however, required for any proposed trials involving xenotransplantation.

2.5.1.2 Clinical Trial Exemption

This is an exemption from the need to hold a Clinical Trial Certificate and this scheme has been available since 1981. It was introduced in an attempt to avoid delay to medical research and has the advantage of statutory timelines. Summary data, under the same headings as for a CTC, are submitted and are assessed by assessors from each of the three disciplines on behalf of the Licensing Authority. If the Exemption is granted, it is valid for a period of three years. If it is refused then the applicant can submit a revised application, taking account of the reasons for refusal, which are always on safety grounds. This process can be repeated as often as is required until an Exemption can be granted. In the event of a refusal, the applicant also has the option of applying for a CTC.

The advantage of the CTX scheme is its speed, since a decision has to be made by the Licensing Authority within 35 days with the possibility of one 28-day extension to this period. The maximum time for determination of a CTX application is therefore 63 days.

2.5.1.3 Doctor's and Dentist's Exemption

This is an exemption which is available to doctors or dentists who are undertaking clinical trials initiated by them and not at the request of a pharmaceutical company. Outline information about the trial is required and a decision is made within 21 days. Where the product to be used is unlicensed and is complex, further information may be requested and the 21-day time period may be extended.

2.5.1.4 Clinical Trials on Marketed Products

Where a clinical trial is proposed with a marketed product then the CTMP scheme can be used. This is a streamlined process based on the fact that there are no quality issues with a product that has already been granted a marketing authorisation. The applicant submits a copy of the trial protocol, provides information on the investigators and, depending on whether or not the applicant is the MA holder, information on the procedures for reporting adverse drug reactions. It is only possible to use this approval for UK marketed products. It does not apply to unauthorised products manufactured specifically for trial nor to products which are licensed only in countries other than the UK.

2.5.2 EU Clinical Trials Directive

With a view to harmonising the conduct of clinical trials across the EU, Directive 2001/20/EEC was finally agreed on 14 December 2000 and was formally adopted in May 2001 with a three year transition period for its implementation.

The EU Clinical Trials Directive contains specific provisions regarding the conduct of clinical trials, including multicentre trials, on human subjects. It sets standards relating to the implementation of good clinical practice and good manufacturing practice, with a view to protecting clinical trial subjects. All clinical trials, including bioavailability and bioequivalence studies, must be designed, conducted, and reported in accordance with the principles of good clinical practice. It proposes the introduction of procedures in the Community that will provide an environment where new medicines can be developed safely and rapidly. The Directive is very detailed and comprehensive in terms of clarifying ethical and scientific standards.

It defines "clinical trial" as any investigation in human subjects intended to discover or verify the clinical, pharmacological, and/or other pharmacodynamic effects of one or more investigational medicinal product(s), and/or to identify any adverse reactions to one or more investigational medicinal product(s), and/or to study absorption, distribution, metabolism, and excretion of one or more investigational medicinal product(s) with the object of ascertaining its (their) safety and/or efficacy, and defines "subject" as an individual who participates in a clinical trial as a recipient of either the investigational medicinal product or a control. Thus, healthy volunteer studies are included.

If the competent authority of the Member State notifies the sponsor of grounds for non-acceptance, the sponsor may, on one occasion only, amend the content of the request to take due account of the grounds given. There are specific measures before the commencement and end or early termination of a clinical trial, including a time limit not exceeding 60 days for Member States to consider a valid request. No further extension to this period is permissible except in the case of trials involving medicinal products for gene therapy or somatic cell therapy or medicinal products containing genetically modified organisms for which an extension of a maximum 30 days is permitted. For these products, this 90-day period may be extended by a further 90 days under certain circumstances. In the case of xenogenic cell therapy no time limit to the authorisation period is allowable. It is important to note that "The Member States may lay down a shorter period than 60 days within their area of responsibility if that is in compliance with current practice", and that "The competent authority can nevertheless notify the sponsor before the end of this period that it has no grounds for non-acceptance."

The Directive contains detailed articles on the conduct of a clinical trial, exchange of information between Member States, EMEA, and the Commission, the reasons and procedures for suspension of the trial by a Member State, and notification of adverse events, including serious adverse reactions.

The Directive lays down specific obligations for the Member States. Many of the particulars have yet to be settled in guidance to be produced by the EC in consultation with the Member States as required by the Directive before it can be implemented in all Member States by 1 May 2004. Most of the procedures and criteria are already part of the current

UK clinical trials practice. Nevertheless, the legislative basis and the procedures involved in initiating clinical trials in the UK will change following the imminent adoption of a new EU Directive relating to the implementation of good clinical practice in the conduct of clinical trials on medicinal products for human use.

2.6   Medicines for paediatric use

It is estimated that over 50% of the medicines used in children have never actually been studied formally for use in children in specifically designed studies. The absence of suitably tested and evaluated medicinal products authorised to treat children has been an issue of concern for some time. Since existing EU medicines frequently do not include information on safe and effective use in paediatric populations, their use is largely "off-label" and may result in significant risks, including lack of efficacy and/or unexpected adverse effects, even death.

A note for guidance on clinical investigation of medicinal products in the paediatric population (CPMP/EWP/462/95) was adopted by CPMP and came into operation in September 1997. Following a round table meeting at the EMEA in 1997 organised by the EC, one of the conclusions at that time was that there was a need to strengthen the legislation, in particular by introducing a system of incentives. An ICH guideline (CPMP/ICH/2711/99) was agreed and subsequently adopted as a European guideline in July 2000 to come into operation in January 2001. This superseded the original CPMP/EWP/462/95 guideline of September 1997. Directive 2001/20/EC on Good Clinical Practice (in clinical trials), which was adopted in April 2001, also takes into account some specific concerns of performing clinical trials in children, and in particular lays down criteria for their protection in clinical trials.

It has been suggested that a new set of legislative provisions may be necessary to achieve the objectives outlined. At a meeting in November 2001, the importance of taking a European-wide approach was stressed which took into account single market considerations and development efficiencies. A consultation paper was issued in February 2002. However, even if there is a clear therapeutic need for the product, there is currently no legal provision for obliging these studies to be performed if the company does not present the product for use in the paediatric population. The paper proposes an obligation for companies to perform paediatric studies as a marketing authorisation requirement, unless the medicine is unlikely to be used for children.

In addition, the CPMP adopted in May 2002 a concept paper on a proposal to develop a "CPMP Points to Consider" document on the evaluation of the pharmacokinetics of medicinal products in the paediatric population and it is anticipated that a draft of this will be released for consultation in early 2003.

Such is the emphasis on the scientific development of medicines for paediatric use that Section 4 of the application for marketing authorisation specifically requires the applicant to state whether or not there is a paediatric development programme.

2.7 Scientific advice

In order to optimise drug development, it often becomes necessary to obtain scientific views ("scientific advice") from the authorities on issues which are not regulatory in nature and which are *not* covered by existing guidelines, or when the applicant is proposing to deviate from these guidelines. Scientific advice also facilitates the evaluation of the dossier, as there are no ambiguities or inconsistencies between Member States. It is particularly important to seek this advice before embarking on Phase III studies.

Applicants are free to solicit advice from individual Member States and they often do. Apart from the FDA, the EU Member States most often consulted are Germany, France, Sweden and the UK. However, it is often important to secure pan-European advice. Article 51 of Council Regulation EEC/2309/93 requires the EMEA to provide the Member States and the institutions of the Community with the best possible scientific advice on any question relating to the evaluation of the quality, the safety, and the efficacy of medicinal products for human or veterinary use: "To this end, the EMEA shall undertake (subsection j) where necessary, advising companies on the conduct of the various tests and trials necessary to demonstrate the quality, safety and efficacy of medicinal products."

The CPMP has established a procedure for companies to obtain scientific advice and this was greatly improved in January 1999. There is also a standard operating procedure (SOP) for the giving of scientific advice by the CPMP for innovative medicinal products (CPMP/SOP/2072/99). The procedure is highly structured to strengthen and to widen the CPMP input and to guarantee the availability of proper expertise.

The Scientific Advice Review Group (SciARG) of the CPMP is the body in charge – it brings forward to the CPMP an integrated view of all the Member States. The membership of SciARG consists of the CPMP members, two members from the Committee for Orphan Medicinal Products (COMP), experts nominated by coordinators appointed by the CPMP for each request, and representatives of different working parties. The SciARG met on the Monday before the CPMP meeting. However, in view of the ever increasing number of requests, SciARG now meets for two days about two weeks before the CPMP meetings.

A presubmission meeting with the EMEA secretariat is encouraged and is free. It is especially advisable if it is the applicant's first experience in seeking a scientific advice, and should usually be scheduled about one to two months before submitting a request. This meeting is valuable for guidance on scientific advice procedure and for help with the structure/content of the request. There is an EMEA Scientific Advice Guidance Document available to the applicants. Having paid the appropriate fees, the applicant should inform the EMEA Secretariat of the intention to submit an application about two weeks before the submission of request.

At the CPMP meeting two coordinators are appointed, to whom the applicant should submit the documentation. These two have a deadline of 20 days by when they should circulate their individual first reports. These are discussed at the next meeting of SciARG and, if there is no need for further discussion, a Joint Report is adopted and the final scientific advice letter is prepared for adoption by the CPMP. If there is a need for further discussion, the areas of disagreement between the coordinators and other members are identified and a decision is made on whether to constitute an expert meeting (and if necessary to do so, when) or request an oral explanation from the applicant. Subsequently, the events follow a highly structured course and by day 90 of the procedure, a final scientific advice is prepared for approval by CPMP.

The CPMP has emphasised repeatedly that scientific advice is not presubmission evaluation of the data available but is intended to provide clarification on issues of science. The plans for adequate development of the drug remain a company responsibility and the scientific advice is *not* binding on either side, especially if there have been significant scientific advances of relevance to the advice in the interim.

Details of guidance for companies requesting scientific advice can be accessed on the EMEA website at http://www.emea.eu.int/pdfs/human/sciadvice/426001en.pdf.

2.8 Procedures for marketing authorisations

The marketing authorisation holder (MAH) must be established within the European Economic Area (EEA), which consists of the EU plus Norway, Iceland, and Liechtenstein.

The applications for national authorisations are submitted to the national competent authority which, in the UK, is the Licensing Authority (LA), whose functions are discharged by the Medicines Control Agency (MCA) of the Department of Health. The LA/MCA are advised by the Committee on Safety of Medicines (CSM), a multidisciplinary scientific body consisting of clinical, preclinical, and pharmaceutical members well known for their expertise in their respective fields. Lay members are also included.

The applications for community authorisations are submitted to the EMEA, based in Canary Wharf, London. The EMEA is advised by the CPMP, a scientific body which consists of two delegates from each

Member State of the EU. These delegates are chosen by reason of their role and experience in the evaluation of medicinal products and they represent their competent authorities and may be accompanied by their experts. In addition to providing objective scientific opinions, these members ensure that there is appropriate coordination between the tasks of EMEA and the work of the competent national authorities, including the consultative bodies. While NASs or innovatory medicinal products *may* use this "centralised" procedure, all medicinal products developed by biotechnological processes *must* go through this "centralised" procedure and can be the subject of only the community authorisations.

2.8.1 UK national authorisations

When an application is received, it is validated to ensure that it is submitted in the correct format, with all requirements for contents and procedure satisfied, and the fees having been paid.

The data are then assessed and an integrated assessment report prepared for discussion at the CSM. It is possible to appoint special member(s) for the day in case of drugs that require unique expertise at the Committee. Following in-depth discussion, the Committee communicates its *provisional* advice to the applicant. This may be a refusal to grant a marketing authorisation and the reasons for this rejection, grant of a marketing authorisation, or, as is more often the case, grant of a marketing authorisation subject to any number of amendments to the SPC and other conditions for data to be provided. If the advice of the CSM is other than in the terms of the application, this is conveyed to the applicant in a Notice under Para. 6(1) of Schedule 2 to the Medicines for Human Use (MA etc.) Regulations 1994 (previously Section 21(1) of the Medicines Act).

In the event of a refusal or a conditional grant, the applicant either accepts the conditions or has a right of appeal. This appeal is supported by additional data or clarification of concerns from data already available.Most or all of the CSM concerns/conditions may (or may not) be resolved and the CSM has no further role after delivering their final advice to the Licensing Authority. If the advice is to reject the application, this is conveyed to the applicant in a Notice under Para. 7(4) of Schedule 2 to the Medicines for Human Use (MA etc.) Regulations 1994 (previously Section 21(3) of the Medicines Act).

If the applicant is still unhappy with refusal or revised conditions, the only option available is an appeal to the Medicines Commission. The Commission will consider only the outstanding issue(s) and their decision is final. If the applicant is still not content with the outcome, the only course open to the applicant is to seek a judicial review in the High Court. The High Court is concerned primarily with ensuring that the due legal processes were adhered to and is not concerned with the science behind the rejection.

Apart from some differences in detail, similar procedures operate for national authorisation in almost all EU Member States.

When an applicant has obtained one national authorisation (within an EU country), any ongoing assessment of that product in other EU Member States is suspended and the first authorisation granted is entered for mutual recognition by all or selected (depending on the applicant) Member States.

2.8.2 Mutual recognition procedure

Information on the mutual recognition procedure can be accessed from the EMEA website on http://pharmacos.eudra.org/F2/pharmacos/docs.htm.

During this procedure, the original competent authority and the applicant act jointly. The applicant submits an application and the updated dossier to each Member State from whom the applicant seeks a marketing authorisation. The original competent authority (now called the Reference Member State, RMS) transmits the assessment report to each Member State (now called the Concerned Member States, CMS), together with the Summary of Product Characteristics (SPC) approved by it.

From then on, each CMS treats the application almost as a national application with the important differences that, first, they deal with the RMS in respect of any concerns, queries or need for clarification, and secondly, the procedure is driven by predetermined immutable deadlines. The mutual recognition procedure is shown in Figure 2.1.

By day 50, all CMSs are required to have communicated their concerns to the RMS. By day 60, the applicant, with the help of the RMS, responds to all CMSs, addressing their concerns and enclosing a RMS-approved revised SPC. At day 75, outstanding issues of major concerns are discussed in a face-to-face meeting, known as the breakout session, between the RMS, CMSs and the applicant. The SPC is still revised further. By day 89 any CMS which still has major public health concerns declares its position and reasons for concerns. The procedure is closed on day 90 with a final revision to the SPC and the applicant having withdrawn the applications from those CMSs (on average one or two) which still have major public health concerns (the applicant has the right to withdraw the applications from objecting Member States). If the applicant refuses to withdraw the application from a CMS which has major public health concerns, the CMS has no choice but to refer the application to CPMP for arbitration. The applicant too is free to refer the application to arbitration if it considers some major objections to be unreasonable. The arbitration procedure has its own timetable.

It is easy to see why an SPC coming out of this procedure is usually a highly effective document in terms of the therapeutic claims allowed, a dose schedule that is carefully scrutinised, and detailed safety information and/or monitoring requirements. In rare instances, the SPC comes out too restricted or unbalanced because of the differences in medical practices and cultures among the Member States.

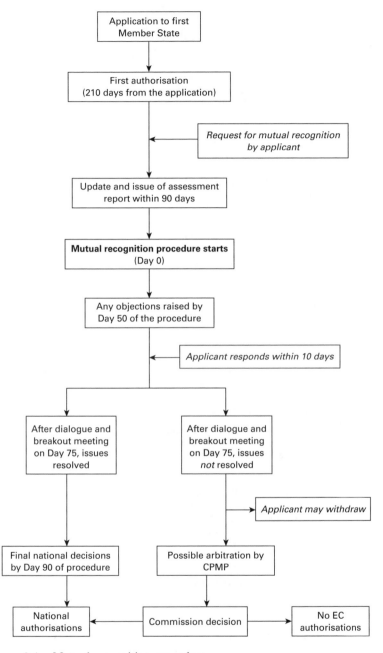

Figure 2.1 Mutual recognition procedure

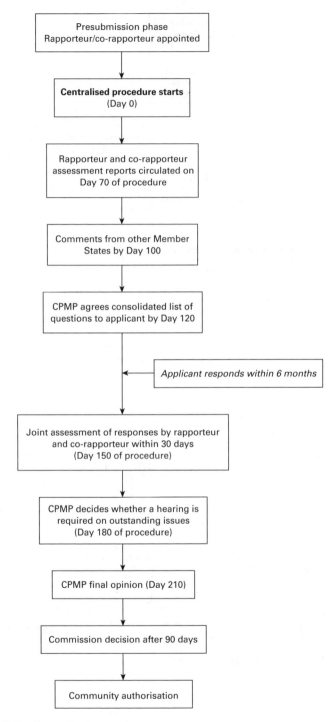

Figure 2.2 Centralised procedure

Once a product goes through the mutual recognition procedure, all its post-approval activities are undertaken by the same RMS and go through this procedure.

2.8.3   Community authorisations

Information on the centralised procedure can be accessed from the EMEA website on http://pharmacos.eudra.org/F2/pharmacos/docs.htm.

Conceptually, this procedure for Community authorisations (known as the centralised procedure) resembles a hybrid of the national procedure and the mutual recognition procedure, with the differences that first, the application is submitted to EMEA; secondly, the product undergoes a detailed assessment by the CPMP before approval in any Member State of the EU; thirdly, the applicant is provided with an opportunity to clarify any issues raised by any of the EU Member States; fourthly, the procedure naturally has an extended time frame but still with predetermined deadlines; and finally, the applicant ends up with an approval or a refusal to market the product in all or any Member States of the EU. The centralised procedure is shown in Figure 2.2.

Through the European Economic Area (EEA) agreement, three European Free Trade Area (EFTA) states – Iceland, Liechtenstein, and Norway – have adopted a complete Community *acquis* on medicinal products, and are consequently parties to the centralised procedure. The only exemption from this is that legally binding acts from the Community, for example Commission decisions, do not directly confer rights and obligations in these countries but first have to be transposed into legally binding acts in these states.

The types of product which fall within the scope of Council Regulation (EEC) No. 2309/93 as amended, are set out in the Annex to that Regulation. For medicinal products falling within the scope of Part A of the Annex, applicants are obliged to use the centralised procedure and send their application to the EMEA. For those falling within the scope of Part B of the Annex, applicants may, at their discretion, also use the centralised procedure. Unlike the previous concertation procedure (Council Directive 87/22/EEC) there is no provision for an application for a Part A medicinal product intended to be marketed in only one Member State to be exempted from the scope of the centralised procedure. Box 2.3 shows the scope of products covered by Parts A and B of this Annex.

In certain cases companies may wish to obtain more than one marketing authorisation for the same medicinal product, through either simultaneous or subsequent applications. A specific procedure has been agreed for this between the EMEA and the EC. Under this procedure, companies should inform both the EMEA and the Commission Services, at the latest four months prior to submission of their intentions, in particular providing the Commission with an explanation of the underlying motives for the multiple

---

Box 2.3 Products covered by Part A and Part B

Part A   Medicinal products derived from biotechnology

Any medicinal product developed by means of one of the following biotechnological processes:

- Recombinant DNA technology
- Controlled expression of genes coding for biologically active proteins in prokaryotes and eukaryotes, including transformed mammalian cells
- Hybridoma and monoclonal antibody methods

Any medicinal product in the composition of which there is a proteinaceous constituent obtained by means of recombinant DNA technology irrespective of whether or not the constituent is an active substance of the medicinal product. This also applies where a recombinant DNA technology step is introduced into the manufacture of a proteinaceous product after the granting of a marketing authorisation.

Part B   Innovative medicinal products

- New active substance (this is also defined further)
- Medicinal products developed by other biotechnological processes which, in the opinion of the EMEA, constitute a significant innovation
- Medicinal products administered by means of new delivery systems which, in the opinion of the EMEA, constitute a significant innovation
- Medicinal products presented for an entirely new indication which, in the opinion of the EMEA, are of significant therapeutic interest
- Medicinal products based on radio-isotopes which, in the opinion of the EMEA, are of significant therapeutic interest
- New medicinal products derived from human blood or human plasma
- Medicinal products the manufacture of which employs processes which, in the opinion of the EMEA, demonstrate a significant technical advance such as two-dimensional electrophoresis under micro-gravity
- Medicinal products intended for administration to human beings, containing a new active substance which, on the date of entry into force of the Regulation, was not authorised by any Member State for use in a medicinal product intended for human use

---

application and their intentions regarding exploitation of any authorisations granted.

At the time of receipt of the letter of intent, the proposed trade name will be checked. However, review of the trade name more than six months in advance of the submission date is also acceptable, although such an early checking will only serve to detect existing objections. This check will be performed by the EMEA in liaison with the national competent authorities, in order to determine whether the name would raise any identifiable public health concern, for resolution one month thereafter.

For applications to be processed via the centralised procedure, the CPMP appoints one of its members to act as rapporteur for the coordination of the evaluation of an application for a marketing authorisation. The CPMP will also appoint a second member to act as co-rapporteur. For line extensions, the CPMP will decide on the need for appointment of a co-rapporteur on a case-by-case basis. All members have equal opportunities to play the role of rapporteur or co-rapporteur, and therefore the CPMP members are invited to express their preference regarding rapporteurships in writing in advance of the meeting at which rapporteurs are appointed. Rapporteurs are usually appointed at every other meeting to facilitate the decision making process as regards (co)-rapporteurships.

Appointments of rapporteur and co-rapporteur are made on the basis of two criteria: first, the preferences expressed by the applicant, and secondly, the preferences of CPMP members based on their expertise. The CPMP will take into account preferences expressed by applicants in selecting rapporteurs, although there is no obligation to follow those preferences. In order to increase the likelihood that the choice of the applicant is followed, the applicant is advised to express three to four preferences for names of members coming from three to four delegations from EU Member States, Norway or Iceland. The membership of the CPMP has been established so that it is a technically expert committee that advises the EMEA. A member of staff of the Human Medicines Evaluation Unit of the EMEA is officially appointed as EMEA project manager, and the applicant is notified of the project manager's identity. The project manager remains responsible for providing procedural guidance during the presubmission phase, coordinating the validation of the application submitted, monitoring compliance with the time frame and coordinating all the activities (between the applicant, EMEA, CPMP and the rapporteurs) with regard to the progression and final determination of the application.

On receipt of a valid application via the EMEA, the rapporteur and the co-rapporteur both prepare their separate detailed assessment reports, which are circulated to the EMEA and all other Member States by day 70 from the start of the procedure. By day 100, rapporteur, co-rapporteur, CPMP members and EMEA receive comments from all other members of the CPMP. A draft consolidated list of questions is prepared by the rapporteur and circulated to the members by day 115. A final consolidated list of questions is agreed by the CPMP on day 120 and communicated to the applicant, and the clock of the procedure is stopped. This consolidated list includes any major public health concerns, points for clarification and changes to the SPC, raised by all the Member States.

The applicant, after seeking clarification from the rapporteur if necessary, responds to these issues (the maximum time allowed for responding is no longer than six months) and the clock is restarted. The rapporteur and co-rapporteur prepare a joint assessment (of responses) report that is circulated by day 150 to all members of the CPMP. The deadline for comments from CPMP members to be sent to rapporteur and co-rapporteur, EMEA, and other CPMP members is day 170. Any issue(s) still outstanding are discussed on day 180 of the procedure at the CPMP. These are communicated to the applicant and may be addressed at a hearing before the CPMP, and a decision is made on whether to issue a positive or a negative CPMP opinion. The deadline for adopting an opinion is day 210 of the procedure. A positive opinion requires an absolute majority (at least 16 positive votes of the potential 30) in support; otherwise a negative opinion is issued. If positive, the CPMP opinion is communicated to the EC for their decision.

A negative opinion may be the subject of an appeal, a procedure that has its own time frame. The EMEA immediately informs the applicant when the opinion of the CPMP is that the application does not satisfy the criteria for authorisation set out in the Regulation. The following documents are annexed and/or appended to the opinion: first, the appended CPMP assessment report stating the reasons for its negative conclusions, and secondly, when appropriate, the divergent positions of committee members, with their grounds. The applicant may notify the EMEA/CPMP of their intention to appeal within 15 days of receipt of the opinion (after which, if the applicant does not appeal, they are deemed to have agreed with the opinion and it becomes the final opinion). The grounds for appeal must be forwarded to the EMEA within 60 days of receipt of the opinion. If the applicant wishes to appear before the CPMP for an oral explanation, this request should also be sent at this stage. The CPMP may decide to appoint a new rapporteur and co-rapporteur, for whom applicants can express their preference, to coordinate the appeal procedure, accompanied, if necessary, by additional experts. Within 60 days from the receipt of the grounds for appeal, the CPMP will consider whether its opinion should be revised. If considered necessary, an oral explanation can be held within this 60-day time frame. Once the CPMP issues a final opinion, it is forwarded (with the required annexes) within 30 days of its adoption, to the Commission, the Member States, Norway, and Iceland and to the applicant, stating the reasons for its conclusion.

The opinion is issued by the CPMP and is transmitted to the EC, which issues a decision that is binding upon all Member States. Once a product goes through the centralised procedure, all its post-approval activities are undertaken by the same rapporteur and go through this procedure.

Information regarding each of the products approved through the centralised procedure (European Public Assessment Report – EPAR) can be obtained via the EMEA website at http://www.emea.eu.int/htms/ human/epar/epar.htm.

2.9   Applications for orphan designation

The definition of what constitutes a "rare" disease varies with the region. The prevalence figure accepted in the EU is no more than 5 individuals per 10 000 of the EU population. In the USA, it is defined as a disease that affects less than 200 000 of the population. This size of population is approximately equal to a prevalence of 7·5 individuals per 10 000 of the US population. The prevalence figures accepted in Japan and Australia are no more than 4·2 and 1·1 individuals respectively per 10 000 of their corresponding populations.

The sponsor proposing to develop a drug for an orphan indication is required to submit an application for the designation of a drug as orphan for a defined clinical entity. To meet the criteria for a successful orphan designation, the applicant should establish:

- that the prevalence of the condition in the EU is ≤ 5 in 10 000 or that the product is unlikely to generate sufficient return on investment
- the life-threatening or debilitating nature of the condition
- the biological plausibility of the use of the drug in the indication proposed
- that no satisfactory methods exist for the treatment of the condition or if there is a product already authorised in the EU, the medicinal product will be of significant benefit.

All claims should be substantiated by references.

The applicants are generally advised to have a presubmission meeting with the secretariat. On receipt of a valid application, COMP appoints an EMEA coordinator and a COMP member as a coordinator (day 0). A joint report is prepared by these two for discussion at the next meeting (day 30). If COMP is satisfied that the criteria are met, a positive opinion is issued. More often, there are issues that require clarification and a list of issues to be addressed or questions is sent to the applicant. The responses are assessed by the coordinators and discussed at the next meeting (day 60). If there are still any outstanding issues, these can be dealt with during an oral hearing on day 90 when an opinion is issued. In case of a negative opinion, the applicant has full appeal rights.

Following its consideration of an application, COMP adopts an opinion which is transmitted to the European Commission, which is responsible for granting a binding decision on the orphan designation status of the drug for the indication concerned. This is similar to the EC decisions on CPMP opinions in respect of a centralised application or a variation.

Products designated as orphan products have automatic access to the centralised procedure but an applicant may opt to take the mutual recognition route. In this event, no withdrawals are permissible, as are possible with the conventional drug application going through this route. Applications for marketing authorisation of orphan medicinal products are evaluated with the same scientific rigour as the normal drugs.

Details about orphan drug legislation, its application, and associated procedures and guidance notes are available at the EMEA website at http://www.emea.eu.int/sitemap.htm.

2.10   Sale and supply of human medicines

Regarding the sale and supply, the natural tendency of medicinal products approved in the UK was a pharmacy sale under the supervision of a pharmacist, unless restrictions were relaxed or tightened. Legislation had already existed in the USA (Durham–Humphrey Amendment of 1951) that defined the kinds of drugs that could not be safely used without medical supervision and restricted their sale to prescription by a licensed practitioner, and in 1958 the FDA published the first list of Substances Generally Recognised as Safe (GRAS). The list contains nearly 200 substances. With a similar objective in mind, the Medicines Commission recommended the appointments of a "Committee on Prescription Only Medicines and Related Matters" and a "General Sales Lists Committee".

In the UK, a significant milestone was reached in 1977 when the work on classification of medicines was completed and the new arrangements provided for three categories according to their safety factor – those available on prescription only (POM), those sufficiently safe to be on general sale to the public through any retail outlet (GSL), and an intermediate category of those which, while not requiring a prescription, should only be sold at pharmacies (P). Under section 59 of the Medicines Act, all new medicinal products containing an NAS (new active substance) and not previously on market are Prescription Only for the first five years. A conscious decision is made for reclassification of each before the five year period expires. This requires updating the Prescription Only Medicines (POM) Order or the General Sales List (GSL) Order.

Restriction of medicinal products to the POM list had been recommended where they contain substances that present a toxicity hazard, are dependence-producing or present a community hazard. In special circumstances and subject to special provisions, a pharmacist is allowed to supply a POM medicine without a prescription when, by reason of some emergency, a doctor was unable to furnish a prescription immediately. This emergency exemption was originally designed to enable diabetic patients to obtain an emergency supply of insulin which, at that time, was a Prescription Only Medicine. The GSL list included products that were pre-packed and could "with reasonable safety" be sold or supplied by retail at shops other than registered pharmacies. These were the products where the hazard to health, the risk of misuse, or the need to take special precautions in handling was small and where wider sale would be a convenience to the purchaser – the concept of "with reasonable safety". Inclusion in no way implied that the product had any therapeutic value. Nor does it imply that no harm could ever come from its use.

2.10.1 Harmonisation across the EU

The supply of medicinal products for human use to the public varied appreciably from one Member State to another, whereas medicinal products sold without prescription in certain Member States could be obtained only on medical prescription in others. Council Directive 92/26/EEC "Concerning the classification for the supply of medicinal products for human use" was adopted as an initial step towards harmonising the basic principles applicable to the classification for the supply of medicinal products in the Community or in the Member States concerned. The relevant articles in Directive 2001/83/EC are 70–75.

Article 1 of Council Directive 92/26/EEC provides two classifications for the supply of medicinal products for human use in the Community:

- medicinal products subject to medical prescription
- medicinal products not subject to medical prescription.

Article 3 provides the criteria for classifying a medicinal product as subject to medical prescription. These are products which are likely to present a danger either directly or indirectly, even when used correctly, if utilised without medical supervision; or are frequently and to a very wide extent used incorrectly, and as a result are likely to present a direct or indirect danger to human health; or contain substances or preparations thereof, the activity and/or adverse reactions of which require further investigation; or are normally prescribed by a doctor to be administered parenterally. Thus a medicinal product that meets these criteria is subject to a medical prescription and a medicinal product that does not meet these criteria is not subject to a medical prescription.

The Directive provides discretion and options to Member States for subcategories for medicinal products which are available on medical prescription only but is silent on the subcategorising of non-prescription products.

There is also an EU guideline (dated 29 September 1998 and in operation since January 1999) on changing the classification for the supply of a medicinal product for human use. Article 3 predetermines the POM products. Therefore, the criteria in Article 3 have been used as a basis for this guideline. This guideline does not address the different restrictions that may be available for medicinal products not subject to a medical prescription, such as available in pharmacies only following initial medical diagnosis, or available on general sale, as the case may be.

Part 2 of this guideline describes the data required for changing the classification. The documentation concerning safety and efficacy in support of an application for a change in the classification for the supply will depend on the nature of the active substance and the extent of any changes to the marketing authorisation. In order to facilitate the evaluation of safety in relation to benefit it should be presented in a logical and concise manner.

2.10.2 Expert Report

In all cases, an Expert Report, which is a critical analysis of the proposed availability of the product without a medical prescription with the dose and indications as stated in the application, must be provided. The expert is expected to take a clear position, defend the proposal in light of current scientific knowledge, and demonstrate why none of the criteria that determine classification for supply subject to a medical prescription applies to the product.

2.10.3 Safety

Safety data are vital in supporting any application for a change in the classification. Such data will cover the following aspects.

- A summary should be given of, or references to, animal studies or studies on humans that show low general toxicity and no relevant reproductive toxicity, genotoxic or carcinogenic properties relevant to the experience/exposure of the product.
- Experience in terms of patient exposure to the substance needs to be considerable and should be outlined. Normally, active substances which are suitable for supply without a medical prescription will have been in widespread use for five years, in medicinal products subject to a medical prescription. However, provided enough data is available, this does not exclude the possibility of an authority accepting a shorter time. Adverse drug reactions to the pharmaceutical form and dose proposed for supply not subject to a medical prescription should in normal conditions be minor and should cease on discontinuing therapy.
- Information should be provided on adverse reactions, including experience of use without medical supervision, for example in another Member State or in a third country.
- Risks of drug interactions should be detailed.
- Consequences concerning misuse, for example use for longer periods than recommended, as well as accidental or intended overdose and the use of higher doses, should be discussed.
- Consequences of the use of the product by a patient who has incorrectly assessed his or her condition or symptoms should be considered.

- The application should consider the consequences of incorrect or delayed diagnosis of a patient's condition or symptoms due to self-medication with the product.

2.10.4 Efficacy

Evidence of the product's efficacy is not normally considered in the application for changing the classification for supply, unless this application also includes changes to the indications or posology. If other parts of the dossier are changed, for example indication, posology or strength, then supporting data should be provided. A suitable time period for treatment of the suggested indication(s) should be justified and given, together with a proposed pack size.

2.10.5 Product information

For a medicinal product classified for supply without a medical prescription, the proposed product label and leaflet are important elements of the application and will be closely examined for comprehensive information and effectiveness in protecting patients from any safety hazards.

Under the Directive, the competent authorities are required to draw up a list of the medicinal products subject, on their territory, to medical prescription, specifying, if necessary, the category of classification. They should update this list annually. The Directive also requires that on the occasion of the five-yearly renewal of the marketing authorisation or when new facts are brought to their notice, the competent authorities should examine and, as appropriate, amend the classification of a medicinal product. Each year, Member States have to communicate to the Commission and to the other Member States the changes that have been made to the list referred to above.

2.11 Communications

Communication with healthcare professionals and the general public is essential to promoting safe and effective use of medicines. Legislation is in place in the EU to ensure not only that these avenues of communications are not abused but also to impose appropriate penalties when the legislative code is breached.

2.11.1 Package information leaflet

The package information leaflets and labels are regulated by Council Directive 92/27/EEC of 31 March 1992 on the labelling of medicinal products for human use and on package leaflets. Article 6 of this Directive requires the inclusion within the packaging of all medicinal products of a leaflet for the information of users. This is obligatory unless all the

Box 2.4 Contents of a package insert leaflet

- Identification of the medicinal product

  - the name of the medicinal product, followed by the common name
  - the pharmaceutical form and/or the strength
  - a full statement of the active ingredients and excipients expressed qualitatively and a statement of the active ingredients expressed quantitatively, using their common names, in the case of each presentation of the product
  - the pharmaceutical form and the contents by weight, by volume or by number of doses of the product, in the case of each presentation of the product
  - the pharmacotherapeutic group, or type of activity in terms easily comprehensible for the patient

- The name and address of the holder of the authorisation
- The name and address of the holder of the manufacturer
- The therapeutic indications
- A list of information which is necessary before taking the medicinal product

  - contraindications
  - appropriate precautions for use
  - forms of interaction with other medicinal products and other forms of interaction which may affect the action of the medicinal product
  - special warnings, taking into account the particular condition of certain categories of users (for example, children, pregnant or breastfeeding women, the elderly, persons with specific pathological conditions)

- Mention, if appropriate, of potential effects on the mental alertness

  - ability to drive vehicles or to operate machinery

- Details of excipients

  - knowledge of which is important for the safe and effective use of the medicinal product and included in the guidelines published

- The necessary and usual instructions for proper use, in particular

  - the dosage
  - the method and, if necessary, route of administration
  - the frequency of administration, specifying if necessary the appropriate time at which the medicinal product may or must be administered
  - depending on the nature of the product, the duration of treatment where it should be limited

- The action to be taken in the case of an overdose
- The course of action to take when one or more doses have not been taken

continued....

- Indication, if necessary, of the risk of withdrawal effects
- A description of the undesirable effects

    - which can occur under normal use and, if necessary, the action to be taken in such a case; patients should be expressly invited to communicate any undesirable effect which is not mentioned in the leaflet to their doctor or to their pharmacist

- A reference to the expiry date indicated on the label, with

    - a warning against using the product after this date
    - where appropriate, special storage precautions
    - if necessary, a warning against certain visible signs of deterioration

- The date on which the package leaflet was last revised

information required by Article 7 is directly conveyed on the outer packaging or on the immediate packaging. Article 7 specifies that the package leaflet shall be drawn up in accordance with the SPC and that it shall include the information in an order which is specified in the Directive. An acceptable package information leaflet is expected to contain the details shown in Box 2.4.

Article 8 requires that the package leaflet must be written in clear and understandable terms for the patient and be clearly legible in the official language or languages of the Member State where the medicinal product is placed on the market. This provision does not prevent the package leaflet being printed in several languages, provided that the same information is given in all the languages used. In order to address this issue of readability, the EU has issued a detailed guideline, dated 29 September 1998, on the readability of the label and package leaflet of a medicinal product for human use and this came into operation in January 1999. This guideline makes recommendations on the print size and type as well as print colour. Regarding the syntax, it recommends that as far as possible, overlong sentences (that is, more than 20 words) should be avoided.

Moreover, it is recommended that lines of a length exceeding 70 characters are not used. Different fonts, upper and lower case letters, length of words, number of clauses per sentence, and length of sentences can all influence readability. A group of bullet points should be introduced with a colon and a single full stop should be placed at the end of the group. A list of bullet points should begin with the uncommon and specific case and end with the common or general case, unless this is inappropriate for the product. A minimum number of words should be used in the bullet points and never more than one sentence. There should be no more than nine items where the bullet points are simple and no more than five when they are complex. Abbreviations should be avoided.

2.11.2 Promotion and advertising

Advertising is regulated by Council Directive 92/28/EEC of 31 March 1992 on the advertising of medicinal products for human use. For the purposes of this Directive, advertising of medicinal products includes any form of door-to-door information, canvassing activity or inducement designed to promote the prescription, supply, sale or consumption of medicinal products. It includes in particular the advertising of medicinal products to the general public, to persons qualified to prescribe or supply them, visits by medical sales representatives to persons qualified to prescribe medicinal products, the supply of samples, the provision of inducements to prescribe or supply medicinal products by the gift, offer or promise of any benefit or bonus, whether in money or in kind, except when their intrinsic value is minimal, sponsorship of promotional meetings attended by persons qualified to prescribe or supply medicinal products, sponsorship of scientific congresses attended by persons qualified to prescribe or supply medicinal products, and in particular payment of their travelling and accommodation expenses in connection therewith.

The Directive has special provisions for advertising to the general public as well as to the health professions.

Member States have an obligation to prohibit any advertising of a medicinal product in respect of which a marketing authorisation has not been granted in accordance with Community law. Member States must prohibit the advertising to the general public of medicinal products for therapeutic indications specified in the Directive. When permissible, all advertising to the general public of a medicinal product has to be set out in a prescribed manner.

All parts of the advertising of a medicinal product must comply with the particulars listed in the SPC. The advertising of a medicinal product should encourage only the rational use of the medicinal product, by presenting it objectively and without exaggerating its properties, and not so as to be misleading.

In respect of advertising to health professionals, there are detailed requirements in respect of provision of information, free samples, and gifts and hospitality as well as the training and duties of medical sales representatives.

Member States have an obligation to monitor advertising and are required to ensure that there are adequate and effective methods to monitor the advertising of medicinal products. Such methods, which may be based on a system of prior vetting, must in any event include legal provisions under which persons or organisations regarded under national law as having a legitimate interest in prohibiting any advertisement inconsistent with the Directive may take legal action against such an advertisement, or bring such an advertisement before an administrative authority competent either to decide on complaints or to initiate appropriate legal proceedings.

Under the legal provisions, Member States must confer upon the courts or administrative authorities powers enabling them, in cases where they deem such measures to be necessary, taking into account all the interests involved and in particular the public interest, to order the cessation of, or to institute appropriate legal proceedings for an order for the cessation of, misleading advertising, or if misleading advertising has not yet been published but publication is imminent, to order the prohibition of, or to institute appropriate legal proceedings for an order for the prohibition of, such publication, even without proof of actual loss or damage or of intention or negligence on the part of the advertiser. Member States must also make provisions for the statutory measures that confer various powers upon the courts or administrative authorities.

The Directive, however, does not exclude the voluntary control of advertising of medicinal products by self-regulatory bodies and recourse to such bodies, if proceedings before such bodies are possible in addition to the judicial or administrative proceedings referred to above.

2.12   Pharmacovigilance

Every Member State has local legislation and obligations for maintaining effective pharmacovigilance and there are criminal, civil, and/or regulatory penalties for non-compliance by marketing authorisation holders.

The legislative framework for pharmacovigilance across the EU is already provided in a number of regulations, directives, and guidelines. These consist of Council Regulation EEC/2309/93, Commission Regulation 540/95, Council Directive 75/319/EEC as amended and Commission Directive 2000/38/EC. Various legislation has been codified in Articles 101–108 of Directive 2001/83/EC. Volume 9 of the Notice to Applicants is a compilation of all the guidelines on pharmacovigilance.

The harmonisation of pharmacovigilance within the EU is a relatively recent process. Not surprisingly, there are significant variations between Member States (and from other major regulatory regions such as the USA and Japan) in terms of reporting requirements generally. Neither are there any consistent requirements for periodic reporting of clinical trials or post-authorisation safety studies. Despite most Member States using Regulation EEC/2309/93 as the basis for expedited reporting, there are still a number of variations between States in terms of reports requiring expedited reporting.

However, rapid progress is being made to eliminate inconsistencies and to harmonise procedures generally. There is an active Pharmacovigilance Working Party (PhVWP) which meets every month, with the Chairman reporting to the plenary meeting of the CPMP. PhVWP has already adopted a number of guidelines. Of particular interest are the following two.

2.12.1 Notice to Marketing Authorisation Holders: Pharmacovigilance Guidelines (CPMP/PhVWP/108/99)

This guideline lays down the roles and responsibilities of the marketing authorisation holders and of the national competent authorities in respect of the products authorised through the national procedures (including the mutual recognition procedure). Also defined are the roles and responsibilities of the Reference Member States (for mutual recognition products) and of the rapporteur and EMEA for centrally approved products. Marketing authorisation holders' role and responsibilities include having a named, qualified person responsible for pharmacovigilance at the EU level, and there may be a need for an additional named person at the national level when this is required.

The duties of the qualified person include:

* the establishment and maintenance of a system for collection, evaluation and collation of all suspected adverse reaction information so that it may be accessed at a single point in the Community
* preparation of reports referred to in Council Directive 75/319/EEC for competent authorities and for centrally authorised products, for competent authorities and EMEA reports referred to in Council Regulation EEC/2309/93
* reporting to the Member State concerned within 15 days of receipt of information on all suspected serious adverse reactions within the Community
* preparation of six-monthly scientific reports and records of all suspected serious adverse reactions for the first two years after marketing, annual reports for the next three years, and thereafter at renewal of the authorisation – these are the Periodic Safety Update Reports (PSURs)
* answering fully and promptly any request from competent authorities for the provision of additional information necessary for the evaluation of the benefits and risks afforded by a medicinal product.

2.12.2 Note for Guidance on Procedure for Competent Authorities on the Undertaking of Pharmacovigilance Activities (CPMP/PhVWP/175/95 Rev. 1)

This guideline lays down the requirements and procedures for national competent authorities regarding the collection, evaluation and management of pharmacovigilance data on medicinal products, however authorised in the community.

Other guidelines adopted by PhVWP are listed below:

- Requirements related to the Electronic Transmission of Individual Case Safety Reports in the Community (ICH M2)
- Note for Guidance on Electronic Exchange of Pharmacovigilance Information for Human and Veterinary Medicinal Products in the European Union (CPMP/PhVWP/2056/99)
- Note for Guidance on the Rapid Alert System (RAS) and Non-Urgent Information System (NUIS) in Human Pharmacovigilance (CPMP/ PhVWP/005/96, *Revision 1*).

The need for more structured monitoring of the post-marketing safety of products approved by centralised and mutual recognition routes, and for a very interactive relationship with other regions and principles for providing the WHO with pharmacovigilance information, has been set out in the following papers:

- Conduct of Pharmacovigilance for Centrally Authorised Products (CPMP/183/97)
- Conduct of Pharmacovigilance for Medicinal Products Authorised through the Mutual Recognition Procedure (Rev. 1)
- Principles of Providing the World Health Organisation with Pharmacovigilance Information (CPMP/PhVWP/053/98).

2.13 Safety referrals to CPMP

The EU has a highly structured legislative framework for resolution of safety related referrals to CPMP – for new applications as well as for products already authorised.

For mutual recognition applications, Article 29 of Directive 2001/83/EC provides that where a Member State considers that there are grounds for supposing that the marketing authorisation of the medicinal product concerned may present a risk to public health, it shall forthwith inform the applicant, the RMS, other CMSs, and the EMEA. The Member State must state its reasons in detail and indicate what action may be necessary to correct any defect in the application.

Article 30 provides for a situation where several applications have been made for a marketing authorisation for a particular medicinal product, and Member States have adopted divergent decisions concerning the authorisation of the medicinal product or its suspension or withdrawal. A Member State, or the Commission, or the marketing authorisation holder, may refer the matter to the CPMP for application of the procedure laid down in Article 32. The Member State concerned, the marketing authorisation holder or the Commission must clearly identify the question which is referred to the CPMP for consideration and, where appropriate, must inform the holder.

Under Article 31, the Member States or the Commission or the applicant or holder of the marketing authorisation may, in specific cases where the interests of the Community are involved, refer the matter to the CPMP for the application of the procedure laid down in Article 32 before reaching a decision on a request for a marketing authorisation or on the suspension or withdrawal of an authorisation, or on any other variation to the terms of a marketing authorisation which appears necessary, in particular to take account of the information collected in accordance with Title IX of the Directive 2001/83/EC. The Member State concerned or the Commission must clearly identify the question which is referred to the CPMP for consideration and must inform the marketing authorisation holder.

Article 32 describes the timelines and the procedures to be followed following a referral. When reference is made to the procedure described in this Article, the CPMP has to consider the matter concerned and issue a reasoned opinion within 90 days of the date on which the matter was referred to it. However, in cases submitted to the CPMP in accordance with Articles 30 and 31, this period may be extended by 90 days. In case of urgency, on a proposal from its Chairman, the CPMP may agree to a shorter deadline.

2.14   Conclusions and Review 2001

For all practical purposes, the most important document is the Summary of Product Characteristics (SPC). Its terms are carefully scrutinised by the competent authority in light of the dossier accompanying the application. The approved SPC sets out the agreed position of the medicinal product as distilled during the course of the assessment process. It is the definitive statement between the competent authority and the marketing authorisation holder and it is the common basis of communication between the competent authorities of all Member States. As such, the content cannot be changed except with the approval of the originating competent authority. The agreed SPC forms the basis for subsequent marketing of the medicinal product and all information which may/should be made available to health professionals and the patients.

Involving as it does the scrutiny of pharmaceutical, preclinical, and clinical assessors from each of the Member States, the Euro-SPC of a NAS (new active substance) is a highly effective document, doing full justice to the efficacy of the product and delineating precise indications and dose schedules for its clinical use while providing all information aimed at or necessary for safeguarding the public.

The marketing authorisation holder needs the approval of the competent authority should it wish to vary the terms of the SPC. Such variations require supporting data.

There are, of course, special provisions when a Member State can suspend or revoke an authorisation where the product proves to be harmful in the normal conditions of use or where its therapeutic efficacy is found to be lacking or where its qualitative and quantitative composition is not as declared. An authorisation may also be suspended or revoked where the particulars in the dossier are incorrect or have not been amended or when the controls on the finished product have not been carried out.

Regarding all activities for the regulation of pharmaceuticals at the EU level, Article 71 of Regulation EEC/2309/93 required that "Within six years of the entry into force of this Regulation, the Commission shall publish a general report on the experience of the procedures laid down in this Regulation, in Chapter III of Directive 75/319/EEC and in Chapter IV of Directive 81/851/EEC". The tender was awarded to a consortium of Cameron McKenna and Arthur Anderson. The general objectives of the review were to provide answers to the following questions.

- Have the Centralised and Decentralised Procedures contributed in a qualitative and quantitative sense to the creation of a harmonised Community market in medicinal products?
- Have these procedures provided a high degree of safety of use for patients? Is the quality of the evaluation carried out in the two procedures of a comparable level?
- Have the availability of the new medicinal products and patients' access to such products been improved by the introduction of the new Community system and are they satisfactory at the present time?
- What are the benefits of the two procedures (cost/benefit ratio)? Are they carried out with sufficient transparency?

The full report from Cameron McKenna, entitled "Evaluation of the Operation of Community Procedures for the Authorisation of Medicinal Products", is a comprehensive and highly constructive document. It can be accessed on the EMEA website at http://pharmacos.eudra.org/F2/pharmacos/docs.htm#news.

All interested parties, such as the national authorities, the EC, and the EFPIA, have considered and discussed the report from Cameron McKenna and have offered their solutions. These have been actively debated and discussed. The EC has now proposed comprehensive reform of the EU pharmaceutical legislation. These proposals can be

---

Box 2.5 Principles and guidelines for GMP

- Quality management: Implementation of quality assurance system
- Personnel: Appropriately qualified with specified duties, responsibilities and management structures
- Premises and equipment: Appropriate to intended operations

Documentation

- Production: According to pre-established operating procedures with appropriate in-process controls, regularly validated
- Quality control: Independent department, or external laboratory responsible for all aspects of quality control. Samples from each batch must be retained for one year, unless not practicable
- Work contracted out: Subject to contract, and under the same conditions, without subcontracting
- Complaints and product recall: Record keeping and arrangements for notification of competent authority
- Self inspection: By the manufacturer of his own processes with appropriate record keeping

---

accessed on the EMEA website at http://pharmacos.eudra.org/F2/review/index.htm.

This involves significant amendments to Directive 2001/83/EC (for human medicines) and Council Regulation EEC/2309/93. During its first reading of the proposed changes to the pharmaceutical legislation, the European Parliament has already approved 144 of the 167 amendments to Regulation EEC/2309/93 and 160 of the 202 amendments to Directive 2001/83/EC. It is anticipated that the European system of the control of human medicinal products will undergo significant changes over the next few years. The result should be an even more robust and efficient system.

2.15 Regulatory activities under national authorities

Essentially, four major activities still remain entirely within the remit of national competent authorities.

2.15.1 Manufacturers Licences

Manufacturers Licences were issued by the UK Licensing Authority from the inception of the Medicines Act to cover all manufacturing operations including those previously embraced by the Therapeutic Substances Act (TSA). The Medicines Inspectorate laid down standards in its *Guide to Good Manufacturing Practice* (GMP), otherwise known as "The Orange Guide". The most recent edition was issued in 1997. Although the issue of Manufacturers Licences remains a national regulatory function, it is governed by the standards set in EC Commission Directive 91/356/EEC, which can be summarised as follows.

The Directive lays down the principles and guidelines of manufacturing practice to be followed in the production of medicines, and requirements to ensure that manufacturers and Member States adhere to its provisions. Manufacturers must ensure that production occurs in accordance with GMP, and the manufacturing authorisation. Imports from non-EU countries must have been produced to standards at least equivalent to those in the EU, and the importer must ensure this. All manufacturing processes should be consistent with information provided in the marketing authorisation application, as accepted by the authorities. Methods have to be updated in the light of scientific advances, and modifications must be submitted for approval.

Good manufacturing standards are enforced by the Medicines Inspectorate of the Medicines Control Agency. The UK has been involved in the Pharmaceutical Inspection Convention (PIC) since its inception and through the Orange Guide set standards which are now reflected in the EU Directives. Articles 111–121 of Directive 2001/83/EC define the obligations of the Member States in respect of supervision and sanctions.

Fees are charged for inspections. Usually, there is mutual recognition of inspections undertaken by countries which are members of the PIC. Membership of the PIC is wider than that of the EU.

2.15.2 Wholesale Dealers Licences

This activity, established under the Medicines Act, still remains wholly within the remit of national authorities but in accordance with Directive 92/25/EEC on the wholesale, distribution of medicinal products for human use (now Articles 76–85 of Directive 2001/83/EC).

There are strict controls and requirements placed on the wholesalers in respect of premises, installations, and equipment for appropriate conservation and distribution of medicines, and for record keeping. They must comply with Good Distribution Practice.

2.15.3 Routes of sale and supply

As stated earlier, the Medicines Act 1968 assumes that in the UK all medicinal products will be sold through a pharmacy unless it is decided by the Licensing Authority that supply of the product should be limited to being dispensed only on a registered medical practitioner's prescription. Such products appear on the POM list and their packaging is marked POM. Similarly, products available through outlets other than pharmacies and designated as GSL products, are listed in the General Sales List and their packaging is marked GSL.

Additional restrictions on supply are imposed by the Misuse of Drugs Act 1971 and the Misuse of Drugs Regulations. Substances that have a potential for abuse are scheduled under three categories, Class A, B and C.

> *Class A* includes: alfentanil, cocaine, dextromoramide, diamorphine (heroin), dipipanone, lysergide (LSD), methadone, morphine, opium, pethidine, phencyclidine, and class B substances when prepared for injection.
>
> *Class B* includes: oral amphetamines, barbiturates, cannabis, cannabis resin, codeine, ethylmorphine, glutethimide, pentazocine, phenmetrazine, and pholcodine.
>
> *Class C* includes: certain drugs related to the amphetamines such as benzphetamine and chlorphentermine, buprenorphine, diethylpropion, mazindol, meprobamate, pemoline, pipradrol, and most benzodiazepines.

The Misuse of Drugs Regulations 1985 define the classes of person who are authorised to supply and possess controlled drugs while acting in their professional capacities and lay down the conditions under which these activities may be carried out. In the Regulations drugs are divided into five schedules each specifying the requirements governing such activities as import, export, production, supply, possession, prescribing, and record keeping which apply to them.

Schedule 1 includes drugs such as cannabis and lysergide which are not used medicinally. Possession and supply are prohibited except in accordance with Home Office authority.

Schedule 2 includes drugs such as diamorphine (heroin), morphine, pethidine, quinalbarbitone, glutethimide, amphetamine, and cocaine and which are subject to the full controlled drug requirements relating to prescriptions, safe custody (except for quinalbarbitone), the need to keep registers, etc. (unless exempted in Schedule 5).

Schedule 3 includes the barbiturates (except quinalbarbitone, now Schedule 2), buprenorphine, diethylproprion, mazindol, meprobamate, pentazocine, phentermine, and temazepam. They are subject to the special prescription requirements (except for phenobarbitone and temazepam) but not to the safe custody requirements (except for buprenorphine, diethylpropion, and temazepam) nor to the need to keep registers (although there are requirements for the retention of invoices for two years).

Schedule 4 includes 33 benzodiazepines (temazepam is now in Schedule 3) and pemoline which are subject to minimal control. In particular, controlled drug prescription requirements do not apply and they are not subject to safe custody.

Schedule 5 includes those preparations which, because of their strength, are exempt from virtually all Controlled Drug requirements other than retention of invoices for two years.

There is no "harmonised" comprehensive legislation to control drugs of abuse under an EU Directive.

2.15.4 Pricing policy

Each Member State of the EU operates its own policy regarding the pricing of pharmaceutical products. In the UK, the primary tool is the Pharmaceutical Price Regulation Scheme (PPRS), which is better described as a profit regulating scheme.

The EC has in the past tried to achieve a harmonisation of prices but this could not be achieved and produced the Transparency Directive (89/105/EEC). The contents of this Directive can be summarised by its various Articles as follows:

Article 1	If the authorities fix prices of the medicinal products, they must comply with the rules of this Directive
Article 2.1	Time limit to comply with rules is 90 days
Article 2.2	Reasons must be given by authorities if the price is other than that sought by the person putting the product on the market
Article 3	Deals with procedures where price increases are sought
Article 4	Imposed price freezes
Article 5	Deals with profit regulation schemes
Article 6	Deals with Limited Lists (Positive lists)
Article 7	Deals with Limited Lists (Negative lists)
Article 8	Classification of products by therapeutic class for inclusion or exclusion
Article 9	Report on the operation of the Directive to be made within two years of its adoption
Article 10	A Committee to be set up
Article 11	Demand that all Member States conform.

Essentially, the Directive allowed Member States to operate whatever scheme they chose provided they operated to "objective and verifiable criteria".

Undoubtedly, in the future steps may be taken to encompass even these activities, which are at present within the remit of each national authority.

3: European regulation of medical devices

CHRISTOPHER HODGES

3.1 Introduction

The regulatory system for medical devices is quite different from that for pharmaceuticals. It does not involve the assessment of a product by a medicines agency or the grant of a marketing authorisation. Instead, the onus of ensuring and declaring that a product conforms to the legal essential requirements is placed on the manufacturer, but in many instances this is subject to approval by an independent technical organisation (known as a *notified body*).

A manufacturer must apply an appropriate *conformity assessment* procedure to their device in order to ensure that it complies with the essential requirements, after which they must certify this fact by completing a *declaration of conformity*. There is usually a choice of conformity assessment procedures open to a manufacturer, depending on a risk-based classification of the class into which the device falls. The two main approaches to conformity assessment are based either on an approved total quality management system audited to ISO 9000 series standard, as customised for medical devices with EN 46000 series standard, or individual product assessment.

The essential requirements relate to the safety in use of the device, including labelling requirements, but are principally expressed in terms of scientific and technical performance characteristics. Efficacy, as such, is not a criterion. Confirmation of conformity must include evaluation of clinical data for many devices, generated from either a compilation of scientific literature or the results of clinical investigations on the product, for which prior ethical and regulatory approval is required. Conformity of a device with the essential requirements is denoted by affixing *CE marking* to the device. CE marking, which must be marked on the device, acts in effect as the passport that authorises the device to be placed on the market and to circulate freely within the European Economic Area (EEA).

The legal obligation is that a product must comply with the relevant essential requirements, but where the manufacturer chooses to apply a national standard that adopts a European harmonised standard (EN series) to an aspect of the product, conformity will be *prima facie* presumed in respect of the aspects of the essential requirements covered by that standard. Other national or international standards do not have this regulatory benefit. Compliance with the essential requirements at the time of placing the device on the market, or declaration of this fact, should mean that the device is safe but it may later transpire that this is not the case. Manufacturers therefore have some post-marketing vigilance requirements. If a marketed device is unsafe, the competent authority of a Member State has power under a safeguard clause in each Directive to take regulatory action to effect the withdrawal of the product from the market in its jurisdiction: the matter is then referred to the Commission and all Member States who then coordinate their actions.

European pharmaceutical regulation has been in existence since the mid-1960s and over three decades has successively extended from control of the requirements for placing a product on the market and the data necessary to justify this, coupled with control on manufacture, to virtually all aspects of dealing with a medicine, including wholesale dealing, advertising, and clinical research. In contrast, systematic regulation of medical devices is more recent and dates from the 1990s. It essentially covers the requirements for placing a product on the market, coupled with aspects of manufacture, labelling, and clinical investigation, but does not cover aspects such as distribution or advertising. The central difference is that many activities with pharmaceuticals require prior competent authority approval, which is not the case with devices.

Before the medical devices Directives came into being, most medical devices were unregulated in most European states. In some states some were regulated (illogically, but this was the only available mechanism) as if they were medicines. Examples of products formerly regulated as medicines in the United Kingdom include: contact lens products; intrauterine contraceptives; certain medicated dressings, surgical ligatures, and sutures; absorbent or protective materials; and dental filling substances.

3.2 Law on specific devices

The EEA law on the marketing of medical devices is governed by three principal Directives which each adopt the Community's scheme for product regulation known as the "new approach".[1] The new approach applies to many product sectors, such as machinery, personal protective equipment, low voltage equipment and electromagnetic compatibility requirements but not to pharmaceuticals or cosmetics. There are three device Directives.

- Directive 90/385/EEC on Active Implantable Medical Devices ("AIMDD") came into force on 1 January 1993 and is mandatory from 1 January 1995. This covers all powered implants or partial implants which are left in the human body, such as a heart pacemaker.
- Directive 93/42/EEC on medical devices (MDD) came into force on 1 January 1995 and became mandatory on 14 June 1998. This covers a wide range of devices ranging from first aid bandages, tongue depressors, and blood collection bags to hip prostheses and active (powered) devices.
- Directive 98/79/EC on *in vitro* diagnostics ("IVDD") came into force on 7 June 2000 and is mandatory from 7 December 2003. This covers products such as pregnancy tests, blood glucose monitoring, and tests for transmissible diseases.

A transitional period is provided under each of these Directives so that during the period from the coming into force of the Directive until it is mandatory, manufacturers may choose whether to apply the Directive to their device or the national rules which were in force immediately prior to the date on which the Directive came into force. From the date a Directive becomes mandatory, a device which is covered by national law implementing that Directive must comply with it.

Under Community law, a Directive is binding on each Member State, which is obliged under the EC Treaty to implement the Directive into its national law. A Member State has the discretion to choose the manner in which the Directive may be implemented so long as the effect of the Directive is achieved under its national legal order. Most Member States transpose Directives into their national law by enacting domestic legislation which follows the text of the Directives closely, if not *verbatim*. However, differences between implementing laws can arise, particularly in relation to enforcement and sanctions for non-compliance, which are aspects only governed by Directives in broad terms so are in any event matters for the national authorities. It is the national law which is directly binding on people, companies, and operations within a particular state, not the Directive. However, since the Directive ultimately governs the national law, people often colloquially refer to the Directive rather than the national law and this approach will be adopted in this chapter. Nevertheless, in any given situation, one must always check the relevant national law and consider, first, what its provisions are, second, to what extent they differ from the Directive and, third, whether any difference constitutes a breach of Community law by the Member State and what consequences might flow, such that the national provision might be unenforceable.

The European and United Kingdom legislation is set out in Table 3.1.

The basic structure, concepts, and terminology of the three Directives on AIMDs, MDs, and IVDs is identical: such differences as exist between them arise out of the different nature of these products. The following

Table 3.1 Summary of European and UK legislation

Device Sector	Directives	UK law
AIMDs	90/385 amended by 93/42	The Active Implantable Medical Device Regulations 1992, SI 1992 No. 3146, amended by the Active Implantable Medical Devices (Amendment and Transitional Provisions) Regulations 1995, SI 1995 No. 1671
MDs	93/42	The Medical Device Regulations 1994, SI 1994 No. 3017
IVDs	98/79	The In Vitro Diagnostic Medical Device Regulations 2000, SI 2000 No. 1315

discussion will therefore focus on the MDD, since this is the central Directive and covers most products. Short sections follow on AIMDs and IVDs. Detailed analysis of the relevant provisions would fill a large book: what is intended here is to highlight the important aspects which should be considered.

The basic purpose of the medical devices Directives, as with all product Directives based on Article 95 (formerly 100a) of the EC Treaty, is to ensure that devices placed on the EEA market ensure *a high level for the protection of safety and health* of patients, users, and others when properly maintained and used in accordance with their intended purpose.[2] The reference to a "high level" of protection should be noted: the standard of safety and protection required by the legislation is significant. Strictly speaking, this high level only applies where a device is properly maintained and used in accordance with its intended purpose. In practice, however, danger arising where a device has not been properly maintained or as a result of misuse would be highly likely to lead to action by the authorities.

Despite the emphasis of the legislation on safety, an equally important basic purpose of the legislation relates to the EEA's commerce and the economy. All Directives have as a basic purpose the creation of a European internal market without internal barriers to trade and with a single harmonised set of laws governing the placing of a product on the market and its free movement within the market.[3]

The intention behind the legislative scheme is that a product should essentially be regulated under a single product-specific regime as a medicinal product,[4] AIMD, MD, IVD, cosmetic,[5] blood or blood product,[6] or personal protective equipment.[7] However, certain other Directives might apply to particular medical devices, including:

- Directive 89/336/EEC on electromagnetic compatibility (the EMC Directive): EMC requirements are included within the essential requirements of the medical device Directives so the EMC Directive only applies to medical devices before the relevant medical device Directive is applicable
- Directive 92/59/EEC (from January 2004 replaced by 2001/95/EC) on general product safety: this applies to all consumer products, some of its obligations apply to medical devices used by consumers (see below).

3.3 Resolution of uncertainties

Since this legislation is extensive, complex, frequently written in generalised terms, and seeks to create an entirely new regulatory system for products that were formerly largely unregulated, difficulties of interpretation or application are bound to arise. Since the Directives constitute a legal system, ultimate authority for interpretation rests with the courts, fundamentally with the Court of Justice of the European Communities in Luxembourg, to which questions of interpretation of Community law may be referred by national courts. A mechanism exists, however, under the medical devices Directives by which measures and interpretations may be formally adopted: in the case of the MDD this is the Article 7 Committee, which is a committee of representatives of Member States chaired by the Commission. Under the Article 7 procedure, the Commission may submit to the Committee a draft of measures to be taken, on which the Committee delivers its opinion based on a weighted majority of representatives. The Commission will adopt the measures envisaged if they are in accordance with the opinion of the Committee. If there is divergence, the Commission then permits a proposal to the Council of Members, which acts by a qualified majority of votes.

Less formal, non-binding procedures also exist. There are frequent meetings between representatives of the Commission, Member States, and notified bodies. The Commission is also assisted by a Working Group of Experts. A sequence of guidance notes have been issued by the Commission (MEDDEV series), by certain competent authorities (such as the UK Medical Devices Agency's Bulletins), arising out of the meeting of notified bodies, by trade associations and others.

3.4 Competent authorities and notified bodies

Each Member State has designated a competent authority, which is the governmental authority responsible for implementing the Directive in that Member State. In the case of the United Kingdom, the competent authority is the Medical Devices Agency (MDA), an executive agency of the Department of Health. From April 2003 the MDA will merge with the MCA and will be known as the Medicines and Healthcare Products Regulatory

Agency (MHRA). The principal function of a competent authority in practice is to ensure the safety and health of patients and users of medical devices.

A competent authority is not involved in the assessment or authorisation for placing on the market of a medical device. As stated above, the legal responsibility in each case rests with the individual manufacturer. However, in many cases the manufacturer is required to obtain independent certification from a third party testing house, called a notified body. Such testing houses are private, commercial enterprises who may apply for and be approved for the purposes of the legislation by the competent authority in their Member State and are then notified within the Community by their approval being published in the Official Journal. Notified bodies may be approved for all devices or only for specific classes of devices. Criteria which they must satisfy in order to be approved are set out in an Annex to the relevant Directive (Annex XI for the MDD). In effect, therefore, notified bodies, although private entities, perform certain delegated regulatory functions. A manufacturer who is required by law to utilise the services of a notified body may choose any notified body within the Community who has the appropriate certification, irrespective of where either of them is located. The relationship between manufacturer and notified body is based on contract even though certain actions of the notified body have regulatory authority.

3.5   What is a medical device?

A medical device is defined as

any instrument, apparatus, appliance, material or other article, whether used alone or in combination, including the software necessary for its proper application intended by the manufacturer to be used for human beings for the purpose of:

- diagnosis, prevention, monitoring, treatment or alleviation of disease
- diagnosis, monitoring, treatment, alleviation or compensation for an injury or handicap
- investigation, replacement or modification of the anatomy or of a physiological process
- control of conception

and which does not achieve its principal intended action in or on the human body by pharmacological, immunological or metabolic means, but which may be assisted in its function by such means.[8]

An accessory is also considered to be a medical device. An accessory is defined as:

an article which whilst not being a device is intended specifically by its manufacturer to be used together with a device to enable it to be used in accordance with the use of the device intended by the manufacturer of the device.[9]

3.5.1 The drug and device borderline

Difficult borderline questions arise in relation to a significant number of products, particularly whether they are to be classified as medicinal products or as medical devices. As a general rule, a relevant product is regulated either under the medical devices Directives or by the medicinal products Directives (MPDs). Normally, the procedures of both Directives do not apply cumulatively. The Commission has issued Guidelines on this drug–device borderline issue[10] and also on what constitutes medical devices, AIMDs, and accessories. In order to decide which regime applies, the relevant criteria are:

- the intended purpose of the product, taking into account the way the product is presented (this is likely to establish if either the MDD or MPD apply, rather than distinguish between the two regimes)
- the method by which the principal intended action is achieved. This is crucial in the definition of a medical device. Typically, the medical device function is fulfilled by physical means (including mechanical action, physical barrier, replacement of or support to organs or body functions). The action of a medicinal product is achieved by pharmacological or immunological means or by metabolism.

The principal intended action of a product may be deduced from:

- the manufacturer's labelling and claims
- scientific data regarding mechanism of action.

Although the manufacturer's claims are important, it is not possible to place the product in one or other category in contradiction with current scientific data. Manufacturers may be required to justify scientifically their rationale for classification of borderline products.

Medical devices may be assisted in their function by pharmacological, immunological or metabolic means, but as soon as these means are not any more ancillary with respect to the principal purpose of a product, the product becomes a medicinal product. The claims made for a product, in accordance with its method of action may, in this context, represent an important factor for its classification as medical device or medicinal product. Examples of medical devices incorporating a medicinal substance with ancillary action include catheters coated with heparin or an antibiotic, bone cements containing antibiotic, and blood bags containing anticoagulant.[11]

3.5.2 Drug–device combinations

The MDD specifies the following approach.[12]

- A device that is intended to administer a medicinal product (for example, an unfilled syringe) is a medical device. The medicinal product itself remains regulated as a medicine.
- If the device and the medicinal product form a single integral product which is intended exclusively for use in the given combination and which is not reusable (for example, a pre-filled syringe), that single product is regulated as a medicine. An application for a marketing authorisation must be made under Directive 65/65/EEC. However, the safety and performance of the device features of the integral product are assessed in accordance with the essential requirements of Annex I of the MDD.
- Where a device incorporates, as an integral part, a substance which, if used separately, may be considered to be a medicinal product and which is liable to act upon the body with action ancillary to that of the device (for example, a heparin-coated catheter), the product is classed as a medical device. However, the medicinal product is to be assessed in accordance with the requirements of Directive 75/318/EEC (replaced by 2001/83/EC). A notified body undertaking conformity assessment on a medical device which incorporates a medicinal substance having ancillary action has a responsibility to consult a national medicines agency about the medicinal substance, to verify its safety, quality, and usefulness by analogy with the appropriate methods specified in Directive 75/318/EEC.

3.6   Classification of devices

The purpose of classification of devices is simply so as to provide options for conformity assessment methods. Under the MDD, medical devices are categorised into four classes, generally according to the degree of risk which they represent. In summary, Class I covers those that do not enter or interact with the body, Classes IIa and IIb are invasive or implantable devices or those which do interact with the body, Class III is for devices that affect the functions of vital organs. Implantables with an energy source are covered by the AIMD Directive. The detailed classification rules are lengthy and are set out in Annex IX of Directive 93/42/EEC. A sequence of rules must be worked through: charts and software are available to assist this.

The classification system uses three basic criteria, in various combinations: duration of contact with the body, degree of invasiveness, and the anatomy affected by the use of the device. Duration is based on continuous use (i.e., uninterrupted actual use) and categorised as transient (<60 minutes), short term (±30 days), and long term (>30 days). Invasive devices penetrate wholly or partly inside the body by way of an orifice or via the surface of the body. A body orifice is a natural opening in the body and includes the external surface of the eyeball and any permanent artificial opening, such as a stoma. Surgically invasive devices penetrate via the surface to the inside of the body by surgical intervention. Implantable devices are surgically invasive devices intended to be totally introduced to the body, to replace an epithelial surface or the surface of the eye and intended to remain in place after the procedure, and also includes those partially introduced surgically invasive devices remaining in place for at least 30 days. The central circulatory system is defined by the following vessels: *arteriae pulmonales, aorta ascendens, arteriae coronarieae, arteria carotis communis, arteria carotis externa, arteria carotis interna, arteriae cerebrales, truncus brachicephalicus, venae cordis, venae pulmonales, vena cava superior, vena cava inferior*. The central nervous system consists of the brain, meninges, and spinal cord. Active medical devices depend on a power source such as electricity for its operation, but not sources of power generated by the human body or gravity.

Non-invasive devices are covered by rules 1 to 4 and include the following classes.

- Class I   for example, ostomy pouches, wheelchairs, eye glasses, incontinence pads, cups and spoons for administering medicines, wound dressings such as cotton wool and wound strips.
- Class IIa   for example, transfusion equipment, storage and transport of donor organs, polymer film dressings, hydrogel dressings.
- Class IIb   for example, haemodialysers, dressings for chronic extensive ulcerated wounds.

Invasive devices are covered by rules 5 to 8 and include the following classes.

- Class I   for example, dressings for nose bleeds, hand held dentistry mirrors, enema devices, reusable surgical instruments.
- Class IIa   for example, contact lenses, urinary catheters, tracheal tubes connected to a ventilator, needles used for suturing, infusion cannulae, dental bridges and crowns.
- Class IIb   for example, urethral stents, insulin pens, devices supplying ionising radiation, prosthetic joint replacements, intraocular lenses, maxillofacial implants.
- Class III   for example, prosthetic heart valves, rechargeable non-active drug delivery systems, absorbable sutures, spinal stents, neurological catheters, temporary pacemaker leads.

Active devices, whilst covered under the above rules, are largely covered by rules 9 to 12 and include the following classes.

- Class I   for example, examination lights, surgical microscopes, wheelchairs, thermography devices, recording, processing or viewing of diagnostic images.

91

- Class IIa   for example, suction equipment, feeding pumps, anaesthesia machines, ventilators, hearing aids.
- Class IIb   for example, lung ventilators, incubators for babies, surgical lasers, x ray sources.

Special rules 13 to 18 govern several hazardous characteristics that may be found in certain devices and require a certain level of control and conformity assessment. Rule 13 deals with devices incorporating a medicinal substance whose action is ancillary to that of the device – Class III, for example, antibiotic bone cements, condoms with spermicides, heparin-coated catheters.

Rule 14 deals with devices used for contraception or the prevention of transmission of sexually transmitted diseases – Class IIb for example, condoms, contraceptive diaphragms, and if they are implantable or long term invasive; Class III, for example, intrauterine devices.

Rule 15 deals with devices for specific disinfecting, cleaning and rinsing and includes contact lens disinfecting, cleaning, rinsing, and hydrating – Class IIb, for example, contact lens solutions, comfort solutions, and devices specifically intended for disinfecting medical devices; Class IIa, for example, disinfectants for use with endoscopes.

Rule 16 classifies non-active devices specifically intended for recording x ray diagnostic images as Class IIa, for example, x ray films.

Rule 17 classifies all devices utilising animal tissues or derivatives rendered non-viable and coming into contact with breached skin as Class III, for example, biological heart valves, porcine xenograft dressings, catgut sutures, collagen implants and dressings.

Rule 18 puts blood bags into Class IIb.

If several rules apply to a device, the strictest rule resulting in the higher classification applies.

It must be reiterated that classification is based on the manufacturer's intended use and thus the listing of devices into classes must be taken as guidance only. No classification system can be perfect and thus the aim is to capture the majority of products whilst recognising that there will always be products that are borderline either between classes or with other product types, such as drugs and cosmetics, and also new innovative products that do not fit the criteria laid down.

3.7   Conformity assessment procedures and CE marking

Depending on the class of the device, a manufacturer may be able to choose between a number of alternative conformity assessment procedures in the assessment of whether a medical device conforms to the essential requirements. Although the rules should be considered in detail in each case,[13] the basic options might be summarised as follows.

- For all products in classes IIa, IIb, and III and AIMDs, *a full quality assurance* system, audited periodically by a notified body (Annex II of the MDD), which includes examination and certification by the notified body of the design dossier of each product covered. The manufacturer must keep documentation on the quality system and the design dossier of each product plus other documentation. The quality system obligations include post-marketing and vigilance aspects. Compliance with Annex II may be achieved (this is not mandatory but is invariably adopted voluntarily) by compliance with the EN 29000 and 46000 series standards, which apply the ISO 9000 series.
- For products in classes IIa, IIb, and III and AIMDs, examination and certification by a notified body of a specimen product (*type examination*: Annex III of the MDD) coupled with a varying degree (partially restricted by product class) of product or production quality assurance (MDD Annexes IV, V, and VI) which ensures that the manufacturing process produces products that conform to the certified type and might involve a quality system for manufacture and final inspection (Annex V), or a quality system for final inspection and testing (Annex VI).
- For products in class I, the manufacturer must have specified technical documentation on the design of the product showing that it conforms to the essential requirements: manufacturing aspects are not covered and a notified body is not involved unless there is a measuring function and/or the product is sterilised. (Annex VII: *EC declaration of conformity*).

In all cases, the specified documentation must be kept for five years after the last product has been manufactured. The Annex VII procedure is also available for class IIa devices if coupled with the Annex IV or V or VI procedure.

3.7.1 Registration

The manufacturer of a class I device or of a custom-made device, or a person who markets a system or procedure pack, must inform the competent authority of the manufacturer's registered place of business and the description of the devices concerned.[14] Such manufacturers who are located outside the EEA must designate persons established within the Community who are responsible for such registration.

3.7.2 Harmonised standards

Manufacturers may voluntarily decide to apply any standard to their product or business. Devices that are in conformity with a national standard adopted pursuant to a harmonised EC standard published in the Official Journal of the European Communities are presumed by Member States to comply with those aspects of the essential requirements which are covered by the standard. Harmonised standards are those adopted by the

EC standards bodies pursuant to a mandate issued by the Commission, in this case the European Committee for Standardisation (CEN) and the European Committee for Electrotechnical Standardisation (CENELEC). A large number of standards are contemplated but may take time to be written and adopted. Standards may be horizontal (covering aspects common to all or a number of product types) or vertical (dealing only with a specific aspect or specific product type). Important harmonised standards exist on the following:

EN 29000 and EN 46000 series quality systems for medical devices
EN 1041 information and labelling for medical devices
EN 980 graphical symbols
EN 10993 series biological evaluation of medical devices
EN 540 clinical investigation of devices
EN 60601 series medical electrical equipment
EN 1441 risk analysis
EN 1174 sterilisation

3.7.3 Custom-made devices

A new device which is specifically made in accordance with a duly qualified medical practitioner's written prescription and which gives, under the practitioner's responsibility, specific design characteristics, and is intended for the sole use of a particular patient is permitted to be marketed without CE marking under provisions referring to custom-made devices.[15] The prescription may be made by any person authorised by virtue of their professional qualifications to do so. Mass produced devices which need to be adapted to meet the specific requirements of the medical practitioner or any other professional user are not considered to be custom-made devices.

The manufacturer must undertake to keep available for the competent authorities documentation on the design, manufacture, and performance of the product so as to allow assessment of conformity with the essential requirements. He must also draw up a statement containing the following information:

- data allowing identification of the device in question
- a statement that the device is intended for exclusive use by a particular patient, together with the name of the patient
- the name of the medical practitioner or other authorised person who made out the prescription and, where applicable, the name of the clinic concerned
- the particular features of the device as specified in the relevant medical prescription
- a statement that the device in question conforms to the essential requirements set out in Annex I of the Directive and, where applicable,

indicating which essential requirements have not been fully met, together with the grounds. The manufacturer must inform the competent authorities of his registered place of business and the description of the devices concerned.

3.7.4 Systems and procedure packs

A number of items are sometimes assembled and marketed together as a particular system or to be used with a particular medical procedure. The individual items might or might not already bear CE marking. Where all the devices bear CE marking and are put together within the intended purposes specified by their manufacturers, a person or manufacturer who puts them together must draw up a declaration stating the following.

- They have verified the mutual compatibility of the devices in accordance with the manufacturers' instructions and have carried out their operations in accordance with these instructions.
- They have packaged the system or procedure pack and supplied relevant information to users incorporating relevant instructions from the original manufacturers.
- The whole activity is subjected to appropriate methods of internal control and inspection.

The system or procedure pack must not bear additional CE marking and must be accompanied by the original manufacturers' information. The declaration must be kept for 5 years.

Where the above conditions are not met, as in cases where the system or procedure pack incorporates devices that do not bear CE marking or where the chosen combination of devices is not compatible in view of their original intended use, the system or procedure pack must be treated as a device in its own right and the appropriate conformity assessment procedure must be followed.

3.7.5 Essential requirements

The essential requirements contained in Annex I of each new approach Directive specify the aspects of safety and performance which must be satisfied at the time at which a relevant product is placed on the market. Essential requirements are stated as principles or as generalised aspects and exclude detailed technical requirements. The scheme of the Community's new approach is that detailed technical aspects are not required as legal obligations but, if they are generally accepted, may be applied voluntarily by manufacturers through being included in official standards.[16] The essential requirements are intended to be comprehensive and all must be

95

satisfied save for those requirements which do not apply to a particular product as a matter of common sense.

The essential requirements in the MDD fall under two headings: general requirements and requirements regarding design and construction. The general requirements include the following provisions.

1. The devices must be designed and manufactured in such a way that, when used under the conditions and for the purposes intended, they will not compromise the clinical condition or the safety of patients, or the safety and health of users or, where applicable, other persons, provided that any risks which may be associated with their use constitute acceptable risks when weighed against the benefits to the patient and are compatible with a high level of protection of health and safety.

2. The solutions adopted by the manufacturer for the design and construction of the devices must conform to safety principles, taking account of the generally acknowledged state of the art. In selecting the most appropriate solutions, the manufacturer must apply the following principles in the following order:

    (i) eliminate or reduce risks as far as possible (inherently safe design and construction)
    (ii) where appropriate, take adequate protection measures including alarms if necessary, in relation to risks that cannot be eliminated
    (iii) inform users of the residual risks due to any shortcomings of the protection measures adopted.

3. The devices must achieve the performances intended by the manufacturer and be designed, manufactured, and packaged in such a way that they are suitable for one or more of the functions as specified by the manufacturer.

4. The characteristics and performances referred to in sections 1, 2, and 3 above must not be adversely affected to such a degree that the clinical conditions and safety of the patients and, where applicable, of other persons are compromised during the lifetime of the device as indicated by the manufacturer, when the device is subjected to the stresses that can occur during normal conditions of use.

5. The devices must be designed, manufactured, and packed in such a way that their characteristics and performances during their intended use will not be adversely affected during transport and storage taking account of the instructions and information provided by the manufacturer.

6. Any undesirable adverse effect must constitute an acceptable risk when weighed against the performances intended.

Section 2 above implies that a manufacturer must carry out a risk analysis. A harmonised standard is available on this topic, EN 1441, which amplifies the methodology for risk analysis, elimination or reduction required by section 2.

The essential requirements regarding design and construction are too extensive to be summarised here. They cover the following headings:

- clinical, physical and biological properties
- infection and microbial contamination
- construction and environmental properties
- devices with a measuring function
- protection against radiation
- requirements for medical devices connected to or equipped with an energy source
- information supplied by the manufacturer (this is discussed further below).

3.7.6 Information supplied by the manufacturer

The general principle is that each device must be accompanied by the information needed to use it safely and to identify the manufacturer, taking account of the training and knowledge of the potential users. This information comprises the details on the label and the data in the instructions for use. A series of 13 particular requirements are specified for inclusion in the label and the same 13 requirements plus a further 15 categories of information must be included in the instructions for use.

As far as practicable and appropriate, the information needed to use the device safely must be set out on the device itself and/or on the packaging for each unit or, where appropriate, on the sales packaging. If individual packaging of each unit is not practicable, the information must be set out in the leaflet supplied with one or more devices. Instructions for use must be included in the packaging for every device. By way of exception, no such instructions for use are needed for devices in Class I or IIa if they can be used safely without any such instructions.

Where appropriate, this information should take the form of symbols. Any symbol or identification colour used must conform to the harmonised standards. In areas for which no standards exist, the symbols and colours must be described in the documentation supplied with the device.

It will be noted that in the above 3 paragraphs, which are quoted verbatim from Annex I, certain flexibility is permitted through use of the words "where appropriate": this is a feature of many of the other essential requirements. The manufacturer is permitted some discretion over compliance with the essential requirements, based on an application of common sense to the circumstances of his particular product.

3.7.6.1 Who is a manufacturer?

A manufacturer is defined as the natural or legal person with responsibility for the design, manufacture, packaging, and labelling of a device before it is placed on the EU market under that manufacturer's own name, regardless of whether these operations are carried out by that manufacturer or on their behalf by a third party. The Directives also apply to those who assemble, package, process, fully refurbish or label a product and in certain other situations.

The intention is that the person (more normally, the company) who assumes the legal responsibility of "manufacturer" need not be the person who assembles the product. One or more of the activities of design, manufacture, packaging or labelling may be subcontracted by the legal manufacturer. The name or tradename and address of the legal manufacturer must appear on the label and instructions for use.[17] In addition, for devices imported into the Community, the label, or the outer packaging, or instructions for use, must contain the name and address of either the authorised representative of the manufacturer established within the Community, or of the importer established in the Community (this is in effect for devices whose importation is not authorised by the manufacturer), or for the person who has the responsibility to register with the competent authorities in the case of class I or custom-made devices.

3.7.6.2 Manufacturers outside the EEA

A non-EEA manufacturer may place a Class I or custom-made medical device or a system or procedure pack on the EU market under their own name provided it has undergone a relevant conformity assessment procedure and bears CE marking, and the competent authorities in the relevant member state have been informed of either

- the manufacturer's registered place of business in that Member State, if they have one, and the description of the device, or
- the registered place of business in that Member State of a person designated by the manufacturer as responsible for marketing the device in the EU, and the category of the device.[18]

In relation to devices in Classes II, IIa, and IIb, a manufacturer must certify conformity personally under the Annex II procedure, but an authorised representative established in the EU may do this in place of the manufacturer under the Annex III and IV procedures.

The functions of an authorised representative are not precisely defined in the Directives save for the IVD Directive, but such a person is explicitly designated by the manufacturer, and acts and may be addressed by authorities and bodies in the Community instead of the manufacturer with regard to the latter's obligations.[19] It would be good practice for the manufacturer to have a written contract recording their relationship.

3.7.7 "Placing on the market" and "putting into service"

The Directives provide that devices may be placed on the market and put into service only if they comply with the requirements laid down in the Directive when duly supplied and properly installed, maintained, and used in accordance with their intended purpose.[20] Devices, other than devices which are custom-made or intended for clinical investigations, which are considered to meet the essential requirements set out in Annex I of the relevant Directive must bear the CE marking of conformity when they are placed on the market.[21]

The CE marking of conformity, as specified in MDD Annex XII, must appear in a visible, legible, and indelible form on the device or its sterile pack, where practicable and appropriate, and on the instructions for use. Where applicable, the CE marking must also appear on the sales packaging. It must be accompanied by the identification number of the notified body responsible for implementation of the relevant conformity assessment procedure. It is prohibited to affix marks or inscriptions which are likely to mislead third parties with regard to the meaning or the graphics of the CE marking. Any other mark may be affixed to the device, to the packaging or to the instruction leaflet accompanying the device provided that the visibility and legibility of the CE marking is not thereby reduced.

The concepts of "placing on the market" and "putting into service" are standard in Community "new approach" Directives. For the purposes of the MDD, they are defined as follows:

- *placing on the market* means the stage of first making available in return for payment or free of charge a device other than a device intended for clinical investigation, with a view to distribution and/or use on the Community market, regardless of whether it is new or fully refurbished
- *putting into service* means the stage at which a device has been made available to the final user as being ready for use on the Community market for the first time for its intended purpose.[22]

The European Commission has issued guidance on these concepts in the context of all "new approach Directives".[23] In essence, a device is placed on the market when it is first put into the stream of distribution or commerce by its manufacturer. A device which is fully refurbished is treated as if it were a new device and must be subject afresh to the requirements of the Directive. Difficulties arise over the definition of what constitutes refurbishment (simple servicing is clearly not included) and aspects such as upgrading.

3.8   Clinical investigation

Confirmation of conformity with the essential requirements must be based on clinical data in the case of:

- (as a general rule) implantable and long term invasive devices falling within Classes IIa and IIb, and all Class III devices under the MDD[24]
- all active implantable devices under the AIMDD.[25]

The adequacy of such clinical data must be based on either:

- a compilation of the relevant scientific literature and, "if appropriate", a written report containing a critical evaluation, or
- the results of all clinical investigations made.

Thus, *evaluation* of the clinical safety and performance is required for all devices, whereas a clinical *investigation* of each device may or may not be necessary (the term "clinical trial" is not used in relation to devices). The Directives give some latitude over the circumstances in which a clinical investigation of a non-CE marked device is required. Guidance issued by the Medical Devices Agency[26] states that an investigation would be required where:

- there is the introduction of a completely new concept of device into clinical practice where components, features, and/or methods of action, are previously unknown
- an existing device is modified in such a way that it contains a novel feature, particularly if such a feature has an important physiological effect; or where the modification might significantly affect the clinical performance and/or safety of the device
- a device incorporates materials previously untested in humans, coming into contact with the human body or where existing materials are applied to a new location in the human body, in which case compatibility and biological safety will need to be considered
- a device, either CE marked or non-CE marked, is proposed for a new purpose or function.

Clinical investigation will also be required where a CE marked device is to be used for a new purpose.

The regime of the Directives is that if clinical evaluation is required, it must be subject to ethical approval in accordance with the principles of the

Declaration of Helsinki.[27] The Directives provide[28] that the purpose of clinical investigation is to:

- verify that, under normal conditions of use, the performance of the devices conform to [those intended by the manufacturer, viz. the device should be designed and manufactured in such a way that it is suitable for the functions specified by the manufacturer]
- determine any undesirable side effects, under normal conditions of use, and assess whether they are acceptable risks having regard to the intended performance of the device.

The Directives also specify the methodology to be adopted in clinical investigations. Adverse incidents occurring in the investigation must be reported to the competent authority. A general requirement in the MDD is:

Clinical investigations must be performed on the basis of an appropriate plan of investigation reflecting the latest scientific and technical knowledge and defined in such a way as to confirm or refute the manufacturer's claims for the device; these investigations must include an adequate number of observations to guarantee the scientific validity of the conclusions.[29]

The primary consideration of a clinical investigation of a device is assessment verification of the manufacturer's claims for the technical performance of the device. Safety considerations are nevertheless relevant in that the clinical investigation should determine and assess any undesirable adverse effects, but the main thrust of the clinical evaluation, and in particular of the conformity assessment by a notified body or the manufacturer to permit marketing, is on technical performance rather than a complete evaluation of safety. It is an essential requirement for marketed devices that "[A]ny undesirable side-effect must constitute an acceptable risk when weighed against the performances intended".[30]

Both the AIMDD[31] and the MDD[32] specify that a manufacturer must submit to the competent authority of the Member State in which the investigation is to be conducted a statement in the specified form (MDD Annex VIII) containing information as detailed as design drawings, manufacturing methods, descriptions, and explanations and the results of calculations and technical tests. For Class II devices and implantable and long term devices in Classes IIa and IIb the investigation may commence either after 60 days unless the authority has objected, or earlier if the authority so authorises, provided a favourable ethics committee opinion is available. For devices other than those just specified, the Member State may authorise immediate commencement after receipt of notification, provided a favourable ethics committee opinion has been issued. A device which is intended for clinical investigation must not bear CE marking.

Compliance with the requirements relating to clinical investigations (AIMDD Annex VII; MDD Annex X) is assisted by adoption of standard EN 540 on "Clinical Investigation of Medical Devices for Human Subjects" which is very similar to pharmaceutical GCP.

Clinical investigation is not required for in vitro diagnostics (IVDs).

3.8.1 In vitro diagnostics

An in vitro diagnostic medical device is defined as any medical device which is a reagent, reagent product, calibrator, control material, kit, instrument, apparatus, equipment or system, whether used alone or in combination, intended by the manufacturer to be used in vitro for the examination of specimens including blood and tissue donations, derived from the human body, solely or principally for the purpose of providing information concerning a physiological or pathological state, or concerning a congenital abnormality, or to determine the safety and compatibility with potential recipients, or to monitor therapeutic measures. For the purpose of this Directive, a specimen receptacle, whether evacuated or not, specifically intended by its manufacturer to contain a specimen for the purposes of in vitro diagnostic examination, is considered to be a device. Products for general laboratory use are not devices unless such products, in view of their characteristics, are specifically intended by their manufacturer to be used for in vitro diagnostic examination.[33]

The IVD Directive follows the same general "new approach" scheme as the other medical devices Directives with the following major differences. IVDs are divided into two classes: Annex II devices and everything else. Annex II devices are themselves divided into List A (high risk) and List B which include the following (each case also including calibrators and control materials).

List A

- Reagents and reagent products for determining the following blood groups: ABO system, Rhesus (C, c, D, E, e) anti-Kell.
- Reagents and reagent products for the detection, confirmation, and quantification in human specimens of markers of HIV infection (HIV 1 and 2), HTLV I and II, and Hepatitis B, C, and D.

List B

- Reagents and reagent products for determining the following blood groups: Anti-Duffy and Anti-Kidd.
- Reagents and reagent products for determining irregular antierythrocytic antibodies.
- Reagents and reagent products for the detection and quantification in human samples of the following congential infections: rubella, toxoplasmosis.

102

- Reagents and reagent products for diagnosing the following hereditary disease: phenylketonuria.
- Reagents and reagent products for determining the following human infections: cytomegalovirus, chlamydia.
- Reagents and reagent products for determining the following HLA tissue groups: DR, A, B.
- Reagents and reagent products for determining the following turmoral marker: PSA.
- Reagents and reagent products, including software, designed specifically for evaluating the risk of trisomy 21.
- The following device for self-diagnosis: device for the measurement of blood sugar.

One of two conformity assessment procedures may be followed for devices covered by Annex II:

- the EC Declaration of Conformity procedure (full quality assurance: Annex IV), or
- the EC type examination procedure (Annex V) coupled with either the EC verification procedure (Annex VI) or the EC Declaration of Conformity (production quality assurance: Annex VII).

All devices other than those covered by Annex II are subject to the EC Declaration of Conformity procedure (Annex III), which does not involve the intervention of a notified body, but which includes supplementary requirements for devices for self-testing, which does involve a notified body (Annex III).

Common Technical Specifications (CTS) are to be adopted by the Article 7.2 Committee (a working group of scientific experts appointed by the member states) which will apply to devices in Annex II List A and, when required, devices in Annex II List B. There is some uncertainty about the circumstances in which the requirement might apply to List B devices. CTS establish appropriate performance evaluation and re-evaluation criteria, batch release criteria, reference methods, and reference materials. If, for duly justified reasons, manufacturers do not comply with the CTS, they must adopt other solutions which are at least equivalent to these specifications. CTS are intended mainly for the evaluation of the safety of the blood supply and organ donations.

Manufacturers shall notify competent authorities:

- for reagents, reagent products, reference and control materials, of information concerning common technological characteristics and/or analytes, as well as any important and subsequent modification, including suspension of marketing authorisation
- for other IVDs, appropriate indications

- for devices in Annex II and devices for self-testing, all data allowing identification and the analytical parameters and, where applicable, for diagnostic products in Annex I.3, results of evaluation of performance in accordance with Annex VIII and certificates of notified bodies.

Clinical evaluation is not appropriate for IVDs but a procedure is specified for performance evaluation studies in clinical laboratories or in other appropriate environments outside the manufacturer's premises (Annex VIII). Manufacturers who place devices on the market under their own name must notify the competent authorities of the Member State in which they have their registered place of business of the address of that registered place of business, the categories of devices as defined in terms of common characteristics of technology and/or analytes, and of any significant change thereto.

3.9 Adverse event reporting: vigilance

All adverse events with medical devices of which the manufacturer becomes aware must be recorded. The detailed legal requirements in relation to recording and reporting are, curiously, more onerous in relation to MDs than AIMDs. However, the Commission's Guidance is that they should be treated the same in practice. In general, a manufacturer of general medical devices should report, and a Member State record and evaluate,

- any malfunction or deterioration in the characteristics and performance of a device, or inadequacy in the labelling, which might lead to, or have led to, the death of a patient or user or to a serious deterioration in their state of health
- any technical or medical reason in relation to the characteristics or performance of a device for the reasons referred to above, leading to systematic recall of devices of the same type by the manufacturer.

Guidance is issued by the European Commission on medical device vigilance[34] which includes an explanation of the difficult concept of when a deterioration in state of health should be considered serious:

- life-threatening illness or injury
- permanent impairment of a body function or permanent damage to a body structure
- a condition necessitating medical or surgical intervention to prevent permanent impairment of a body function or permanent damage to a body structure.

Regulatory data is (to be) stored on a European Database on medical devices accessible only to competent authorities. This will include data on registration, certificates issued or withdrawn, and vigilance data.[35]

3.10 General Product Safety Directive

Directive 92/59/EEC imposes general product safety (GPS) obligations on producers and distributors (as defined) of products "intended for consumers or likely to be used by consumers".

The obligations on producers are that they must:

- place only safe products on the market
- provide consumers with the relevant information to enable them to assess the risks inherent in the product throughout the normal or reasonably foreseeable period of its use, where such risks are not immediately obvious without adequate warnings, and to take precautions against those risks
- adopt measures commensurate with the characteristics of the products which they supply, to enable them to be informed of risks which these products might present
- take appropriate action including, if necessary, withdrawing the product in question from the market to avoid these risks.

Other obligations apply to distributors of consumer products. The GPS obligations apply in the absence of other specific rules of Community law governing the safety of such products. It is clear that the obligations under the medical device Directives cover producers' obligations which arise under the GPS Directive numbers 1 and 2 above and possibly also the post-marketing obligations 3 and 4. Manufacturers are obliged, for example, under MDD Annex II, to undertake to their notified body that they will institute and keep up to date a systematic procedure to review experience gained from devices in the post-production phase and to implement appropriate means to apply any necessary corrective action. This undertaking includes an obligation to notify the authorities of reportable adverse events. Whatever the strict legal position on whether GPS obligations do or do not apply to medical device manufacturers, their general principles should be followed as a matter of prudence and for product liability reasons.

The GPS obligations are to be amended and significantly extended from January 2004 under Directive 2001/95/EC. A major extension relates to post-marketing obligations on a producer to notify the authorities if they have placed a dangerous product on the market, and to take appropriate action to safeguard consumers.

3.10.1 Recall

A manufacturer may have a number of post-marketing obligations arising under either the medical devices legislation and/or the GPS legislation, and under product liability or negligence law. The precise legal provisions constitute a somewhat incomplete matrix, although the UK Medical Devices Agency has issued guidance on the subject of recall (defined to include the return, modification, exchange, destruction or retrofit of a device) which covers in general terms the circumstances in which a recall might be appropriate and how it should best be implemented.[36]

3.10.2 Enforcement and sanctions

The medical device Directives authorise Member States to take enforcement action against medical devices which prove to be unsafe. The specific powers, offences, sanctions and penalties are subject to the discretion of Member States. Accordingly, these matters are provided for under national legislation and practice. It must be remembered that relevant national provisions may be found not only within national legislation implementing the relevant medical device Directive but also in other provisions such as general consumer protection, trade descriptions or criminal legislation. Where a Member State invokes the "safeguard clause" under a medical device Directive, removing a product from the market on grounds of safety, a mechanism must be followed under which the Commission and other Member States are notified, the position discussed, and a unified approach taken by the authorities.

Enforcement provisions are generally of two types: first, powers to investigate and take action against a product and, secondly, offences which may be committed by individuals for breach of which they may be prosecuted by the authorities and subject to criminal sanctions. In the United Kingdom, for example, the first category of provisions arise under the product-specific Regulations and Part II of the Consumer Protection Act 1987. The offences are as specified in the product-specific Regulations. There is a considerable variation between Member States in the number and wording of criminal offences which may be committed and in the penalties which might be imposed.

Different national agencies have different practices on what action they may take when faced with dangerous products. The UK Medical Devices Agency, for example, operates a practice of issuing a sequence of three advisory notices to UK health services, for which the criteria for the various safety warning categories are as follows.[37]

- Hazard Notices are issued:

  - in cases of actual death or serious injury, or where death or serious injury would have occurred but for fortuitous circumstances or the timely intervention of health care personnel (or a carer)

- where the medical device is clearly implicated
- where immediate action is necessary to prevent recurrence.

• Device Alerts are issued:

  - in cases where there is the potential for death or serious injury, or there may be implications arising from the long term use of the medical device
  - where the medical device is likely to be implicated
  - where the recipient is expected to take immediate action on the advice.

• Safety Notices are used to recommend or inform:

  - where action by the recipient will improve safety
  - where it is necessary to repeat warnings on long standing problems
  - to support or follow up manufacturers' field modifications.

References

1　Council Resolution of May 7, 1985 on a new approach to technical harmonisation and standards, OJ 1985 No. C 136/1, 4.6.85.
2　Directive 93/42/EEC, recitals 2, 3, and 5 and Article 2.
3　For example, Directive 93/42/EEC, recital 1.
4　Directive 65/65/EEC as amended and related Directives.
5　Directive 76/768/EEC as amended.
6　A Directive or Directives will be forthcoming on these products.
7　Directive 89/686/EEC as amended.
8　Directive 93/42/EEC, Article 1.2(a); Directive 90/385/EEC, Article 1.2(a).
9　Directive 93/42/EEC, Article 1.2(b).
10　*Drug/Device Borderline Issues*, European Commission, MEDDEV 2.1/3 rev. 5 February 1998.
11　Draft Commission Guidelines, MEDDEV 14/93 rev. 2.
12　Directive 93/42/EEC, Recital 6 and Article 1.3 and 1.4.
13　Directive 93/42/EEC, Article 11.
14　Directive 93/42/EEC, Article 14.
15　Directive 93/42/EEC, Articles 1.2(d), 12.6 and Annex VIII.
16　Council Resolution of December 21, 1989 on a global approach to conformity assessment, OJ 1989 No. C10/1, 16.1.90.
17　Directive 93/42/EEC, Annex I, paragraph 13.1.
18　Directive 93/42/EEC, Article 14.
19　Directive 98/79/EC, Article 1.2(g).
20　For example, Directive 93/42/EEC, Article 2.
21　For example, Directive 93/42/EEC, Articles 17 and 3.
22　Directive 93/42/EEC, Article 1.2(h) and (i) as amended by Article 21 of Directive 98/79/EC.
23　*Guide to the Implementation of Directives Based on the New Approach and the Global Approach*, European Commission, 2000.
24　Directive 93/42/EEC, Annex X and Article 15.
25　Directive 93/42/EEC, Article 9, Annex 2 para. 4.1 and Annex 3 para. 3.
26　*Guidance Notes for Manufacturers or Clinical Investigations to be carried out in the UK*, Medical Devices Agency, September 1996.
27　Directive 93/42/EEC, Annex 7, para. 2.2 and Directive 93/42/EEC, Annex X, para. 2.2.
28　Directive 93/42/EEC, Annex 7 and Directive 93/42/EEC, Annex X.
29　Directive 93/42/EEC, Annex X, Requirement 2.3.1.

30 Directive 93/42/EEC, Annex I, Requirement 6.
31 Directive 93/42/EEC, Article 10.
32 Directive 93/42/EEC, Article 15.
33 Directive 98/79/EC, Article 1.2(b).
34 *The Medical Devices Vigilance System: European Commission Guidelines,* Medical Devices Agency, undated.
35 Directive 93/42/EEC, Article 14a.
36 Medical Devices Agency, *Guidance on the Recall of Medical Devices,* 2000.
37 Medical Devices Agency, *Safety Notices,* 2001.

4: The supply of unlicensed medicines for particular patient use

JOHN O'GRADY, AMANDA WEARING

4.1 Introduction

The use by the medical profession of medicines with no current marketing authorisation and of authorised medicines outside the terms of their marketing authorisation raises various regulatory issues. Leaving aside use in a clinical trial, such products are also used to treat the particular clinical needs of individual patients. This is known variously as "named patient", "particular patient", or "compassionate use" supply. The first of these terms is misleading because there has never been any requirement to identify a particular patient; for the purposes of this chapter the term "particular patient supply" is used instead.

Supply on a particular patient basis encompasses various categories of unauthorised use of medicinal products. A product may be unauthorised because it has been specially formulated for use; it may be at the clinical trial stage of development, but be requested by doctors for use outside a trial; it may have been authorised previously and then withdrawn from the market for commercial reasons, or because of safety, efficacy or quality concerns; or it may be authorised currently, but for a different indication or patient population, or in a different country.

This chapter describes the regulatory framework covering the supply of medicinal products on a particular patient basis. This framework is the outcome of the balancing by the regulators of two important but conflicting principles. On the one hand, there is the need to ensure that patients are not exposed to any unnecessary risks, hence the extensive legal framework regulating the placing on the market of medicinal products. On the other hand, there is the desire to respect the clinical freedom of medical practitioners to determine the most appropriate treatment for their patients.

4.2 Legal framework

4.2.1 EU law

There is only limited EU legislation dealing with the supply of medicinal products for particular patient use and there were no relevant provisions prior to 1989. Article 3 of Directive 65/65/EEC sets out the general rule that a medicinal product must have a marketing authorisation before being placed on the market. However, Article 2.4 (as amended by Directive 89/341/EEC) provides an exception from this general rule:

> A Member State may, in accordance with legislation in force and to fulfil special needs, exclude from Chapters II to V [which set out the requirements for applying for a marketing authorisation] medicinal products supplied in response to a *bona fide* unsolicited order formulated in accordance with the specifications of an authorised health professional and for use by his individual patients on his direct personal responsibility.

This provision allows Member States if they wish (there is no obligation to do so) to make national arrangements for the supply of unlicensed medicines for particular use, but only in the very limited circumstances specified by the Directive. As part of the 2001 review process, the European Commission recently issued proposals to regulate the compassionate use of medicinal products falling within the scope of Regulation 2309/93/EC (the centralised procedure). However, these proposals are unlikely to come into force for several years.

4.2.2 UK law prior to 1 January 1995

The UK legislation has for many years permitted particular patient supply in specified circumstances. The original provisions date back to the early 1970s. Under section 7(2) of the Medicines Act 1968, it was necessary to hold a product licence in order to sell, supply, export or import a medicinal product, or to procure those activities, or the manufacture or assembly of the product. However, various exemptions from the licensing requirements, including those relating to particular patient supply, were provided for in the Act and in related statutory instruments. The most important exemptions were contained in sections 9 and 13 of the Act, the Medicines (Exemption from Licences) (Special and Transitional Cases) Order 1971,[1] the Medicines (Exemption from Licences) (Special Cases and Miscellaneous Provisions) Order 1972[2] and the Medicines (Exemptions from Licences) (Importation) Order 1984.[3]

4.2.3 1995 onwards

Significant changes to the legal basis for the exemptions, rather than to their scope, were introduced by the Medicines for Human Use (Marketing Authorisations Etc.) Regulations 1994,[4] which came into force on 1 January 1995. These Regulations disapply much of the Medicines Act for "relevant medicinal products", including section 7 (and consequently all exemptions relating to section 7). Relevant medicinal products are defined in the 1994 Regulations as those medicinal products for human use to which Chapters II to V of Directive 65/65/EEC apply. This broad definition includes most medicinal products. The exceptions are medicinal products for clinical trial use, products prepared in a pharmacy in accordance with a pharmacopoeial formula for direct supply to a patient, intermediate products, registered homeopathic products, non-industrially produced herbal remedies, and some products which are not medicinal products within the meaning of the Directive but which by Order have been made subject to control under the Medicines Act 1968. For products designated under such an Order, the old provisions on particular patient supply are still applicable. In practice, there are very few such products.

Regulation 3(1) of the 1994 Regulations states that no medicinal product may be placed on the market or distributed by way of wholesale dealing unless it has a marketing authorisation. This replaces the product licence requirement in section 7 of the Act. The exemptions to this requirement are provided for by Regulation 3(2) and Schedule 1 to the Regulations. They permit supply for individual patients and also enable practitioners to hold limited supplies of stocks of unauthorised medicines. The provisions apply equally to doctors and dentists.

4.3   Scope of exemption

The supply of unlicensed medicinal products for individual patients is governed by paragraph 1 of Schedule 1 to the Regulations. The text closely follows the wording of Article 2 of Directive 65/65/EEC:

> Regulations 3(1) shall not apply to a relevant medicinal product supplied in response to a *bona fide* unsolicited order, formulated in accordance with the specification of a doctor or dentist and for use by his individual patients on his direct personal responsibility, but such supply shall be subject to the conditions specified in paragraph 2.

The conditions specified in paragraph 2 are:

- The product is supplied to a doctor or dentist, or for use in a registered pharmacy, hospital or health centre under the supervision of a pharmacist, in accordance with paragraph 1.
- No advertisement relating to the product is issued with a view to being seen generally by the public in the UK, no such advertisement, by means of any catalogue, price list or circular letter, is issued by any person involved in the manufacture, sale or supply of the product, and the sale or supply is in response to a *bona fide* unsolicited order.

- The manufacture and assembly of the product is carried out under conditions which ensure that the product is of the character required by, and meets the specifications of, the doctor or dentist.
- Written records of manufacture and assembly are made, maintained and kept available for inspection by the licensing and enforcement authorities.
- The product is manufactured, assembled, or imported into the EU by the holder of the authorisation referred to in Article 16 of Directive 75/319/EEC (for products manufactured or assembled in the EU, a manufacturer's authorisation; for products imported in finished form into the EU, a wholesale dealer's (importation) licence).
- The product is distributed by way of wholesale dealing by the holder of a wholesale dealer's licence.

Paragraph 3 extends the exemption to the supply of product for limited stocks, subject to a number of conditions.

- (a) The medicinal product is specially prepared by a doctor or dentist, or to his order, for administration to one or more patients of his. Where that doctor/dentist is a member of a practice group working together to provide general medical or dental services, the proposed recipients can be the patients of any other doctor or dentist in that group; or
- (b) The manufacture/assembly of such stocks is procured by a registered pharmacy, a hospital or health centre, where this is done by or under the supervision of a pharmacist.
- The product is manufactured and assembled by the holder of the appropriate licence (see above).
- Only limited stocks of such products are held: no more than 5 litres of fluid and 2·5 kilograms of solid of all such products per doctor or dentist.

Paragraph 4 sets out an exemption in certain circumstances for medicinal products not requiring a prescription for sale or supply, which are prepared by or under the supervision of a pharmacist and are sold or supplied to a person exclusively for use by him or her in the course of his or her business for the purpose of administration to one or more persons.

Paragraph 5 contains an exemption for radiopharmaceuticals prepared from an authorised kit, generator or precursor in respect of which there is a marketing authorisation in force, subject to certain conditions.[5]

Paragraph 6 requires any person selling or supplying a relevant medicinal product to maintain, for a period of at least five years, records showing:

- the source from which that person obtained the product
- the person to whom, and the date on which, the sale or supply was made
- the quantity of each sale or supply

- the batch number of the product sold or supplied
- details of any suspected adverse reaction to the product sold or supplied of which he or she is aware. This does not require suppliers to search the literature for reports concerning the substance, however.

Paragraph 7 requires that person to notify the licensing authority of any such suspected serious adverse reaction and to make available for inspection at all reasonable times the records referred to in the previous paragraph.

4.4 Particular issues

4.4.1 Advertising

Paragraph 2(b) of the Schedule makes it clear that no advertisement or representation may be issued to encourage the sale or supply of medicinal products for particular patient use. Sale or supply must be in response to a *bona fide* unsolicited order from the doctor. While the paragraph prohibits issuing catalogues, price lists, and circulars referring to relevant medicinal products, it does not prohibit the advertising of a specials manufacturing facility, provided no specific products are mentioned. A manufacturer may also respond to an enquiry as to whether or not a particular product could be supplied.

This raises the question of whether the Schedule prevents the supplier giving the doctor at the time of supply purely factual, technical information on the use of that product. Since the rationale for particular patient supply is that the doctor has requested the product of his own accord and is acting on his direct personal responsibility, it would seem reasonable to assume that he or she is familiar with its use and should not need any further information. On the other hand, particularly where there are known to be significant risks associated with the use of the product, it may be prudent to issue safety information to minimise the product liability exposure of the supplier. It seems unlikely that the Medicines Control Agency (MCA) would consider this to be advertising, although no formal guidance has been issued on this point. If a company does decide to provide such information, it must ensure that the wording cannot be said to be an invitation to the doctor to order further supplies of the product, since that would arguably amount to soliciting subsequent orders, in breach of the Regulations.

In addition to the specific prohibitions set out in the Regulations, companies should also have in mind the more general provisions against the advertising of unauthorised medicinal products. It is a criminal offence under regulation 3(1) of the Medicines (Advertising) Regulations 1994[6] to issue an advertisement for a relevant medicinal product in respect of which there is no marketing authorisation in force, and under regulation 3A to issue an advertisement which does not comply with the particulars listed in the summary of product characteristics. These Regulations implement Directive 92/28/EEC on the advertising of medicinal products for human use. Corresponding restrictions on the availability of promotional materials also appear in the ABPI Code of Practice.

4.4.2 Quantity

The Regulations do not expressly impose any limit on the amount of medicinal product the company may supply for use by the doctor's individual patients under paragraph 1 of the Schedule. In view of the specific provisions on stock set out in paragraph 3 (a total of 5 litres of fluid and 2·5 kilograms of solid of all such products per doctor or dentist), it is likely that supply under paragraph 1 should be limited to a reasonable course of treatment for a specific patient for whom the doctor is prescribing the product. Companies should always be suspicious of large orders from doctors and should enquire as to why such large quantities are being sought.

4.4.3 Doctor's specification

Supply must be "formulated in accordance with the specification" of a doctor or dentist. Strictly, this means that the product should be made up, or imported, in accordance with the doctor's specification and must not be manufactured in advance of any order being received, unless that product is already on the market in a country from which it is being sourced. As a matter of practice, it is rarely the case that a product is formulated in response to a detailed specification provided by a doctor.

4.4.4 Special needs

Directive 65/65/EEC requires that supply should be to "fulfil special needs". Curiously, this condition is omitted from paragraph 1 of Schedule 1 to the UK Regulations and it is necessary to consider whether this omission has any significance. The prevailing view is that the Regulations should be interpreted in a manner consistent with the Directive and that the exemption should only be available where there is no equivalent product containing the same active ingredient already authorised and on the market in the UK. This view has recently been endorsed in the Guidance Note issued by the MCA.[7]

It is then necessary to review the meaning of "special needs". It is difficult to see how such needs can exist where there is a licensed version of the product on the market for the physician to use. However tempting it may be for medical institutions to save costs by requesting an unlicensed version of a licensed product, economic needs will never be special needs in this context. This accords with the rationale of Directive 65/65/EEC, which requires only authorised medicinal products to be placed on the market unless exceptional circumstances apply.

The more difficult question arises where the product to be manufactured differs in some way from the licensed version. The Guidance Note issued by the MCA states that unlicensed products which are the "pharmaceutical equivalents" of available licensed medicinal products will not be permitted. A medicinal product will be regarded as a "pharmaceutical equivalent" where it contains the same amount of the same active substance, in the same dosage form, and it "meets the same or comparable standards considered in the light of the clinical needs of the patient at the time of use of the product". In the light of this guidance, a different formulation of an authorised substance (for example, for children, the elderly or those with an allergy to a particular excipient) would probably satisfy the principle of fulfilling special needs.

4.4.5 Manufacture overseas

The Medicines (Exemption from Licences) (Importation) Order 1984 set out additional conditions to be complied with in the case of unauthorised medicinal products imported for particular patient supply but, as noted above, that Order was disapplied by the 1994 Regulations. There were no provisions in the 1994 Regulations to parallel the 1984 Order and consequently the controls on imported unlicensed products were reduced to the level of those on products manufactured in the UK. This was clearly the result of an oversight, and additional controls were reinstated in February 1999 by the Medicines (Standard Provisions for Licences and Certificates) Amendment Regulations 1999.[8]

The Regulations introduce a number of amendments into Schedule 3 (standard provisions for wholesale dealer's licences) of the Medicines (Standard Provisions for Licences and Certificates) Regulations 1971.[9] The 1999 Regulations reproduce the relevant wording from Directive 65/65/EEC (including the reference to "special needs"). Supply of an "exempt imported product" falling within the scope of this wording is only permitted provided certain conditions are complied with.

- At least 28 days prior to each importation, the licence holder must give written notice to the licensing authority, together with certain specified details relating to the product, the quantity to be imported and the manufacturer/assembler/supplier.
- If, within 28 days of acknowledgement of receipt of the notice, the licensing authority notifies the licence holder that the product should not be imported, the licence holder must comply with this notification; if, within this period, he has received notification that the product may be imported, he may proceed with the importation.
- In addition to the usual record keeping requirements for wholesale dealers, the authorisation holder must keep records of the batch number of the product and of any adverse reaction of which the holder becomes aware.

115

- The licence holder may import on each occasion no more than is sufficient for 25 single administrations or for 25 courses of treatment not exceeding three months; the licence holder must not import more than the quantity referred to in the notice.
- The licence holder must inform the licensing authority forthwith of any matter coming to the holder's attention which might reasonably cause the authority to believe that the product can no longer be regarded as safe for administration to human beings or as of satisfactory quality for such administration; the licence holder must cease importation or supply if a written notice is received from the licensing authority requiring cessation.
- The licence holder must not issue any advertisement, catalogue, price list or circular, or make any representations, relating to the exempt imported product.

4.4.6 Labelling

Confusion remains on the rules covering the labelling of unauthorised medicines. Special provisions were contained in regulation 11 of the Medicines (Labelling) Regulations 1976.[10] The Medicines for Human Use (Marketing Authorisations Etc.) Regulations 1994 disapplied the 1976 provisions, but did not introduce replacement provisions for medicinal products without a marketing authorisation. In the absence of further legislation on this point, many companies are continuing to label their products on a voluntary basis in compliance with regulation 11 of the 1976 Regulations.

4.4.7 Charging for supply

The Regulations do not deal with this point. Companies may charge doctors for products supplied to them on a particular patient basis. There are no general Department of Health restrictions on levels of price or price increase, as the Pharmaceutical Price Regulation Scheme only governs products with a marketing authorisation.

4.4.8 Other types of authorisations

The Schedule only provides exemptions from the requirement to hold a marketing authorisation. Other activities involved in the supply of medicines on a particular patient basis need to be carried out under the appropriate authorisations.

4.4.8.1 Manufacturer's licences

Section 8(2) of the Medicines Act 1968 requires those involved in the manufacture or assembly of a medicinal product to hold a manufacturer's licence. In fact, Schedule 1 to the 1994 Regulations requires the manufacturer/assembler in the UK of an unlicensed product for particular patient supply to hold a particular type of manufacturer's licence (a manufacturer's "specials" licence). It should also be noted that section 23 of the Act prohibits the manufacture of a medicinal product unless that product has a marketing authorisation or is exempt from the marketing authorisation requirement.

4.4.8.2 *Wholesale dealer's licences*

Section 8(3) of the Act requires those involved in the wholesale dealing of a medicinal product to hold a wholesale dealer's licence. If the product is imported from another Member State, a wholesale dealer's licence will be required. If it is imported from a country outside the EU, a wholesale dealer's (importation) licence will be required. Schedule 1 to the 1994 Regulations confirms that these provisions apply equally to particular patient supply.

4.4.9 Clinical trials

The widest use of unlicensed medicinal products is in the course of clinical trials. It is important to distinguish between clinical trial use and particular patient use, as very different rules govern these different types of use.

Sections 31–39 of the Medicines Act, which set out the general provisions governing the conduct of clinical trials in the UK, are unaffected by the 1994 Regulations. The Act provides that a clinical trial must be authorised before taking place, either by the terms of the marketing authorisation of the product involved, or by a clinical trial certificate ("CTC") (sections 31(3) and 35(1)). Exemptions, allowing use in clinical trials in other circumstances, are contained in the Medicines (Exemption from Licences) (Special Cases and Miscellaneous Provisions) Order 1972[2] (exemption for trials initiated by doctors and dentists – "DDX" scheme), the Medicines (Exemption from Licences) (Clinical Trials) Order 1995[11] and the Medicines (Exemption from Licences and Certificates) (Clinical Trials) Order 1995[12] (exemption for company initiated trials – "CTX" scheme). Both of these exemptions are subject to certain conditions, such as notification to the MCA.

These restrictions do not currently cover Phase I clinical trials, which are excluded from the scope of the Medicines Act by section 130(4). However, such trials come within the scope of the Directive 2001/20/EC on good clinical practice in the conduct of clinical trials, and further amendments to the UK legislation will be necessary when the Directive is implemented.

In contrast with the position of the manufacturer involved in particular patient supply, section 35(2) of the Act currently exempts from the requirement to hold a manufacturer's licence the manufacturer or assembler of products for the sole purpose of clinical trial use.

Trials initiated by a pharmaceutical company are sometimes continued for an open extension period. This is permissible, provided there are genuine scientific reasons for continuing the study (rather than commercial reasons, such as attempting to create demand for the product) and that the appropriate regulatory clearance has been obtained. If the company does not wish to do this, it would be open to the doctor to request further supplies of the product, but the company must not invite him to do this. Any further supply to the doctor would then need to comply with the provisions regarding particular patient supply, unless the doctor decided to carry out his own trial under a DDX.

It is clear from the above that the distinction between supply for use by particular patients and supply for use in a clinical trial is important, particularly since the rules in the latter case are stricter, and companies must be certain about the basis upon which supply of unlicensed products is made. Various factors are relevant in determining the basis of supply, such as the purpose of the administration (particular patient supply is concerned with treatment; clinical trials are concerned with testing the effects of treatment), the number of patients being treated (although section 31 of the Act makes it clear that a trial may be very small, consisting of "one or more patients") and the degree of organisation and co-ordination between the physicians treating patients.

4.5 Product liability issues

Paragraph 1 of the Schedule states that the supply of the unlicensed product must be for use by a doctor's or dentist's individual patients, on his or her direct personal responsibility. Doctors should be aware of the product liability implications of using such products.

The leaflet MAL 30, issued by the MCA to give guidance on the provisions of the legislation affecting doctors and dentists, states that:

> It should be remembered that a practitioner prescribing an unlicensed medicine does so entirely on his own responsibility, carrying the total burden for the patient's welfare and, in the event of an adverse reaction, may be called upon to justify his actions. Under these circumstances it may be advisable for the practitioner to check his position with his medical defence union before prescribing such unlicensed products.

In theory, the practitioner, as a professional person, is able to assess the risks and potential benefits to his patient, and to decide that the balance lies in favour of the use of a particular unauthorised product. A company receiving a request from that practitioner will therefore assume that the doctor will exercise reasonable care and skill in using the product, in a way that avoids causing injury to his patients. However, the principle that supply is the doctor's sole responsibility does not provide companies with total protection against liability where a patient is injured by treatment with an unlicensed product.

Companies should therefore respond with great care to requests for unlicensed products from practitioners, bearing in mind that there is no legal obligation to comply with such requests. If they do not act with caution, companies risk becoming involved in a negligence claim, or in a product liability action under the Consumer Protection Act 1987 for supplying a defective product (one which does not provide the safety that persons are entitled to expect, taking account of all the circumstances, including the information supplied).

Where a company suspects that the product is to be used in a way that is not safe for patients, its duty to those patients may involve warning the doctor that it considers the proposed use to be hazardous and, if necessary, refusing or terminating supply. While there is no general obligation to provide product information with unlicensed medicines (and, as noted above, the use of promotional material is prohibited), from the standpoint of product liability, the provision of basic safety information about the product is a sensible precaution.

At the operational level, manufacturers must apply proper care and rigorous quality controls during production, to ensure that unlicensed medicinal products that they supply are of the highest quality. They must also have in place proper systems for dealing with requests for particular patient supply and for keeping all the necessary records.

Companies are advised to have in place a standard operating policy for dealing with requests for particular patient supply, even though this can never act as a guarantee against a patient making a claim at a later stage. As part of this, it is useful to have a standard physician consent form, highlighting the unlicensed status of the product and reminding the requesting physician that he or she has a personal responsibility for his or her use of the product.

In Guidance Note 14, the MCA states that hospital trusts, health authorities and independent hospitals should have clear policies on the use of unlicensed medicines, explaining liability considerations and requiring all those involved in the supply chain to ensure that the unlicensed status of a product is communicated and fully understood.

Doctors are, of course, under an obligation to inform their patients adequately about proposed treatments, but a company may be concerned that a patient may not know that he or she is being treated with an unlicensed medicine. One option would be for the company to provide a form for patients to sign, recording their consent to treatment with the unauthorised product. As a matter of English law, such a consent form could not exclude the manufacturer's liability for personal injury for negligence or under the Consumer Protection Act 1987.[13] Nevertheless, it might be helpful in qualifying the patient's expectations of safety from the product.

4.6 Conclusion

There are compelling pragmatic reasons for allowing the supply of unauthorised medicines for particular patient use. Doctors are able to select the treatment that they consider most appropriate for each patient, even though that treatment may not have a marketing authorisation. Companies are permitted to respond to requests for such products, provided that they, and the doctors, comply fully with the provisions of the Medicines for Human Use (Marketing Authorisations Etc.) Regulations 1994. Where the product in question can cause serious adverse reactions or requires very careful monitoring, the company must ensure that it takes particular care, in order to avoid liability in negligence or under the strict liability provisions of the Consumer Protection Act 1987. Any failure to comply with the 1994 Regulations would be regarded unfavourably in any such litigation.

References

1 The Medicines (Exemption from Licences) (Special and Transitional Cases) Order 1971 (SI 1971/1450).
2 The Medicines (Exemption from Licences) (Special Cases and Miscellaneous Provisions) Order 1972 (SI 1972/1200).
3 The Medicines (Exemption from Licences) (Importation) Order 1984 (SI 1984/673).
4 The Medicines for Human Use (Marketing Authorisations Etc.) Regulations 1994 (SI 1994/3144).
5 Medicines (Administration of Radioactive Substances) Regulations 1978 (SI 1978/1006).
6 The Medicines (Advertising) Regulations 1994 (SI 1994/1932).
7 Medicines Control Agency. Guidance Note 14: The supply of unlicensed relevant medicinal products for individual patients. London: MCA, 2000.
8 The Medicines (Standard Provisions for Licences and Certificates) Amendment Regulations 1999 (SI 1999/4).
9 The Medicines (Standard Provisions for Licences and Certificates) Regulations 1971 (SI 1971/972).
10 The Medicines (Labelling) Regulations (SI 1976/1726).
11 The Medicines (Exemption from Licences) (Clinical Trials) Order 1995 (SI 1995/2808).
12 The Medicines (Exemption from Licences and Certificates) (Clinical Trials) Order 1995 (SI 1995/2809).
13 Unfair Contract Terms Act 1977, Section 2; Consumer Protection Act 1987. Section 7: The Unfair Terms in Consumer Contracts Regulations 1994, Schedule 3, paragraph 1(a).

5: Controls on NHS medicines prescribing and expenditure in the UK (a historical perspective)

JOHN P GRIFFIN, JANE R GRIFFIN

5.1 Introduction

There is a well-defined system of pharmaceutical distribution in the UK which is controlled by a licensing system covering manufacture, wholesale and retail supply. For every medicinal product there has to be a product licence (PL) or marketing authorisation (MA), and the product may only be manufactured (or imported) and distributed for sale in accordance with that licence. In addition, manufacturers are required to hold a manufacturer's licence and those who deal in medicines wholesale must hold a wholesale dealer's licence. An important factor in the control of the manufacture of human medicines in the UK is the activities of the Medicines Inspectorate of the DoH. Premises are inspected before a manufacturer's licence is granted, and at regular intervals thereafter. Withdrawal of licences and, rarely, prosecutions can result if standards are not maintained. In this respect DoH gives detailed guidance regarding good manufacturing practice (GMP).

The distribution of medicines from manufacturer to retailer is mainly a private function, the wholesaler covering their costs and earning their profit through the margin allowed in the retail price. The wholesale dealer's licence, among other things, seeks to ensure adequate record keeping in case a batch of medicines has to be recalled.

In the UK prescriptions are required for all medicines supplied under the National Health Service (NHS) and for all prescription-only medicines. Prescriptions may only be written by a doctor or dentist registered in the UK.

The UK NHS is financed primarily out of taxation and is available to all permanent residents. Most people are registered with a general medical practitioner (under contract with the NHS and paid mainly on a capitation basis), who provides primary care and is the normal route of referral to hospital and specialist services, whether in the NHS or the private sector. A small minority of the population obtain some or all of their medical treatment privately, mainly through insurance schemes.

As part of primary care, general practitioners are free to prescribe virtually any medicine they consider desirable for the patient, with the exception of medicines in certain therapeutic categories covered by the 1985 and 1992 Selected List restrictions (see below).

In some mainly rural areas the doctor may also dispense the medicines prescribed, but more usually the patient takes the prescription to a community pharmacist, also under contract with the NHS, who dispenses the medicines and claims reimbursement at predetermined rates. Unless they are exempt, patients pay a prescription charge at the time of dispensing.

From April 1985, within certain therapeutic categories, general medical practitioners have been restricted in the medicines they may prescribe under the National Health Service to those included in a limited list. The excluded medicines are generally those that can be purchased directly by the patient without a prescription, i.e. minor analgesics, but also include some prescription items, such as benzodiazepine sedatives and tranquillisers. The principle underlying this economy measure is that, in theory, for the therapeutic categories concerned, the only medicines prescribable at National Health Service expense should be those that meet a real clinical need at the lowest cost. The list will remain under review by an expert advisory committee, the Advisory Committee on National Health Service Drugs. For medicines no longer available under the National Health Service but for which a prescription is necessary, it is open to the doctor to prescribe these and to the patient to pay for them privately. These measures have, for all practical purposes, introduced a "need clause" into British drug regulations.

The prescribing practices of general practitioners are monitored. After dispensing, the prescriptions are sent to one central point for authorisation of reimbursement, and thus it is possible to analyse each practitioner's prescribing habits and costs (PACT). A summary is sent to each practitioner, together with a note of the area and national averages. If a practitioner's costs are significantly different from the average this may be discussed with him or her by a doctor from the Regional Medical Service of the DoH.

5.2   The National Health Service and Community Care Act 1990

Until 1 April 1991 the key features for the procurement of medicines in the Family Practitioner (general practitioner) Service (FPS) were as follows: general practitioners (GPs) were independent contractors to the Family Practitioner Committees (FPCs) with freedom to prescribe without cash constraints. The FPCs reported directly to Department of Health (DoH) and were responsible for paying GPs for the provision of primary healthcare services. A small group of Regional Medical Services Officers (RMSOs) reported directly to the DoH and were responsible for ensuring economical prescribing of medicines by GPs. The non-dispensing GP was not involved in the procurement of medicines. The pharmacist bought and dispensed the product and was reimbursed by the Prescription Pricing Authority (PPA) on behalf of FPCs. The Regional Health Authority (RHA) had responsibility for hospital budgets, including hospital medicines, but no responsibility for the FPS.

Under the system introduced by the National Health Service and Community Care Act 1990 the Government set an overall budget for GP prescribing, putting a cash restraint on the FPS medicines bill for the first time. The RHAs took over responsibility for the FPCs. Each RHA received a share of the overall drug budget and was responsible for allocating the budget to the newly named Family Health Service Authority (FHSA, formerly FPC). The FHSA set indicative amounts for medicines for each GP and was responsible for monitoring GPs' prescribing against that set amount.

In these circumstances the main concern of FHSAs was to stay within their budget. They had little incentive to tackle the problem of underprescribing, whereby GPs could give better patient care by spending more on medicines. Medical audit and FHSA visits were likely to be directed at high-spending practices rather than low-spending ones. After all, it must be borne in mind that one of the declared objectives of the original White Paper "Working for Patients" was to exert "downward pressure" on the NHS Medicines Bill. This Act operated in tandem with the other measures that have been taken since the inception of the NHS in 1948 to control NHS medicines expenditure.

5.3   The problem of the rising NHS medicines bill

The costs of health care are rising in all developed countries, and despite the fact that in the UK since the inception of the NHS in 1948 the cost of pharmaceuticals has been hovering at about 10% of the total, it has been the target of successive governments for savings. This is because health spending is made up of 70% fixed costs, which are difficult to change, and 30% variable costs. Pharmaceutical expenditure is one-third of the variable cost element and is judged to be an obvious target for reduction and control. However, in the last few years there has been a major increase in the proportion of the NHS budget spent on medicines, from 10·3% in

1990–1991 to some 13·1% in 1997–1998. Although there has been a significant increase in the average net ingredient cost of each prescription, the major cause of the rise has been an increase in the annual number of prescriptions, from some 400 million to 600 million for the UK over the last 10 years. Much of this increase has been due to the demands of an ageing population.

The methods used to control NHS medicines expenditure have been on both the supply side by attempting to reduce costs and the demand side by attempting to restrict volume. The ten distinct measures taken by successive UK governments since 1948 to attempt to do this will be reviewed in chronological order.

5.4 Prescription charges for NHS medicines

Prescription charges were first introduced in the UK in 1952, and are collected by the pharmacist when a doctor's prescription is dispensed. The money collected is *not* offset against the cost of the medicines prescribed but is allocated to the cost of running the pharmaceutical services. (The prescription charges levied in 1994 funded only 6% of the cost of pharmaceutical services.) Prescription charges should therefore be regarded as a revenue-raising exercise rather than a genuine co-payment for medicines dispensed.

In 1948 when the National Health Service was established by the then Minister of Health, Aneurin Bevan, during the Labour Government of Clement Attlee, all prescriptions were supplied free of charge. A charge of 1s 0d (£0·05) per prescription, irrespective of the number of items, was eventually introduced in 1952. Shortly after this the charge was changed to 1s 0d (£0·05) per item on the prescription.[1,2]

For a short period between 1965 and 1968, under the Labour government of Harold Wilson, prescription charges were abolished. In 1968, however, charges were reintroduced and the concept of exemptions was introduced.

In 1971, when the prescription charge was £0·20, the proportion of prescriptions that were exempted was 52% of the total; of these, 32% were for the elderly (men over 65 and women over 60) and 20% were for non-age related reasons. In 1995, 89% of prescriptions were exempt from charge, 45% on grounds of age, which means that 44% of prescriptions were exempt from charge for non-age related reasons.

The list of grounds for exemption from a prescription charge in the UK is extensive. The social grounds are low income, children below the age of 16 years, people in full-time education up to 19 years of age, pregnant women and women in the puerperium following either a live or still birth, old age (women over 60, men over 65, but since October 1995 men over 60), and war pensioners.

In addition, for social policy reasons, since July 1975 prescriptions for oral contraceptives have also been exempt from charges. The medical grounds for exemption from prescription charge are diabetes mellitus, diabetes insipidus, hypopituitarism, hypothyroidism, hypoparathyroidism, hypoadrenalism, myaesthenia gravis, epilepsy and permanent fistula, for example colostomy, ileostomy. In addition, police personnel can claim back from their employing authority any prescription charge they incur.

There are illogicalities in the system, as a patient who is exempt from paying a prescription charge gets all medicines free, even if the prescription is for the treatment of an illness unrelated to the medical condition for which the exemption has been allowed. For example, a millionaire with diabetes mellitus would be exempt from a prescription charge for a bottle of aspirins, whereas a patient with a chronic medical condition not on the exemption list would have to pay a charge for medicines prescribed for his or her chronic condition, for example rheumatoid arthritis, parkinsonism or hypertension. (This can to some extent be mitigated by purchase of an annual prescription season ticket, which for a flat sum covers the cost of all prescription charges for medicines and devices for the ensuing 12 months.)

In the 23 years from 1979 to 2002 there were annual increases in the prescription charge, from £0·20 per item to £6·20 per item. The government has attempted to use this tax to raise revenue and as an unsuccessful deterrent to patients demanding a prescription at each visit to their doctor. As about 85% of prescriptions are exempt from charge this latter objective has been deemed to be ineffective. This has been largely due at times to high levels of unemployment – at times in excess of 3 million – during this period, which also has also meant that the unemployed and their families have been exempt from prescription charges. In addition, unemployment also contributes to or is associated with ill health and demands for health care.[3]

In October 1995 the European Court of Justice in Luxembourg ruled on equal treatment for men and women regarding the age at which they should be exempted from paying an NHS prescription charge. Until then the exemption from the prescription charge had been linked to state pensionable age of 60 years for women and 65 for men. Men are now exempt from the age of 60, at an estimated cost in 1995 of £30 million per year for lowering the age and £10 million for refunds for those men between 60 and 65 years who had paid for a prescription in the preceding three months.[4]

Another criticism of the current level of prescription charges is that in 1994 nearly 60% of prescribed medicines could either be purchased from a pharmacist for less than the prescription charge, or had a net ingredient cost (NIC) less than the prescription charge.

Both physicians and economists have called for reform of the prescription charge exemptions for both social and medical conditions.[5-7] It has been pointed out that if the exemptions were reduced from 89% to 55% – the

125

level that applied when they were first introduced – and the charge actually reduced to £2·50 per item, then £250 million per annum extra could be collected at the 1995 prescribing level of 500 million items per year.[5] Changes in the current system would not only have to be logical but politically acceptable, and there are no indications that the political will to introduce changes is growing.

Rationalisation of the exemptions from prescription charges and a variation of the current season ticket scheme linked to annual registration with a general practice have been proposed.[6,7]

In conclusion, charges for NHS prescriptions should be regarded as a tax rather than co-payment for the medicines prescribed. They have been inefficient as a deterrent on the demand side owing to the high level of exemptions. The application of the principle of exemption has led to legal action before the European courts on grounds of sex discrimination. Furthermore, a potential legal challenge exists on the grounds of social inequities and unfairness in selecting certain illnesses as worthy of exemption but not others, and is under consideration by patient pressure groups.

5.5   The Pharmaceutical Price Regulation Scheme (PPRS)

The prices of medicines sold to the National Health Service are controlled in the UK by the Pharmaceutical Price Regulation Scheme (PPRS),[8,9] negotiated periodically every five to six years by the Department of Health (DoH) with the Association of the British Pharmaceutical Industry (ABPI), for example in 1979, 1986, 1993 and 1999. The PPRS controls the maximum – *but not guaranteed* – profits that pharmaceutical companies make on the capital they have invested in plant for research, development and manufacturing for sales made to the NHS. (Capital employed by the individual companies is allocated between that devoted to NHS sales and that for non-NHS sales and exports.)

The scheme was proposed in 1957 in an attempt by the pharmaceutical industry to stave off more draconian measures by the government of the day. It was known as the voluntary price regulation scheme (VPRS), but was neither voluntary nor a price regulation scheme. It was a profit regulation scheme. By the mid-1970s its name had been changed to the Pharmaceutical Price Regulation Scheme (PPRS), but it still retained a level of inaccuracy even until the 1993 agreement. However, the most recent negotiation between the DoH and ABPI in 1999 was in effect no longer a voluntary agreement because of the statutory powers and penalties behind it. This leaves a lot less room for negotiation and flexibility. The 1999–2004 PPRS, which is in accordance with the provisions of the Health Act 1999 Section 33, leaves no room for uncertainty. It changes the status of the PPRS and makes it more formulaic.[16]

The scheme applies to all companies supplying NHS medicines prescribed by medical or dental practitioners or nurses qualified to prescribe. Generic medicines, whose price is determined by the Drug Tariff, are excluded, as are the over-the-counter (OTC) medicines, and sales of medicines derived from private (non-NHS) prescriptions.

5.5.1 Annual financial returns

Each company with sales to the NHS of more than £1 million per annum has to supply financial information and those with sales of between £1 million and £25 million will have to supply full audited accounts. Companies with NHS sales greater than £25 million will have to submit a full annual financial return (AFR). Products with NHS sales of greater than £100 000 and £500 000 will have to be specifically identified. These annual returns cover the overall sales to the NHS and the costs incurred, such as research and development expenditure, manufacturing costs, general administrative costs, promotional expenditure and capital employed. (Details of *specific* product costs or sales are not required.)

5.5.2 Profitability

The reasonableness of the maximum return on capital (ROC) earned by individual companies on home sales of NHS medicines is a matter for negotiation within a published range of 17% for level 1 and 21% for level 2, having regard to the nature and scale of the company's relevant investment and activities, and associated long-term risks.

5.5.3 Margin of tolerance

The allowable returns on capital will be associated with a margin of tolerance (MOT). Companies will be able to retain profits of up to 140% of the level 2 (21%) ROC target calculated by reference to level 2 allowances. Companies will not be granted price increases unless they are forecasting profits less than 50% of their level 1 (17%) ROC target calculated by reference to the level 1 allowances.

The MOT will not be available to a scheme member for any year in which it has had a price increase agreed by the Department. Where a scheme member exceeds its level 1 target profit for a year in which it has received a price increase, all profits above the level 1 target will be repayable. Where a price increase is agreed by the Department in the second half of a year the Department may decide that the MOT will not be available to a scheme member for the year following the increase.

If the Department's assessment of an AFR shows profits in excess of the MOT, it will negotiate one or more of the following:

- price reductions, during the accounting year following that covered by the return, to bring prospective profits down to an acceptable level, on the basis of available forecasts
- repayments of that amount of past profits which is agreed to exceed the MOT
- a delay or restriction of price increases agreed for the company, or both.

5.5.4 Profitability of companies with small capital base in UK

Prior to the 1999 PPRS companies with a negligible capital base in the UK had their profits assessed on a return on sales basis, which ranged from 3·75 to 4·25%.

Scheme members will now be able to include capital employed in their AFR on the basis of its inclusion in UK statutory accounts, by injection or by imputation in the transfer price. This will enable some companies that have been assessed as return on sales (ROS) companies under the 1993 scheme to be assessed as ROC companies under this agreement.

Alternatively, for scheme members whose AFR home sales exceed their average assessed home capital employed (excluding any capital imputation from the transfer price) by a factor of 3·5 or more, a target rate of profit will be set by dividing the ROC target rate by a factor of 3·5. The assessment of the returns of scheme members who elect for the ROS option will take account of the MOT on transfer price profit.

These changes in the 1999 PPRS have been introduced to enable the Department of Health to control transfer pricing arrangements, which ABPI has long resisted.

5.5.5 The export disincentive

Profits allowed on sales of prescription medicines in the UK are limited to a target return on assets related to UK sales.

Manufacturing assets used for NHS products are normally allocated between home sales to the NHS and exports pro rata to cost of sales. Costs must be computed on a fully allocated basis, i.e. overheads are spread on a consistent basis between home and export products.

The effect of an increased proportion of exports is to allocate an increased proportion of the manufacturing assets to exports and, by definition, a reduced share to the UK. Thus the asset base on which target UK profit is computed is reduced.

At the same time an increased proportion of exports will allocate an increased proportion of annual fixed manufacturing overheads to export sales and hence a reduced proportion to UK NHS sales. The effect of this will be to reduce the cost of sales charged to the UK, with a consequent increase in profit.

The effect of these two factors constitutes a double disadvantage for any company wishing to increase its proportion of exports, as its UK NHS asset base is reduced and at the same time its national UK profits are increased.

For a company below its target rate of return this will reduce the price increase it can apply for, and if it is over its target return it will increase the amount it pays back to the DoH or the amount by which it will have to reduce prices.

This disincentive is particularly relevant for large tender business where multinationals typically have several manufacturing sources they can consider. Increasingly they are placing the business in countries where the impact of the domestic market is either cost neutral or has a cost-positive impact.

The export disincentive is becoming increasingly relevant in the context of the single European market, where the number of manufacturing facilities is being reduced by many multinationals and those that remain acquire substantial export business within the Community.

Under the most recent revision of the PPRS, the DoH will allocate 7·5% of the net value of each company's non-research and development fixed assets and its manufacturing infrastructure costs to its NHS sales before the balance is apportioned between home and export sales.[17]

5.5.6 Pricing of major new products

New products introduced following a major application for a product licence from the United Kingdom Licensing Authority may be priced at the discretion of the company on entering the market. This will have to take account of costs of research and development and the competition in the marketplace.

5.5.7 Promotional expenditure

Allocated expenditure by companies on product promotion is limited. The aggregate sales promotional allowance will be set as a percentage of *total* industry NHS sales. The distribution of the aggregate between individual companies is made on the basis of a formula agreed between the DoH and ABPI, for example, in the 1999 agreement promotional expenditure was allocated between three component parts.

1. Basic allowance of £464 000 per company
2. A percentage of NHS sales allowance of 3% for level 1 and 6% for level 2
3. An individual product servicing allowance of £58 000 for three products, £46 000 for a further three products, £35 000 for a further three products, and a £23 000 allowance for the 10th and subsequent products. These allowances only apply to products with NHS sales greater than £100 000 per annum. These figures, agreed in October 1999, are subject to adjustment based on level of inflation.

5.5.8 Research and development expenditure

Under the 1999 revision of the PPRS each company's research and development expenditure allowance will be 20% (level 2) of the company's sales to the NHS for assessing profitability under the scheme (however, a maximum of 17% (level 1) will be allowed for assessing applications from companies seeking a price increase).

For a maximum of 12 in-patent active substances, each with an individual sales level to the NHS of £500 000 or more, a company will be able to add 0·25% of total NHS turnover to their PPRS research and development allowance for each such active substance. Thus a company could achieve a maximum allowance of 23% of NHS sales as its research and development allowance.[16]

5.5.9 Assessment of the PPRS

The weaknesses of the PPRS are clear from the above outline. These are first, the export disincentive, which discourages pharmaceutical companies from sourcing export orders from UK manufacturing sites, so that multinationals with several alternative sourcing arrangements will avoid using the UK. This is clearly disadvantageous for both jobs and UK balance of payments.

The promotional formula and the capping of allowable promotional expenses operate in favour of the pharmaceutical companies with large existing sales to the NHS, and to the disadvantage of small companies or companies wishing to start up business in the UK.

The cap on allowable research and development costs to 20% of NHS sales is a disincentive to conducting research in the UK at levels above this. Small and middle-sized companies are penalised more than the pharmaceutical giants by this provision. It also favours companies who have products in patent being sold to the NHS "but whose current pipe-line may be weak, no financial provision is made to encourage companies with a strong pipe-line to bring them forward more effectively other than an offer of 'jam tomorrow'". The position of companies marketing "in-patent" products that have been licensed from other companies rather than their own research is unclear.

A number of non-UK European-based companies have criticised the rate of return on capital (ROC) on the basis that it favours companies with a large capital base in the UK and could therefore be regarded as an incentive to invest in the UK, which is contrary to European Union legislation.

The same group of companies have regarded the PPRS as discriminatory, as companies with a significant capital investment in the UK have their profits determined as return on capital base, whereas others which have a large investment in the European Union as a whole may operate in the UK as sales companies only. In this situation these companies are treated on a percentage profit on sales, which are less favourable terms.

Some US-owned companies with large UK operations have been particularly vociferous in their criticism of the PPRS.

In terms of curtailing NHS expenditure on medicines the effectiveness of the PPRS is more difficult to assess: it has the power to restrict price increases and "claw back" excess profits, and the opportunities for the Department of Health to enforce these powers has been increased in the 1999 revision of the PPRS. The amount of money "clawed back" from companies each year has been insignificant in the past compared to the overall medicines expenditure, but this will change.

In general, the pharmaceutical industry would regard the freedom to price new products without awaiting the outcome of protracted negotiations – which can delay marketing for months or even years in some EU countries – as a major advantage that counterbalances the system's many faults. This freedom is maintained in the 1999 revision of the PPRS. The pharmaceutical industry will cling to this advantage of the PPRS in particular, and to the scheme in general, on the principle "cling to nurse for fear of worse". The real question is, can PPRS survive long term in the post-Maastricht European climate?[10]

5.6   The Drug Tariff

The Drug Tariff operated by the Department of Health was the first reference price system. Introduced in the early 1950s, the tariff price represents the price that the Prescription Pricing Authority operates on when reimbursing pharmacists and dispensing doctors for the cost of materials dispensed, whether drugs, dressings or devices. The average price for each generic formulation is determined as an average of the prices of the largest four or five manufacturers for each generic formulation (generics in the UK being generally unbranded). The community pharmacist who dispenses the prescribed generic is reimbursed at the tariff price. The pharmacist therefore does not purchase generic preparations from manufacturers whose price is above the tariff price. This effectively forces a downward price spiral for generics, as their tariff price was originally determined on a yearly basis but is now done as frequently as each month.

The prices of generic medicines must inevitably rise in the near future as manufacturers move to produce patient packs, which will be required to contain patient information leaflets. Under EC legislation bulk containers will almost inevitably be phased out of production (except perhaps for hospital use).

5.7   Contract purchase of medicines from cheap sources

In the early 1960s, when Enoch Powell was Minister of Health in Macmillan's Conservative government, the Department of Health bought large quantities of tetracycline from Poland for NHS hospital use. This was found to be clinically ineffective and of substandard quality; a public outcry in the medical press followed. The cheap drugs exercise was not repeated, but bulk hospital purchase at competitive contract prices continues, and this leads to wide discrepancies between the hospital price and the price charged to prescriptions written in the primary healthcare sector.

5.8   Generic substitution

Generic substitution was raised as a means of reducing the NHS medicines bill in the Greenfield Report of 1983, but was not implemented.

5.9   Enforced price reductions

In December 1983, the then Health Minister announced measures to cut industry profits and reduce the NHS medicines bill, then running at £1·3 billion per year, by £100 million. In November 1984 further measures were taken by reducing the return on capital allowed under the PPRS from 25% to a range of 15–17%. ROC was raised to 17–21% in two stages under the 1986 renegotiation of the PPRS. In the 1993 renegotiation of the PPRS the ROC was left unchanged, but a price reduction of 2·5% on pharmaceuticals was enforced. This was negotiated by ABPI to be achieved by a 2·5% reduction overall on each company's products, but could be modulated by taking a larger reduction on some products than on others. The alternative to price reductions was for companies to present the Department of Health with a cheque equivalent to 2·5% of its sales to the NHS, a solution accepted but not favoured by the Department of Health, as these moneys disappeared into Treasury Funds and so did not offer any real advantage to the Department.

In the 1999 PPRS negotiations, as part of the agreement the DoH imposed a 4·5% price reduction on sales to the NHS. This was equivalent to a loss of sales by the industry of £200 million. Because the 1999 revision of the PPRS permits companies to modulate these enforced price reductions across their product range, it could be expected that companies would do so in such a way that competition from parallel-traded products would be reduced, maximum price reductions being applied to those products that were currently being most affected by parallel trade.

5.10   Limited or selected lists

The first limited list proposals were announced in November 1984 and proposed that a list of 31 products was adequate to meet "all clinical needs in the seven therapeutic areas of indigestion remedies, laxatives, analgesics, cold and cough remedies, vitamin preparations, tonics and benzodiazepines". In the event, when the proposals became operational in April 1985 the initial list had been expanded to 129 products, and later to

160 products. The remaining products reimbursable on the NHS could only be dispensed if prescribed by their generic as opposed to their brand names.

The saving from the original limited list exercise in its first year of operation was claimed to be £75 million, and Ministers of Health over the next ten years have been unable to quantify what, if any, savings took place in subsequent years, despite a series of Parliamentary Questions seeking this information.

If 10% of patients previously receiving prescriptions for an antacid were prescribed an H_2 antagonist such as cimetidine or ranitidine, this claimed saving would not have been achieved. The growth in the H_2 antagonist market was rapid at this time, and some of this growth must have been due to such escalation of prescribing.

In November 1992 the Secretary of State for Health announced the extension of the limited list procedure to 10 further therapeutic categories, namely antidiarrhoeals, appetite suppressants, treatments for allergic disorders, hypnotics and anxiolytics, treatments for vaginal and vulval conditions, contraceptives, treatment for anaemia, topical antirheumatics, treatments for ear and nose conditions, and treatments for all skin conditions. These measures were announced despite repeated undertakings by a series of Conservative Secretaries of State for Health that the government had no intention of extending the limited list, and despite the fact that the Department of Health remains unable to quantify the savings achieved from the limited list exercise in the original seven categories.

The second limited list operation affecting 10 therapeutic categories announced in November 1992 became an exercise to reduce the prices of products to preconceived "reasonable levels", these being delegated by Health Ministers to the Advisory Committee on NHS Drugs chaired by a Department of Health official and having outside members from the medical and pharmaceutical professions. The achievement of this exercise has been to inveigle a number of companies into agreeing price reductions in exchange for their product's continuing to be prescribable in the NHS. This exercise has therefore amounted to a reference price system with a non-transparent method of fixing the price. It is therefore probable that the second phase of the limited list operation was in breach of the Transparency Directive (89/105/EEC). (The price reductions achieved under this exercise were not permitted to be counted towards the 2·5% overall price reduction imposed as part of the 1993 PPRS agreement.)

The Advisory Committee on NHS Drugs, when examining oral contraceptives as one of the classes involved in the second phase of the limited list exercise, formed a preliminary position that the more expensive third-generation oral contraceptives should be precluded from availability on NHS prescription on grounds of cost. The outcry from women's groups, family planning practitioners and the medical profession was such that these proposals were never implemented.

5.11   The indicative prescribing scheme and general practitioner fundholding

The indicative prescribing scheme (IPS) and general practitioner fundholding were both introduced in 1991. These schemes were described by Whalley and co-workers in *PharmacoEconomics* in 1992 and 1995, including the various incentives offered to both fundholders and non-fundholders to reduce their prescribing costs by allowing a proportion of the "savings" to be used on other projects in the practice.[11,12] Their effects were summarised by Whalley as follows:

> The IPS has generally failed to control the rise in drug costs because of unrealistic targets, organisational difficulties (including the lack of adequate data to set budgets properly) and because there was neither incentive nor penalty to encourage compliance on the part of the general practitioner (GP). The IPS stresses cost containment, and makes little allowance for the consideration of quality or appropriateness of prescribing.
>
> GP fund holding, in contrast, has reduced the rate of rise of drug costs in participating GP practices, although it has not actually reduced drug costs ... Although there is a commitment on the part of the government to encourage and make use of data about economic evaluations of drug therapy and other medical interventions, so far the emphasis has been exclusively on cost containment.

5.12   The development of primary care groups

The Labour government elected in May 1997 committed itself to abolishing the concept of fundholding practices. This was not because of any fundamental disagreement with the concept of primary care commissioning per se, but rather because of the inevitable "two-tierism" in service provision between fundholders and non-fundholders that resulted. In December 1997 the government produced its own White Paper entitled *The New NHS – Modern. Dependable.* When this document was first published it seemed to be signalling a new direction, but however much of the content could be described largely as a repackaging of existing (Conservative) policy, psychologically it felt different. The evolution of primary care groups can clearly be traced back to the fundholding initiative begun in 1991. Halpen expressed the opinion of many NHS commentators when he wrote:

> The Government use of PCGs as a mechanism for managing primary care is no more than a continuation of the policies of the previous government. Although GP fundholders revelled in their initial freedoms, it is clear that the move towards total purchasing (in whatever guise) was a clear precursor of PCGs.

However, the Labour government has clearly stamped its mark on PCGs and essentially the changed philosophy behind them. The following quote from the White Paper summarises some of their thinking as follows:

[PCGs] will have control over resources but will have to account for how they have used them in improving efficiency and quality. The new role envisaged for GPs and community nurses will build on some of the most successful recent developments in primary care. These professionals have seized opportunities to extend their role in recent years ... Despite its limitations, many innovative GPs and their fund managers have used the fundholding scheme to sharpen the responsiveness of some hospital services and to extend the range of services available in their own surgeries. But the fundholding scheme had also proved bureaucratic and costly. It has allowed development to take place in a fragmented way, outside a coherent strategic plan. It has artificially separated responsibility for emergency and planned care, and given advantage to some patients at the expense of others. So the government wants to keep what has worked about fundholding but discard what has not.

There are a couple of key differences between fundholding and PCGs. First, the unified budget. The White Paper did not set out much detail about the implications and consequences of a unified budget, but its importance should not be underestimated. Its implications for general practice and the NHS as a whole are probably only equalled by the clinical governance initiative (Royce). The government perceive the unified budget and clinical governance as the principal vehicle by which the long-standing problems of successive governments – cost constraint and medical practice variation – can be tackled. As Majeed and Malcolm, writing in the *BMJ*, concluded:

The main factor behind the introduction of unified budgets is the belief that making general practitioners accountable for cost as well as the quality of health care will prove an effective method of tackling many of the problems facing the NHS.

Another key difference is that fundholding was always vulnerable to the charge that it was creating a two-tier NHS, but there is no opt out clause for general practices with the development of PCGs. Together with the unified budget, this means that resource decisions taken by one practice in a PCG have a direct impact on others. They are no longer islands, and practices have to be concerned with how well the PCG is doing as a whole and with any poorly performing practices within it, as the bottom line is that a PCG can be dragged down by them.

This helps to explain why GP involvement makes or breaks the Labour government's reforms. It boils down to simple economics: GPs, principally through their referral and prescribing decisions, commit the vast majority of PCGs' (and consequently NHS) resources. Ultimately, under the new

NHS reforms it is the GP who will have to take responsibility for limiting (and in many cases reversing) the growth in prescribing costs and hospital expenditure.

5.13 Changing the legal status of medicines from prescription only to over-the-counter availability

Speaking at the Annual Pharmaceutical Conference on this matter in November 1993, Dr Brian Mawhinney, the UK Minister for Health, stated that self-medication "encourages people to be more interested in and committed to their own health; [and] it empowers individuals with greater freedom to determine for themselves what medicines they will use".

The theoretical advantages to the government are clear. First, by switching more medicines from being prescription only (POM) to over-the-counter (OTC) or pharmacy sale (P) and encouraging patients to self-medicate, it might be anticipated that the country's medicines bill would be reduced. Second, by encouraging patients to purchase their own medicine it obviates the need for a GP consultation, the main object of which was to obtain a prescription. However, although many items are available considerably cheaper than the prescription charge, approximately 89% of prescription items were dispensed free. Thus there is little incentive for most patients to purchase their medicines over the counter.

In June 1997 DGIII of the European Commission circulated a consultation document entitled "A Guideline on Changing the Classification for the Supply of a Medicinal Product for Human Use". The objective of this was to ensure that the route of sale will be the same in all member states of the European Union. The grounds for making decisions on route of supply are based on safety considerations, and for medicines for purchase directly by the patient stringent requirements for information are proposed. (The Commission document does not consider economic grounds for change of status.)[13]

5.14 Encouragement to prescribe generically

A number of the above government initiatives have resulted in changing doctors' prescribing habits towards a greater use of generic formulations. Doctors are currently happier to prescribe generics as they have become more convinced of their quality. "This was probably not unrelated to the fact that in the year ending August 1993, 80% of generic medicine sales in the UK originated from subsidiaries of the 4 multinational manufacturers Rhône Poulenc Rorer, Hoechst, Fisons and Ivax."[14]

In 1993 the overall shape of the NHS market by value of products dispensed was as follows: generics accounted for 11% by value and over 41% by volume; prescriptions for medicines still within patent accounted for 26% by value but only 7% by volume. The bulk of the NHS prescription market, 63% by value and 52% by volume, was made up of active substances that were out of patent but still being prescribed by brand name.

In 1993, 7% of the 530 million prescriptions dispensed were for products in patent. On the basis of these products coming off patent, the Department of Health believed that by the year 2000 60% of prescriptions would be dispensed generically. In a reply to a question in the House of Commons the Minister of Health stated that for 1994–1995 more than 50% of GP prescriptions dispensed in England and Wales were written generically, with GP fundholders writing 55·3% by generic name and non-fundholders 50·5%. However, the highest figure recorded by the Office of Health Economics was 46% for the year 1998.

Overall, government policies have been directed towards cheap drugs and a drive towards generic prescribing, and this has been successful to a very large extent. It is, however, unfortunate that this policy has deterred doctors from prescribing newer in-patent products.

5.15 The National Institute for Clinical Excellence (NICE)

The National Institute for Clinical Excellence (NICE) was established as a Special Health Authority in April 1999. In establishing NICE, the Labour government hoped to improve standards of patient care and reduce inequalities in access to innovative treatments (postcode prescribing).

NICE was to achieve these aims by providing guidance to the NHS on the effectiveness and cost of clinical interventions. This would be done by appraising new and existing technologies, developing disease-specific clinical guidelines and by supporting clinical audit. Perhaps unsurprisingly, it is the work of NICE in the technology appraisals arena which has dominated its work programme since 1999 and generated the most controversy both within and outside the UK.

For details of the Institute's work and their procedures, the NICE website is a useful source of material (http://www.nice.org.uk/).

The selection of a technology for appraisal is undertaken by the Department of Health and the National Assembly of Wales.

5.16 The European Transparency Directive

Under Directive 89/105/EEC "Relating to transparency of measures regulating the scope of national health insurance systems"[15] all measures introduced by national governments to control expenditure on medicines will have to be compatible with EU rules.

The Directive applies to *any* national measures to control price or restrict the range of products covered by national health insurance systems. The specific articles of the Directive cover the various schemes operational within the Community and demands that objective and verifiable criteria are met in their implementation (see Section 2.15.4, p. 81).

The Transparency Directive does not lay down a requirement for harmonisation of procedures, nor does it imply a need to harmonise prices within the Community, and even if harmonisation of prices were achieved the Directive does not mean that there would be harmonisation of Health Service reimbursement.

As long as price differences exist between Member States of the European Community, parallel importing or parallel trading of medicinal products from Member States with lower prices to those with higher prices will take place. In fact, parallel trading in medicinal products could be called importation of another Member State's price constraints. The European Commission and Member States' Health Authorities not only condone but covertly encourage parallel trading. This creates considerable problems for pharmaceutical companies. The UK Department of Health claws back a percentage of the reimbursement due from the Prescription Pricing Authority to reduce the windfall profits made by pharmacists buying cheaply from parallel traders.

At present healthcare systems remain a national prerogative and are subject to national rather than European controls, but operated within the broad scope of the Transparency Directive. However, future changes in the direction of greater pan-European harmonisation can be envisaged.

5.17 Supply of controlled drugs

Special arrangements apply to the prescribing of drugs of dependence in the UK under the provisions of the Misuse of Drugs Act 1971. Drugs controlled include cocaine, dipipanone, diamorphine (heroin), methadone, morphine, opium, pethidine, phencyclidine, lysergide (LSD), amphetamines, barbiturates, cannabis, codeine, pholcodine, and certain drugs related to the amphetamines, such as chlorphentermine and diethylpropion.

For all controlled drugs, prescriptions must be signed and dated by the prescriber and the following particulars included in the prescriber's own handwriting: name and address of patient, form and strength of preparation as appropriate, total quantity in both words and figures, and dose.

Only medical practitioners who hold a special licence issued by the Home Secretary may prescribe diamorphine, dipipanone or cocaine for addicts; other practitioners must refer the addict to a treatment centre. This stipulation only applies to addicts and does not preclude the prescription of diamorphine or cocaine for the relief of pain due to organic disease or injury (see also Section 2.15.1, pp. 78–81).

5.18   International comparisons

The effectiveness of various measures to contain expenditure on medicines in the UK can only be assessed in the context of the situation in other European Union countries. Table 5.1 gives data for the total expenditure on health care as a percentage of gross domestic product (GDP), expenditure on medicines as a percentage of total healthcare spend, the national pharmaceutical industry's research and development expenditure in euro-millions, the general price index and the medicines price index nationally compared to a European price of 100, and the national pharmaceutical consumption per capita expressed as defined daily doses (DDD). These comparisons are based on OECD Health Data 2000.

The UK is seen from these figures to be a country with a comparatively low per-capita consumption of medicines, to have a high medicines price index and a strong pharmaceutical research base, therefore the various measures to contain medicines expenditure would appear to have had their greatest impact on the demand side.

Three of the four countries with the highest industry research and development spend have the highest medicines price index. France is the exception in this respect but has the highest per capita level of medicine consumption. Expressed in another way, the three largest spenders on health care as a percentage of GDP are France, Switzerland and Germany, which are three of the four countries where the pharmaceutical industry invests most in research and development.

Conversely, in countries where the population is relatively small and where individual consumption of medicines is low and pharmaceutical industry investment is also low, the government is able to enforce low prices for medicines. These countries are typified by the Netherlands, Norway, Finland and Denmark. Sweden, where there is significant pharmaceutical research, is atypical of the rest of Scandinavia and the medicines price index and medicine consumption are approximately the European average.

It would appear that national governments' desires to impose draconian measures to control pharmaceutical prices and/or consumption is modulated by financial/fiscal necessity not to damage its national researched-based industry. Balancing such conflicting demands has been the key to the strength of the PPRS scheme as it was in its inception. It remains to be seen whether this has been retained or lost following the 1999 revision, which now has a legal basis.

Table 5.1 Healthcare expenditure and medicines expenditure as % GDP and comparative cost of medicines (OECD Health Data 2000 and 2001)

Country	Medicine prices according to a model in which 100 sets the average price for the year 2000	Pharmaceutical expenditure per head in US$ for the year 2000	Spending on healthcare as % GDP, in ( ) spending on medicines as % GDP	
Austria	98	277	8·2	(1·2)
Belgium	93	318	8·8	(1·4)
Denmark	101	174	8·4	(0·8)
Finland	95	221	6·8	(1·0)
France	94	446	9·3	(1·7)
Germany	114	283	10·3	(1·3)
Greece	71	—	8·4	(1·4)
Italy	93	307	7·9	(1·7)
Japan	—	361	7·5	(1·3)
Netherlands	108	224	8·7	(1·0)
Norway	94	183	8·5	(0·9)
Portugal	92	—	—	—
Spain	84	238	7·0	(1·5)
Sweden	103	220	7·6	(1·2)
Switzerland	133	214	10·4	(0·8)
United Kingdom	126	229	6·9	(1·1)
USA	—	451	12·9	(1·4)

Acknowledgements

This chapter is based in part on a review article by JP Griffin: "A Historical Survey of UK Government Measures to Control the NHS Medicines Expenditure from 1948–1995", published in *PharmacoEconomics* 1996;10:210-24 and has been expanded and updated.

References

1 Office of Health Economics. *Compendium of Health Statistics, 9th edn.* London: Office of Health Economics, 1998.
2 Prescription Pricing Authority Annual Reports, 1994/5.
3 Griffin JR. *The Impact of Unemployment on Health.* Briefing No 29. London: Office of Health Economics, 1993.
4 Warden J. Men can have free prescriptions at 60. *BMJ* 1995;311:1118.
5 Griffin TD. Patient contribution to the cost of prescribed medicines in Europe. In: Griffin JP, O'Grady J, Wells FO, eds. *The Textbook of Pharmaceutical Medicine,* 2nd edn. Belfast: Queens University, 1995:581–94.
6 Griffin JP. Increasing cost of medicines. *Lancet* 1993;341:1156–7.
7 Green DG, Lucas DA. *Medicard: A Better Way to Pay for Medicines.* London: Institute of Economic Affairs Health and Welfare Unit, Choice in Welfare No 16, 1993.
8 Department of Health. *The Pharmaceutical Price Regulation Scheme.* London: HMSO, 1993. Reference number Det DH 004643, 9/93.
9 ABPI. *A Guide to the Pharmaceutical Price Regulation Scheme (PPRS).* London: Association of the British Pharmaceutical Industry, 1993.
10 Griffin JP. The pros and cons of the PPRS. *Scrip* 1997;October:11–13.
11 Bligh J, Whalley T. The UK indicative prescribing scheme. *PharmacoEconomics* 1992;2: 137–52.
12 Whalley T, Wilson R, Bligh J. Current prescribing in primary care in the UK. *PharmacoEconomics* 1995;7:320–31.
13 European Commission Director General III. *A Guideline on Changing the Classification for the Supply of a Medicinal Product for Human Use.* 12 July 1997.
14 Walker R. Generic medicines: reducing cost at the expense of quality? *PharmacoEconomics* 1995;7:375–7.
15 European Commission Directive 89/105 EEC. Relating to transparency of measures regulating the scope of national health insurance systems. *Official Journal of the European Communities* 1989.
16 *The Pharmaceutical Price Regulation Scheme.* ABPI and Department of Health. www.doh.gov.uk/pprs.htm
17 Butler S. Will PPRS R and D benefits compensate for price cut in UK? *Scrip* 1999; 2457:4.

Recommended further reading on NHS Reforms

Halpen S. Doctoring the truth? Milburn lets the cats out of the bag. *Br J Health Care Mgt* 1998;4:426.
Majeed A, Malcolm L. Unified budgets for primary care groups. *BMJ* 1999; 319:772.
Royce R. *Primary Care and the NHS Reforms: a manager's view.* London: Office of Health Economics, 2000.
Secretary of State for Health. *The New NHS: Modern. Dependable.* London: The Stationery Office, 1997.

6: The regulation of therapeutic products in Australia

JANICE HIRSHORN, DEBORAH MONK

6.1 Introduction

The Commonwealth Therapeutic Goods Act 1989 (the Act) sets out the legal requirements for the import, export, manufacture, and supply of therapeutic goods in Australia. It is supported by the Therapeutic Goods Regulations and various Orders and Determinations. The aim of this legislation is to provide a national framework for the regulation of therapeutic goods in Australia, so as to ensure their quality, safety, efficacy, and timely availability.

The Therapeutic Goods Administration (TGA), as part of the Commonwealth Department of Health, has responsibility for administering the Act. It applies a risk management approach to therapeutic goods regulation, which is intended to ensure public health and safety whilst minimising the regulatory burden and associated costs.

The TGA carries out a range of assessment and monitoring activities to ensure that all therapeutic goods available in Australia are of an acceptable standard:

- pre-market evaluation and approval of registered products intended for supply in Australia
- licensing of manufacturers in accordance with international standards under Good Manufacturing Practice (GMP)
- post-market monitoring, through sampling, adverse event reporting, surveillance activities, and response to public enquiries
- development, maintenance, and monitoring of the systems for listing of medicines
- the assessment of medicines for export.

The term "therapeutic goods" includes prescription medicines, non-prescription medicines, complementary medicines, and medical devices. The TGA also develops and implements national policies and controls for chemicals, gene technology, blood, and blood products.

A product's "risk" is determined by a number of factors, including whether:

- the medicine contains a substance scheduled in the Standard for the Uniform Scheduling of Drugs and Poisons (SUSDP)
- the medicine's use can result in significant adverse effects
- the medicine is used to treat life-threatening or very serious illnesses
- there may be any adverse effects from prolonged use or inappropriate self-medication.

The scheduling of drugs is performed under State and Territory (henceforth referred to as State) legislation controlling access to medicines, but is coordinated at a national level to ensure uniformity except in exceptional circumstances.

All therapeutic goods must be entered as either "registered" goods or "listed" goods on the Australian Register of Therapeutic Goods (ARTG) before they may be supplied in or exported from Australia, unless they are exempt under the legislation.

Prescription medicines are medicines considered as having a higher level of risk. They must be registered on the ARTG, and the degree of assessment and regulation they undergo is rigorous and detailed, with sponsors being required to provide comprehensive safety, quality, and efficacy data. They contain ingredients included in Schedule 4 (prescription) or Schedule 8 (controlled drugs) of the SUSDP, or are specified products such as sterile injectables. Biologics fall into the same overall approach – they are not handled separately.

Non-prescription medicines are medicines considered as having a lower level of risk than prescription medicines. They still must be registered on the ARTG, but undergo a lesser degree of evaluation. They contain ingredients included in Schedule 2 (pharmacy-only) or Schedule 3 (pharmacist-supervised supply) of the SUSDP. Non-prescription medicines have frequently been termed "over-the-counter" (OTC) medicines, and include analgesics, cough and cold products, and sunscreens.

Complementary medicines (also known as "traditional" or "alternative" medicines) include vitamin, mineral, herbal, aromatherapy, and homeopathic products. They may be registered or listed on the ARTG, depending on their ingredients and the claims made. Most complementary medicines are listed.

Medical devices also are required to be registered or listed if not exempt. The specified categories of implantable and other higher risk devices that require registration, rather than listing, must undergo a more comprehensive evaluation process.

All medicines and devices supplied solely for export are listed (not registered) on the ARTG.

For a new medicine to obtain public subsidy for patients in the community, the sponsor must successfully apply for the product to be included in the Commonwealth Government's Pharmaceutical Benefits Scheme (PBS). Data are required on relative cost and effectiveness, and the scrutiny of this information according to prescribed criteria is described as the "fourth hurdle" – in addition to quality, safety, and efficacy – that medicines must overcome to be readily available to the Australian public.

The Commonwealth Government has agreed in principle to establish a joint regulator for therapeutic goods in Australia and New Zealand, to begin operating in 2004. Subsidy arrangements through the PBS and other mechanisms have been specifically excluded from these discussions.

6.2. The history of prescription medicine regulation

6.2.1 Quality, safety, and efficacy

The Commonwealth Department of Health was established in 1921, but most health-related activities at that time remained the responsibility of the States. The current name is the Department of Health and Ageing but its description frequently changes, so throughout this chapter the Department will be called the Department of Health and the relevant Commonwealth Government Minister will be called the Minister for Health.

The Commonwealth Therapeutic Substances Act 1937 gave the Minister for Health power to control the import and export of substances declared to be therapeutic substances in the *Commonwealth Gazette*.

The Therapeutic Substances Act 1953 repealed the 1937 Act and gave the Commonwealth control of the import into Australia and interstate trading of therapeutic substances and controlled therapeutic substances (drugs of addiction). It came into operation in 1956 and was administered by the Therapeutic Substances Branch of the Department of Health. In 1959 the National Biological Standards Laboratory (NBSL) was established, to test therapeutic products imported into Australia or supplied under the PBS for compliance with quality and manufacturing standards, largely based on the British Pharmacopoeia.

In the wake of the thalidomide tragedy, the Australian Drug Evaluation Committee (ADEC) was established in 1963 as a statutory committee to advise the government on the regulation of drugs intended for marketing in Australia. The Adverse Drug Reaction (ADR) reporting scheme and the Adverse Drug Reactions Advisory Committee (ADRAC) were also introduced. Furthermore, Commonwealth legislation was reviewed to give the Commonwealth powers to require companies to submit specified data to establish the quality, safety, and efficacy of imported therapeutic goods.

The resultant Therapeutic Goods Act 1966 provided the basis for the regulation of pharmaceuticals in Australia for over 20 years. The "Guidelines for Preparing Applications for General Marketing or Clinical Investigational Use of a Therapeutic Substance" outlined information requirements for applications. Provision was also made for special Australian standards to apply where appropriate.

Some States had separate arrangements which covered the few locally manufactured products sourced from local active ingredients, as the Commonwealth's jurisdiction was limited to imports, exports and goods crossing State borders (although the last power was thought unlikely to sustain a prosecution if taken to court).

A Code of Good Manufacturing Practice (GMP) was introduced in the late 1960s, covering principles and practices to be followed in the manufacture of therapeutic goods in Australia. It still relied, however, upon State legislation and personnel for its enforcement.

The Customs (Prohibited Imports) Regulations were amended in 1970 to enable the Department of Health to further control importation through import permits for drug products.

The drug evaluation guidelines (known from 1976 as the NDF4 Guidelines) gradually became more detailed and were supplemented by appendices on specific issues such as bioavailability studies and bioequivalence. Rules were also introduced to address agency concerns that companies might manipulate the system, for example, by seeking review of data contained in a clinical trial application for a product that was already the subject of a general marketing application, thereby achieving speedier evaluation.

A revised clinical trial application evaluation scheme introduced in 1983 aimed for a response time of 45 working days for Phase I and early Phase II trials, and 80 working days for Phase II and Phase III trials, but in practice it took an average of 10 or 11 months from submission of data to receipt of written approval.

A Clinical Trial Exemption (CTX) scheme was introduced in Australia in 1987, with the intention of encouraging clinical trial activity. However, in addition to the aforementioned TGA restrictions, which required all clinical trials of an active substance under way in Australia to be completed before the review of a general marketing application relating to that substance, the specified data package included requirements unique to Australia, and the 60 working day review period compared with a 35 calendar day review under the UK CTX scheme.

Australia's drug evaluation system was increasingly criticised due to the "drug lag" in availability of new and improved products in Australia, compared with other countries with well-regarded regulatory systems. Several government inquiries recommended streamlining and making better use of overseas experience. The pharmaceutical industry repeatedly expressed concern about the unique requirements that had led to significant delays in both the submission of applications and obtaining marketing approval, for example, requiring individual patient data (required in the USA but not in Europe) to be presented by parameter (uniquely to Australia) instead of by subject (as required in the USA).

By the late 1980s, it had also become clear that reliance on a combination of Commonwealth and State legislation was not the best way to ensure that desired standards were met. There were many complaints about loopholes and lack of uniformity. The way forward came from an unexpected source – a court case which confirmed that the Commonwealth Government has powers over all corporations, and thus these powers could be used in relation to therapeutic goods matters even if they occurred within one State.

The Therapeutic Goods Act 1989 and Regulations came into effect on 15 February 1991, giving the Commonwealth more clearly defined regulatory authority. It changed the focus of control over therapeutic goods from the point of importation to the point of supply of the goods.

The Act applies to:

- all corporations who supply or manufacture medicines for supply (regardless of where) in Australia
- unincorporated parties who supply or manufacture medicines for supply in Australia outside their own state or territory
- all parties (whether incorporated or unincorporated) who supply medicines under the PBS
- all parties (whether incorporated or unincorporated) who import or export medicines.

Supportive State legislation is required only to cover activities of persons within one State, and specified areas (such as some aspects of labelling, packaging, distribution, and fair trade) that are the responsibility of State governments.

Fees and charges were also introduced – through the Therapeutic Goods Act 1989 and Therapeutic Goods (Charges) Act 1989, respectively, and associated Regulations.

Pressure increased for the TGA to "free up" the regulatory system for prescription medicines. In particular, the 1990 report by the Australian National Council on AIDS Working Party on the Availability of HIV/AIDS Treatments recommended that a notification scheme be introduced for clinical trials of unapproved products that had already been approved by respected agencies overseas.

In March 1991 the Commonwealth Government announced the introduction of an alternative clinical trial system. The Clinical Trial Notification (CTN) scheme was introduced in May 1991, following recognition of the negative effects of discouraging trials of investigational drugs – on patients (who were unable to access possible treatments for potentially life-threatening illnesses) and on pharmaceutical industry investment in research and development (R&D) in Australia. The Government also announced a major review of drug evaluation processes in Australia.

Professor Peter Baume's report, *A question of balance: Report on the future of drug evaluation in Australia"*,[1] was released in July 1991, with a commitment from the Commonwealth Government to speedily implement all 164 recommendations in the stated time frames.

Key aspects were:

- the retention of Australian sovereignty in deciding which drugs might be marketed in Australia
- recognition that considerable streamlining of drug evaluation procedures could be achieved
- acceptance that international harmonisation was a concept whose "time had come", and that considerable benefit could flow from improved cooperation with other comparable developed companies
- recognition that no drugs were totally risk free, and that the need for a system of controls relating to the quality, safety, and efficacy of therapeutic goods must be balanced against the more recently highlighted need for timely availability
- recommendations for reorganisation of the TGA and its advisory committees, with a new management plan and increased emphasis on performance
- provision of a timeline for Australia to bring about the reform of its drug evaluation processes within the next two years.

Recommendations were also made to streamline the CTX scheme for clinical trials and continue the CTN scheme, with further assessment in the future.

Professor Baume noted that, in 1990, the TGA process of evaluation of new chemical entities (NCEs) was taking approximately twice as long as its own target time of 16½ months.

Following the Baume Report, changes were made to the Act and Regulations to introduce specific target evaluation times, together with a fee penalty of 25% if a decision on an application is not made within the specified period.

The statutory time frames led to a major reorganisation of TGA processes to focus on meeting them, and complex measuring arrangements were introduced to ensure that only "TGA working days" were included in the calculations. "The clock" is stopped whenever questions are raised with the product sponsor, and only restarted when no queries are outstanding.

New data requirements came into force from 1993 that closely aligned Australian marketing applications with those in the European Community (EC). The "Australian Guidelines for the Registration of Drugs – Volume 1:

Prescription and Other Specified Drug Products" (AGRD1) specified that the document to support a prescription drug registration application should be compiled in accordance with the current version of "The Rules Governing Medicinal Products in the European Community" Volumes II and III with Addenda and supplementary "Notes for Guidance" published by the Committee for Proprietary and Medicinal Products (CPMP), and also described specific administrative requirements for registration applications in Australia.

Information about the overseas status of the product was also now sought as part of an application. The list of countries mentioned in this context in the AGRD1 included members of the Pharmaceutical Evaluation Report (PER) Scheme, other EC countries and the USA. Expert Reports also began to be utilised in the evaluation of applications.

At 30 June 2001 the ARTG included 9830 registered medicines (5078 of which were Schedule 4 and Schedule 8 medicines), 18 018 listed medicines and 5091 export-listed medicines – a total of 32 939 medicines. It should be noted that this number reflects the separate inclusion of each strength, dosage form, and brand as a distinct therapeutic good. There are also 24 955 medical devices on the register, some of which are "grouped", and some of which would be termed diagnostic products in other countries.

It is a requirement under the Act that a sponsor takes responsibility for each therapeutic good that is imported, exported, manufactured or supplied in or from Australia. The sponsor must be a corporation or person within Australia. Sponsors must be able to substantiate all claims made by them about their therapeutic products. At 30 June 2001 there were 2026 sponsors of therapeutic goods on the ARTG.

6.2.2 Fees and charges

The Therapeutic Goods Act 1989 and Therapeutic Goods (Charges) Act 1989, respectively, and associated Regulations stipulate the fees and charges payable to TGA for applications, GMP inspections and annual licences. When fees and charges were first introduced in 1991 they were intended to cover 50% of the costs attributable to the TGA's responsibilities under the Therapeutic Goods Act, including those deemed to be "for the public good". It took some time to reach those levels – in 1992–93 only 28% of the TGA's relevant costs were covered.

By July 1996 the 50% target was reached, and the Commonwealth Government announced that fees and charges would increase over the following three years to raise industry's contribution to the Government's therapeutic goods programme from 50% to 75%. In 1997 the Government announced that the TGA would be required to recover 100% of its operating costs from 1998/99.

In 2001–2002 the overall revenue raised by the TGA from fees and charges is expected to be AUD$45·2 million, of which the prescription medicines sector contributes approximately 60%.

Fees apply to almost all evaluation activities undertaken by the TGA – not only to the review of general marketing applications but also to minor marketing-related matters, clinical trial applications and notifications, and GMP evaluations and inspections in Australia or overseas, but not to ADR assessments.

Unlike the EU and the USA, where there is a single fee for "major" and "minor" applications, in Australia evaluation fees are calculated according to the number of pages of data submitted with an application. Fees are determined for different types of data (chemistry, pharmaceutical and biological data; preclinical (pharmacotoxicological) data; clinical data) and bands of page count, for example 1–25 pages, 26–300 pages etc. The review of clinical data attracts the highest rate.

In 2001–02 the total evaluation fee to register a new chemical or biological entity for a submission containing page counts in the highest bands was AUD$221 730. Sponsors are required to pay 75% of the evaluation fee together with their application. The balance of 25% of the evaluation fee is payable when the TGA completes the evaluation within the legislated time frame. There is no application fee but, if an application is withdrawn before it is accepted for evaluation, a screening fee of 10% of the evaluation fee up to a maximum of AUD$5000 applies.

Annual charges apply to maintaining each product on the ARTG. The annual charge for continuing registration of a prescription medicine is AUD$1010. Annual charges also apply to manufacturing licences.

6.2.3 Availability to the community

The authority for the Commonwealth Government to provide pharmaceutical benefits was introduced in the 1940s. Prior to that, except for the Federal scheme covering war veterans, health care was the province of the States.

The National Health Act 1953 together with the National Health (Pharmaceutical Benefits) Regulations introduced the current framework for the operation of the PBS.

The Pharmaceutical Benefits Advisory Committee (PBAC) was established under Section 101 of the National Health Act to give advice to the Minister for Health about products to be made available as pharmaceutical benefits. The Minister is required to consider the PBAC's advice but is not required to follow its recommendations. The initial criteria for inclusion of new products on the PBS were comparative safety and efficacy.

Initially 139 "lifesaving and disease preventing drugs" were provided under the scheme without charge to pension recipients and their dependants. By 1960 the scheme had expanded to include a wider range of drugs, and supply to the general public with some co-payment. PBS listing continued to be based primarily on medical considerations.

A non-statutory body called the Pharmaceutical Benefits Pricing Bureau (PBPB) was established in 1963 to make recommendations to government on the pricing of PBS-listed medicines.

Escalation of costs led to multiple measures to limit the increase in PBS expenditure, including the introduction of an authority system for new drugs from 1988. Co-payments were eventually also introduced for concessional patients – for disadvantaged patients in 1989 and for pensioners in 1990. Details of the early history of the PBS and the myriad of subsequent changes can be found in *A History of the Pharmaceutical Benefits Scheme, 1947–1992*.[2]

Amendments to the National Health Act in 1987 introduced the additional requirement for the PBAC to consider cost and effectiveness. Sponsors were encouraged to provide cost-effectiveness substantiation from 1991, and from 1 January 1993 it became mandatory to include pharmacoeconomic analyses in listing applications – the "fourth hurdle".

In 1988 the PBPB was replaced by the (also non-statutory) Pharmaceutical Benefits Pricing Authority (PBPA). The PBPA was required to review the prices of items on the PBS and consider items recommended by the PBAC for listing, taking eight factors in account. Factor (f) – the level of activity being undertaken by the company in Australia – was not to be considered in the price determination of each item, but through a separate allocation of funds to the companies which were successful in their proposals under the Pharmaceutical Industry Development Program (the Factor (f) program).

When the Factor (f) program concluded in 1999, it was followed by the Pharmaceutical Industry Investment Program (PIIP). Both schemes were intended to partially compensate participating companies for the price suppression imposed by the government in exercising its monopsony purchasing powers under the PBS. The PIIP funds of AUD$300 million over five years are fully committed, to nine companies who successfully applied for funding in return for increased R&D and/or production value-adding activity in Australia.

The overwhelming importance of gaining PBS-listing in order to achieve widespread availability and use of a prescription medicine in Australia is evident from information published by the Australian Institute of Health and Welfare (AIHW).[3]

In 1998–99 there were 128·4 million community PBS prescriptions – 109·1 million (85·0%) to concessional patients and 19·3 million to general patients. In addition, about 45 million prescriptions did not attract a subsidy – 35 million below the co-payment threshold and 10 million "private" prescriptions, i.e. prescriptions for drugs not listed on the PBS or Repatriation Pharmaceutical Benefits Scheme (RPBS), for which the consumer pays the full cost of the medicine. Thus 74·0% of prescriptions were for items subsidised through the PBS. Analysis of 1997–98 data shows that the Commonwealth Government contributed AUD$2783 million (82·4%) to the benefit-paid pharmaceuticals and individuals paid the remaining AUD$593 million. Total Commonwealth Government expenditure on non-hospital pharmaceuticals was AUD$5335 million – AUD$3377 million on benefit-paid pharmaceuticals and AUD$1958 million on other non-hospital pharmaceuticals. Thus over 60% of government expenditure on non-hospital pharmaceuticals in 1997–98 was for PBS-listed products. Public hospital expenditure on pharmaceuticals was about AUD$611 million.

In calendar year 2001, Commonwealth Government expenditure for PBS prescriptions was AUD$4049·6 million and patient contributions were AUD$770·1 million, i.e. government expenditure contributed 84·0% of the cost of PBS prescriptions. Concessional cardholders represented 79% of that government expenditure. A total of 150·9 million PBS prescriptions were processed.

Although eligibility for PBS is restricted to Australian residents and visitors from those countries with which Australia has a Reciprocal Health Care Agreement – currently, the UK (including Northern Ireland), Ireland, New Zealand, Malta, Italy, Sweden, the Netherlands, and Finland – this was not strictly enforced. From May 2002, proof of eligibility by means of a Medicare card or passport has been an absolute requirement for the subsidy to be applied, and it is anticipated that this will have some effect on government PBS expenditure. However, measures announced by the Commonwealth Government in the 2002 budget to alter the balance between government and patient contributions could have an even more pronounced effect.

The Government has also decided to introduce a series of programmes aimed at "preventing the unnecessary use of PBS-subsidised medicines" and "reinforcing the commitment to evidence-based medicine". These include "a more detailed consideration process" for new PBS listings, ensuring greater compliance by doctors with PBS prescribing requirements, and the enhancement of PBS restrictions, to reduce prescriptions supplied to individuals in breach of PBS conditions. It also intends to strengthen measures to reduce pharmacy fraud, and further encourage the use of generics.

The Schedule of Pharmaceutical Benefits currently includes more than 600 drug substances in almost 1500 different forms and strengths (items) supplied as almost 2500 different drug products (brands). Restrictions apply to approximately 800 of the items, and about 300 require authority prescriptions.

6.2.4 National Medicines Policy

The Australian National Medicines Policy aims to establish an appropriate balance between health, economic, and industry objectives. It has four central elements:

- timely access to the medicines that Australians need, at a cost individuals and the community can afford
- medicines meeting appropriate standards of quality, safety, and efficacy
- quality use of medicines
- maintaining a responsible and viable medicines industry.

Although these goals are not enshrined in legislation, they have become increasingly accepted by successive governments as a sound basis for informed policy decisions.

The Australian Pharmaceutical Advisory Council (APAC) provides the primary forum for the engagement of all stakeholders in discussion, debate, and resolution of issues arising from the application of the National Medicines Policy, facilitating cooperation between stakeholders and addressing specific issues brought to it for deliberation.

Other groups focus on particular aspects, such as greater dissemination of information about the quality use of medicines.

6.3 Marketing applications for prescription medicines

Prescription medicines and certain other high risk medicines such as injections are evaluated for inclusion on the ARTG by the Drug Safety and Evaluation Branch (DSEB) of the TGA. The types of medicines that are evaluated by the DSEB are described in Schedule 10 to the Therapeutic Goods Regulations. Usually medicines containing new active substances are evaluated by the DSEB for inclusion on the Register as registrable goods. However, a sponsor can submit a justification for an alternative route of evaluation of a new active substance by another Branch of the TGA as a non-prescription medicine, for example where there is experience with the active ingredient in non-prescription medicines in other countries. Guidelines for providing such a justification are available on the TGA website at www.health.gov.au/tga.

6.3.1 Applications for registration

The sponsor of a therapeutic good is responsible for submitting an application to the TGA for registration of the goods and, once the goods are registered, for compliance with conditions of registration such as reporting any adverse drug reactions.

As previously mentioned, Australia has closely aligned its data requirements for the registration of prescription medicines with those of the European Union (EU). The intention is that a sponsor may submit a dossier compiled in accordance with EU technical guidance and data requirements to the TGA. The AGRD1 describes certain administrative requirements and provides technical guidance in addition to EU technical guidance, relevant to applications for registration in Australia.

Where registration is being sought for a new drug to treat a life-threatening illness or to treat a condition for which no satisfactory alternative therapy exists, the TGA will accept the application in either US or EU format.

The TGA has advised that it will accept applications in the format of the International Conference on Harmonisation (ICH) Common Technical Document (CTD). Thus, if a sponsor prepares a dossier in the CTD format for submission in the EU, this will be also accepted in Australia. The acceptance of the CTD format in Australia is expected to be incorporated in the revised AGRD1 currently under development.

The TGA will currently accept dossiers in an electronic format, in addition to hard copy, following discussion with the sponsor. The TGA has been monitoring international developments in relation to applications in electronic formats and is expected to adopt any agreed international standard arising from the ICH process.

There is a formal process for consultation with the pharmaceutical industry on the adoption of each EU guideline in Australia. Australia has adopted the majority of guidelines published by the CPMP without amendment. Guidelines that have not been adopted usually concern labelling or the content of the Australian Product Information (PI) document. All of the EU guidelines that have been adopted or not adopted in Australia are listed on the TGA website. Any changes or additional comments on an EU guideline agreed between the industry and TGA are also published on the TGA website.

6.3.2 Categories of application

There are three categories of applications relating to prescription medicines.

Category 1 applications are defined as being those that do not meet the requirements of Category 2 or 3 applications. Essentially, Category 1 applications are those that include clinical, preclinical or bioequivalence data, such as applications to register goods containing a new active ingredient, a new generic product, a new strength, dosage form or route of administration.

Category 2 applications are defined as those that include clinical, preclinical or bioequivalence data for which there are two evaluation reports from "acceptable countries", where the submission is already approved. The evaluation reports must be independent (not based on each other) and the product must be identical in Australia and the "acceptable countries", in respect to formulation, directions for use, and indications. The countries identified as "acceptable" for the purposes of providing evaluation reports are currently Canada, Sweden, the Netherlands, the UK, and the USA. As the availability of evaluation reports would assist the TGA to evaluate an application, Category 2 applications are subject to shorter legislated evaluation times. However, as most sponsors submit applications for registration in Australia at the same time, or shortly after, they are submitted in the "acceptable countries", it is rare for two evaluation reports to be available to qualify for a Category 2 application. Hence almost no Category 2 applications are submitted.

Category 3 applications seek changes to the pharmaceutical data of goods already included on the ARTG, which do not need to be supported by clinical, preclinical or bioequivalence data. Examples of Category 3 applications include changes to the specifications of the active ingredient, change of shelf life or storage conditions, and change of trade name.

It is a condition of registration that, with limited exceptions, no changes may be made to registered goods without prior approval from the TGA. An exception is that some narrowly specified changes to pharmaceutical and manufacturing aspects may be made without prior approval, as outlined in Appendices 7 and 8 of AGRD1. A number of general and specific conditions must be complied with under the "self-assessable" changes provisions. These are primarily the proper validation of any change and the notification of the change to the TGA.

6.3.3 Evaluation time frames

The Therapeutic Goods Regulations specify time frames for completion of the evaluation of Category 1, 2, and 3 applications in "working days", which excludes weekends and public holidays.

Category 1 applications are required to be:

- accepted for evaluation, or rejected, in 40 working days from receipt of the application and the application fee
- evaluated in 255 working days from the date of acceptance.

Category 2 applications are required to be:

- accepted for evaluation, or rejected, in 20 working days from receipt of the application and the application fee
- evaluated in 175 working days from the date of acceptance.

Category 3 applications are required to be approved or rejected or to have an objection raised within 45 working days of receipt of the application, or payment of the evaluation fee, whichever is the later day. There is no application acceptance period. If an objection to the application is raised, the applicant may respond and provide further information or data. A further 30 working days from receipt of this response is then allowed for consideration of the response before the application must be approved or rejected.

Under Section 31 of the Therapeutic Goods Act, the TGA may request a sponsor to provide additional information or seek clarification of information provided in a submission. Fee penalties apply only if the statutory evaluation period is not met. The evaluation times do not include the time frames for initial acceptance or rejection of an application or the time taken by the sponsor to respond to TGA Section 31 requests. They apply to each application as an absolute criterion, i.e. not as an average performance target. The TGA has almost invariably met the legislated time frames.

In addition, in 2000 the TGA undertook to target the following *mean* evaluation times for different subtypes of Category 1 applications:

- new chemical entities – 150 working days
- new generics, except "own generics" – 100 working days
- new indications – 160 working days
- Product Information (PI) changes – 90 working days
- other Category 1 applications – 130 working days.

In 1999 the average elapsed time from submission of an application to registration, for a NCE, was approximately 17 months.

6.3.4 Confidentiality of submissions

Sponsors routinely require that data contained in their applications remain confidential. If another party requests access to such data under the provisions of the Commonwealth Freedom of Information Act 1982 (FOI Act), the Department of Health will consult with the sponsor to establish whether release of the information is possible, and enable the sponsor to request a review by the Administrative Appeals Tribunal (AAT) of any decision made by the TGA to release the information.

The TGA will not comply with demands for undertakings of confidentiality which seek to limit the lawful use or release of information by the TGA. The TGA will not accept confidentiality statements from sponsors that seek to prohibit the evaluator's access to Departmental records of prior applications, and the accumulated knowledge and experience gained from the evaluation of previous applications. Examples of acceptable confidentiality statements are provided in AGRD1.

6.3.5 Data exclusivity

In 1998 an amendment to the Therapeutic Goods Act was enacted introducing data exclusivity provisions. Under a new Section 25A, the TGA must not use "protected information" about other therapeutic goods when evaluating therapeutic goods for registration. Protected information is information lodged with an application to register goods containing a new active ingredient that is not currently and has never been included in the ARTG. Such information is protected for five years from the date of registration of the goods containing the new active ingredient. Thus products containing new actives are given five years' data exclusivity.

155

At the time the data exclusivity amendments were being discussed, the pharmaceutical industry sought to extend the provisions to protect data relating to new indications, new dosage forms or routes of administration, but was unsuccessful.

The data exclusivity arrangements are primarily of interest to sponsors of products that are not otherwise protected by patent. A sponsor of a generic product may avoid the need for TGA to refer to protected information by submitting a full Category 1 application for registration, including preclinical and clinical data, although this would be unusual.

6.3.6 Orphan Drug Program

The Australian Orphan Drug Program was introduced in 1998. Through a cooperative arrangement with the US Food and Drug Administration (FDA), it intended to improve access to treatments for rare diseases in Australia by utilising US orphan drug evaluations as the basis for Australian approvals, where possible. It also waived evaluation fees for new medicines or indications designated as "orphan".

In order to be designated as an orphan drug in Australia, the prevalence of the disease to be treated is required to be equal to or less than 2000 affected individuals or, if the drug is a vaccine or in vivo diagnostic agent, the persons to whom the drug will be administered in Australia are equal to or less than 2000 per year. The prevalence limit in Australia is considerably lower than other countries' orphan drug programmes, both in absolute terms and as a proportion of the population.

Also, whereas the US Orphan Drugs Program offers several incentives to sponsors to bring drugs to treat rare diseases to market, such as a period of market exclusivity, tax credits for clinical research costs, clinical research grants, and waiver of FDA evaluation fees, the Australian Program offers a 100% reduction of the evaluation fee for a designated orphan drug but no research incentives. The TGA Guideline does state that an orphan drug will be granted five years' market exclusivity, which can be shared by a clinically superior product, but this exclusivity is not supported by any legislation.

Since the Australian program commenced, 42 drugs have been designated as orphan drugs. By the end of 2001, sponsors had lodged applications for marketing approval for 33 of these, and 17 of 20 that had reached their conclusion were approved. Seven of these have been successful in obtaining government funding, as highly specialised drugs or under the life-saving drugs program. Three drugs have been considered and rejected by the PBAC on the grounds of unacceptable cost-effectiveness. The others have not yet sought subsidy or are yet to be considered.

In practice, there have been few opportunities for the TGA to utilise a review by the FDA. Of 215 orphan drugs granted marketing approval in the USA, only 63 have not already been approved for marketing in

Australia or do not have an equivalent in Australia. Of these, a recent review stated that not more than a dozen would represent a significant gap in what has been approved for marketing in Australia, and most of these would fall into the category of "like to have" rather than "need to have because there is no alternative". The review recommended a number of changes to the Australian Orphan Drug Program, primarily focusing on increasing the incentives for sponsors to bring orphan drugs to market by offering greater surety of obtaining public subsidy under the PBS. The full review report is available from the TGA website.

6.3.7 Priority evaluations

The DSEB may allocate priority evaluation to applications for registration of important new medicines. The current criteria for priority evaluation are:

- the active ingredient is a new chemical entity; and
- the drug is indicated for the treatment or diagnosis of a serious, life-threatening or severely debilitating disease or condition; and
- there is clinical evidence that the drug may provide an important therapeutic gain.

Priority evaluation status does not give a definite, shorter evaluation period. Rather, the application is simply moved ahead in the queue of applications under evaluation.

6.3.8 Good Manufacturing Practice

It is a requirement of the Therapeutic Goods Act that all steps in the manufacture of a prescription medicine, including the manufacture of bulk active drugs and finished pharmaceutical products, are performed in manufacturing facilities of acceptable standards. An updated list of manufacturing principles established under the Therapeutic Goods Act is available from the TGA website.

Manufacturing sites within Australia must comply with the Australian "Code of GMP for Medicinal Products". In line with harmonising Australian regulatory requirements with international standards, Australia adopted the Pharmaceutical Inspection Cooperation Scheme (PIC/S) "Guide to Good Manufacturing Practices for Medicinal Products" in August 2002, with a twelve month transition period. Annex 1 of the EU GMP Guide relating to the manufacture of sterile medicinal products and Annex 13 relating to the manufacture of investigational medicinal products have also previously been adopted as Australian manufacturing standards. The ICH GMP Guide for Active Pharmaceutical Ingredients has also recently been adopted.

The standard of any steps of manufacture and quality control conducted outside Australia must also be shown to be acceptable for the inclusion of therapeutic goods on the ARTG. The TGA document "Standard of Overseas Manufacturers" specifies what is regarded as acceptable evidence of GMP standards, and is available on the TGA website. The TGA will accept GMP certification only from countries where it is satisfied that the standard of GMP inspection is equivalent to GMP inspections in Australia.

Australia and the EC have entered into a Mutual Recognition Agreement (MRA) on conformity assessment of medicinal products. The TGA will accept a certificate of GMP compliance of a manufacturer issued under this MRA by the official inspection services of the EU countries. This follows on from Australia's work over many years with the Pharmaceutical Inspection Convention, now known as the Pharmaceutical Inspection Cooperation Scheme.

6.3.9 The evaluation process

Details of requirements for the registration of prescription medicines are contained in the AGRD1, which is only available in entirety in hard copy at this time. However, the revised AGRD1, currently under development, will be available from the TGA website in due course. In the meantime, several Appendices are available electronically, including up-to-date details of EU guidelines that have or have not been adopted in Australia.

Submissions to register new prescription medicines in Australia undergo a two stage process of evaluation by the DSEB – application acceptance and evaluation.

Prior to submitting an application for registration there is an opportunity for a sponsor to have a presubmission meeting with TGA delegates to discuss the application. Presubmission meetings are strongly recommended for complex applications, where there is some uncertainty as to whether the data package to be submitted will meet all Australian regulatory requirements, and for orphan drugs and literature-based submissions.

An application is screened for acceptance by the Application Entry Team of the DSEB. Although primarily intended to be an administrative check that the application is in the required format, the three main Parts (chemical, pharmaceutical, and biological data; preclinical data; clinical data) are also briefly reviewed by the relevant evaluation sections to ensure that there are no major omissions of data.

Once an application has been accepted for evaluation the Pharmaceutical Chemistry Evaluation Section, Toxicology Section, and Clinical Evaluation Units evaluate the Parts 2, 3, and 4 data, respectively. For applications relating to products of biological origin, a second copy of the Part 2 data is also evaluated by the TGA Laboratories (TGAL) Branch, which evaluates aspects such as laboratory methodology, method validation, and shelf life.

There are currently five clinical evaluation units, each headed by a senior medical officer and supported by pharmacists. Applications are distributed amongst the five evaluation units based on the therapeutic area of the drug under evaluation. The DSEB contracts a number of external clinical evaluators who are specialist medical practitioners in the medical condition that the proposed new drug is intended to treat. External evaluators may also be contracted to evaluate the Part 3 data. The head of the clinical evaluation unit coordinates the evaluation and makes the final decision on marketing approval as a delegate under the Therapeutic Goods Act.

From receipt of an application until a final decision on an application, a DSEB evaluator may request additional information or clarification from the sponsor under Section 31 of the Act. During the period from issuing a Section 31 letter and receipt of responses to all questions, the clock is stopped and the elapsed time is not counted towards the TGA's statutory evaluation time frames. If several Section 31 requests overlap, the periods are not additive but the clock remains stopped until the final question is answered. A sponsor is given a time frame in which a Section 31 request should be answered. Justification for an extension of time may be discussed with the evaluator. If a sponsor considers that a Section 31 request is unreasonable they can discuss this with the delegate who issued the request. If the sponsor is unable to resolve the matter with the delegate, it may seek review by the Standing Arbitration Committee.

At the conclusion of evaluation of the Parts 2, 3, and 4 data the evaluators prepare an evaluation report for each part. The evaluation reports are sent to the sponsor as they are received to allow comments to the delegate. Once the three evaluation reports are finalised, the delegate evaluates the reports and prepares an overview of the evaluation and a proposed decision for consideration by ADEC, which are also provided to the sponsor. The sponsor is given 10 working days from receipt of the overview and proposed decision to provide a response and submit any additional comment on the application to ADEC. This "pre-ADEC response" is limited to six A4 pages.

6.3.10 Submission of new data

Two classes of new data may be submitted after an application has been accepted – additional data and supplementary data.

Additional data are data identified at a presubmission meeting that TGA agrees to accept during the course of an evaluation at a predetermined date, such as the results from an ongoing clinical study.

Supplementary data are clinical or preclinical data submitted at the initiation of the sponsor, after it has received either or both of the Part 3 and Part 4 evaluation reports. The sponsor must notify its intention to submit supplementary data within five working days of receipt of the last evaluation report. Only one submission of supplementary data is permitted for each of Parts 3 and 4, unless otherwise agreed by the TGA in writing.

Supplementary data will not be accepted after commencement of the pre-ADEC process, which is signified by the issuing of the delegate's overview and recommendation. Acceptance of supplementary data is at the discretion of the TGA and is dependent upon mutual agreement to a "clock stop".

Up to 60 working days is allowed for all additional data and fees to be presented to the TGA following the sponsor's notification of intent; and up to 135 days may be taken for evaluation of the supplementary data after all data and fees have been received by the TGA.

6.3.11 Australian Drug Evaluation Committee (ADEC)

ADEC makes medical and scientific evaluations of drugs referred to it by the Minister or the Secretary, and gives advice to the Minister or Secretary in relation to the import, export, manufacture and distribution of therapeutic goods. It is important to note that ADEC has an advisory function and is not the final decision maker. The TGA delegate is guided by ADEC's advice but may make a decision contrary to ADEC's recommendations.

ADEC comprises six or seven "core" members – eminent practising physicians, pharmaceutical scientists, and pharmacologists – who attend each meeting. There are up to 20 "associate" members whose expertise is drawn on as appropriate to the applications under consideration at a particular meeting. ADEC members adhere to strict guidelines on competing interests, which effectively exclude a member from proceedings if they have any pecuniary interest in a pharmaceutical company whose product is under consideration or in any competitor company. Participation in company-sponsored clinical trials must also be declared, but may not necessarily exclude the member from proceedings. The ADEC "Competing Interest Guidelines" are available from the TGA website.

ADEC is supported by specialist sub-committees, which currently include the Pharmaceutical Subcommittee (PSC) and ADRAC.

ADEC meets six times a year for two-day meetings in February, April, June, August, October, and December. For each application it receives the sponsor's covering letter, all evaluation reports, the delegate's overview and proposed decision, and the sponsor's pre-ADEC response. ADEC makes recommendations on applications referred to it for advice. This recommendation, termed an ADEC resolution, is sent to the sponsor five working days after the ADEC meeting. Ratified minutes of the meeting in which the resolution is made are available only after the next ADEC meeting, whereafter all positive recommendations relating to applications for registration are published in the *Commonwealth Gazette* and are posted on the TGA website. Occasionally significant recommendations relating to a class of drugs or the content of the PI document are also published.

Not all prescription medicine applications are referred to ADEC. Category 3 applications and some Category 1 applications may be dealt with entirely by the DSEB.

6.3.12   Post-ADEC and the delegate's decision

Following consideration by ADEC, if the delegate proposes to approve the application he or she will communicate with the sponsor to address any outstanding issues, and the final PI will be negotiated. Once all outstanding matters are resolved, a marketing approval letter is issued by the delegate, which states the Conditions of Registration, together with the approved PI. A Certificate of Registration is also issued detailing the information included on the ARTG. The annual registration charge is payable following registration.

If the delegate proposes to reject the application, a letter is sent to the sponsor advising of this intent, giving the reasons for the decision. A sponsor may appeal the initial decision of the delegate.

6.3.13   Appeals against marketing application decisions and Section 31 requests

Under Section 60 of the Therapeutic Goods Act, appeal mechanisms are available to sponsor companies to challenge decisions made by officers of the TGA. Previously, an ADEC recommendation that a marketing application for a new product should not be approved could only be appealed to ADEC.

The decision of the Secretary or delegate is called an initial decision. If the sponsor wishes to appeal an initial decision it must do so within 90 calendar days of receiving advice of that decision. The appeal of the initial decision is directed to the Minister, who generally appoints the TGA Principal Medical Adviser to act as a delegate in considering that appeal, and the decision on the appeal must be issued within 60 days. The outcome of this stage is called a reviewable decision. Reviewable decisions are so called because they may be appealed through the AAT. Eligible appeals to the AAT are defined in the Act and must be made within 28 calendar days of receiving advice on the Minister's decision. This process has been used only a few times since 1991 and can be relatively complex and time-consuming, and potentially expensive. Restrictions have been added over the years that strictly delineate the information that may be considered and the grounds for a successful appeal by this route.

The Baume Report led to the introduction of a non-statutory, additional appeals mechanism at the early stages of the marketing application evaluation process. A three-person Standing Arbitration Committee (SAC) was established to consider sponsor challenges to TGA requests under Section 31 of the Act for additional information which they considered to be unreasonable. Although this was used occasionally to good effect in subsequent years, these issues are now usually handled without the need for formal arbitration by the SAC.

6.3.14 Product Information (PI)

The PI is the summary of the outcomes of the evaluation for registration, in the same way as the Summary of Product Characteristics (SPC) forms the basis for prescribing in the EU. It is intended to provide appropriate information to health professionals for the safe and effective use of the product, and is negotiated between the delegate and sponsor following the ADEC meeting, taking into account ADEC's recommendations. Once approved by the delegate, the sponsor may not change any aspect of the PI without prior approval from the TGA, except in specific circumstances such as safety-related changes. Unlike the SPC, the PI is not subject to five-yearly review, although this has been proposed.

Safety-related changes to the PI that may be made by the sponsor without prior approval are those that reduce the patient population or add a warning, precaution, contraindication or adverse event. They must be notified to the TGA within five days of implementation and the date of each safety-related change must be listed in the PI in addition to the TGA approval date.

Non-safety related changes to the PI may only be made by the sponsor without approval if they are minor editorial matters such as changes to headings or relocation of text or a change consequent to self-assessable change made in accordance with AGRD1. These changes must also be notified to TGA within five working days.

For PI changes that require approval, DSEB accepts three main types of submission:

- conventional submissions, containing full study reports of clinical trials
- literature-based submissions
- hybrid submissions, comprising a mix of conventional and literature-based data.

The type of submission considered by DSEB to be appropriate for a PI update depends on the regulatory and clinical history of the drug in Australia and overseas, with special reference to the UK, USA, Sweden, Canada, and the Netherlands. Submissions based on company sponsored clinical trials are usually required for drugs marketed for less than 5 years, whereas any of the three types of submission can be used for drugs marketed for more than 10 years. Drugs marketed for between 5 and 10 years will be considered on a case-by-case basis, but it is generally expected that either a conventional or hybrid submission will be submitted.

Published preclinical (Part 3) and clinical (Part 4) data may be used for either a literature-based submission or as the literature-based component of a hybrid submission. However, published reports rarely include sufficient validation information for pharmaceutical chemistry (Part 2) data to be accepted in the form of published literature. Conventional Part 2 data may accompany literature-based Part 3 and/or Part 4 data.

Full guidelines on the preparation of literature-based submissions are available from the TGA website.

6.3.15 Paediatric indications

It is recognised internationally that there is a lack of information from proper investigations of the use of medicines in children, and a lack of availability of paediatric-specific formulations, leading to medicines being used outside their approved indications and, at times, being reformulated by pharmacists to make them more suitable for use by children.

The TGA has endeavoured to encourage the submission of paediatric data packages by offering fee reductions for products that are not commercially viable or whose supply is in the public interest, waiving fees for orphan drugs and indications, and by accepting literature-based submissions. The TGA has also adopted internationally recognised ICH/EU guidelines dealing with paediatric data generation and facilitating the extrapolation of data from one patient population to another.

Sponsors are encouraged to consider whether their products are likely to be used in children and, if so, to discuss with the TGA how to make paediatric formulations available and to update PIs with information on paediatric use.

6.3.16 Consumer Medicine Information (CMI)

Since 1993, all new prescription products (including changes to existing products that lead to a "new" entry on the ARTG) must also have a Consumer Medicine Information (CMI) document, referred to in the Therapeutic Goods Regulations as a Patient Information Document. The content of the CMI must be consistent with the PI and contain the information described in Schedule 12 to the Regulations. CMI is also required for pharmacist-only (Schedule 3) medicines approved for registration since mid-1995, in accordance with Schedule 13 to the Regulations.

Enormous effort has been invested in CMI development in Australia, with the aim of producing highly useful and usable information for consumers. Guidelines called "Writing about medicines for people" (the Usability Guidelines) are in their second edition, providing guidance to sponsors on how to prepare CMIs with highly consistent usability. Unlike the EU, Australian sponsors are not required to provide the CMI as a pack insert but may distribute the documents in a form that enables the CMI to be given to a person to whom a product is administered or dispensed. A system has been developed for electronic distribution of CMIs, so that they may be printed by doctors or pharmacists from their computer software, but this is not yet fully operational.

6.3.17 Post-marketing responsibilities

The standard conditions of registration require the sponsor to inform the TGA of any adverse drug reactions and safety alerts related to their product of which they become aware. The requirements for reporting adverse drug reactions occurring in Australia or overseas are described in Appendix 20 to AGRD1, which is available on the TGA website.

For spontaneous reports of reactions occurring in Australia, serious reactions (whether expected or unexpected) should be reported immediately and in no case later than 15 calendar days from receipt of the report. Other reactions occurring in Australia should be reported on request or as line listings in a Periodic Safety Update Report (PSUR).

Reports of reactions occurring in other countries are not required to be routinely submitted to the TGA. However, any significant safety issue or action that has arisen from an analysis of foreign reports, or has been taken by a foreign regulatory agency, must be reported to the TGA within 72 hours.

Australia has harmonised its requirements for post-marketing reports with those of the CPMP/ICH "Guideline on Periodic Safety Update Reports (CPMP/ICH/228/95)". The timing and frequency of provision of PSURs has also been harmonised with the CPMP/ICH requirements. Thus an Australian sponsor may submit PSURs prepared to meet international regulatory requirements to the TGA. Post-marketing reports must be provided annually until the period covered by such reports is not less than three years from the date of the Australian marketing approval letter. No fewer than three annual reports are required. If a PSUR is not available, the Australian sponsor must prepare a post-marketing report.

Another condition of registration is that a product recall (or similar regulatory action) in any other country, that has relevance to the quality, safety, and efficacy of the goods to be distributed in Australia, must be notified to the TGA immediately. Other conditions of registration include conditions related to the sampling and testing of products and manufacturing premises.

6.3.18 Products of gene technology

The Commonwealth Gene Technology Act 2000 came into force in 2001, introducing a national scheme for the regulation of genetically modified (GM) organisms in Australia. The legislation regulates some GM products, but only where the products are not regulated by an existing agency. Thus, therapeutic goods that contain GM organisms or are products of GM organisms continue to be regulated by the TGA.

The Gene Technology Act requires the Gene Technology Regulator to be notified by other regulators such as the TGA about GM products approved for sale in Australia. For example, if the TGA approves a genetically modified medicine for sale in Australia, this must be entered in the centralised, publicly available database of all GM organisms and GM products.

6.3.19 Recalls

Recalls are handled by the Australian Recall Coordinator within the TGA according to the voluntary Uniform Recall Procedures for Therapeutic Goods, in conjunction with the States. The Australian Recall Coordinator also liaises with the Commonwealth Minister responsible for Consumer Affairs in relation to safety-related recalls of therapeutic goods, which must be notified within 48 hours, in accordance with the Trade Practices Act 1974. A mandatory recall of faulty goods may be enforced where safety is involved.

6.3.20 Counterfeit goods and tampering

Amendments were made to the Therapeutic Goods Act in mid-2000 to make it a specific offence to supply counterfeit therapeutic goods in Australia.

Also new offences were introduced under the Act for tampering with therapeutic goods or continuing to supply goods that may have been tampered with, and for failing to notify the TGA of any knowledge of actual tampering or threats associated with tampering.

6.3.21 Trans-Tasman Mutual Recognition Arrangement

The Trans-Tasman Mutual Recognition Act 1997, developed under the policy of Closer Economic Relations between Australia and New Zealand, came into force in 1998. The Act is intended to enhance trans-Tasman trade by allowing goods available in one country to be acceptable in the other (and also recognise professional qualifications in both countries). A special exemption for therapeutic goods was immediately granted in recognition of the differences between the Australian and New Zealand regulatory systems. The special exemption must be renewed annually, until the two countries' therapeutic goods agencies' resolve the need for special exemption.

The Health Ministers in Australia and New Zealand agreed that harmonisation of regulatory requirements for therapeutic goods is the best option under the Trans-Tasman Mutual Recognition Arrangement, and the TGA and the New Zealand Ministry of Health have developed options for resolving the special exemption in consultation with the industry, consumers, medical, and pharmacy professions. The proposal to form a single joint therapeutics regulatory agency, which would be responsible for implementing regulatory controls over the import, manufacture, and supply of therapeutic goods in both countries, has evolved during these consultations, and the Australian Government has accepted this proposal in principle.

Policy development for the single joint agency is under way and, if the proposals proceed successfully through further public consultations, legislation establishing the new agency will be presented to both Parliaments during 2003, with the agency commencing operation in 2004.

165

6.4 Listing on the PBS – the "fourth hurdle"

Applications for listing a product on the PBS are generally submitted by the pharmaceutical company sponsor, which has the data required to support the application, to the Pharmaceutical Benefits Section of the Department of Health. However, submissions from medical bodies, health professionals or members of the public may also be considered.

A product may not be listed on the PBS until marketing approval is granted. However a sponsor may apply for PBS listing once the TGA delegate has recommended to ADEC that the product be granted marketing approval. Thus, consideration of a listing application can to some extent overlap with the final stages of evaluation of an application for marketing approval.

Products may not be subsidised under the PBS for unapproved indications. Some approved indications may not be subsidised.

6.4.1 The PBAC process

The PBAC assesses applications for listing on the PBS for reimbursement against criteria specified in the National Health Act 1953. These criteria include safety and efficacy compared to other available treatments including non-drug therapies, and comparative cost-effectiveness.

The current "Guidelines for the Pharmaceutical Industry on Preparation of Submissions to the PBAC including Major Submissions involving Economic Analyses" were published in 1995, and are available through www.health.gov.au/pbs (PBS website), together with the "Application to List" form (commonly referred to as PB11).

Section 1 of the Guidelines establishes the context of the submission. It asks for a description of the drug, its use on the PBS and the therapies that will be co-administered or substituted. Section 2 asks for the best available evidence on the clinical performance of the drug, including the scientific and statistical rigour of randomised trials, and a preliminary economic evaluation based on evidence from the randomised trials. Section 3 describes when extrapolation beyond the preliminary economic evaluation may be made and how adjustments can be made in a modelled economic evaluation. Section 4 requests a financial analysis from the perspective of the PBS and government health budgets.

The Guidelines must be followed for major submissions to the PBAC to:

- list a new drug on the Schedule of Pharmaceutical Benefits
- request a significant change to the listing of a currently restricted drug (including a new indication or a derestriction)
- enable a review of the comparative cost-effectiveness of a currently listed drug in order to change a PBAC recommendation to the PBPA or its therapeutic relativity or price premium

- list a new formulation or strength of a currently listed drug for which a price premium is requested.

The Guidelines are interpreted in a very prescriptive manner, and have been the subject of ongoing discussion. Improved outcomes that are difficult to quantify, such as "indirect" benefits, are accorded a low weighting. Also large head-to-head comparative studies with adequate power to yield significant differences may be required before superior outcomes are regarded as proven. An interim document to accompany the Guidelines came into effect in June 2000 and introduced changes relating to the selection of randomised trial evidence from the literature and other searches, and the presentation of modelled economic evaluations. It is available from the PBS website.

On receipt of a major application for listing, the PBAC Secretariat forwards the application to the Pharmaceutical Evaluation Section (PES). The PES evaluates these applications together with three external groups from academic institutions contracted for this work. The PES provides an evaluation report to the Economic Sub-Committee (ESC) of the PBAC. The ESC reviews and interprets the economic analyses and advises the PBAC on these analyses.

The sponsor receives a PES evaluation report approximately two and a half weeks prior to the PBAC meeting at which the application will be considered. The sponsor's response to the overview and commentary must be sent to the PBAC Secretariat within one week and is provided to the PBAC along with the ESC advice and the PES's overview and commentary.

As with ADEC, conflict of interest guidelines are strictly applied to PBAC and its sub-committees. The membership of the PBAC was revised in early 2001, allowing for a greater range of expertise to be included, and restrictions on the length of term that members may serve were introduced. Amid some controversy, a member with pharmaceutical industry experience was included, in addition to medical practitioners and members with pharmacy and consumerist backgrounds.

The PBAC meets four times a year, in March, June, September, and December. In making its recommendations, the PBAC receives advice from the ESC and may also receive input from the Drug Utilisation Sub-Committee. Positive recommendations for listing are published on the PBS website.

If an application for listing is successful, the PBAC recommends the maximum quantity to be dispensed on each prescription and the number of repeat prescriptions. The PBAC may also recommend prescribing restrictions – an Authority Required item requires prior approval from the Health Insurance Commission (HIC), obtained by telephone or post, and Restricted Benefit items may only be prescribed for specified therapeutic uses.

6.4.2 Appeals against decisions on PBS listing applications

The National Health Act does not include the option for PBAC recommendations to be appealed to the AAT. Generally the only avenue is for the applicant to appeal to the PBAC.

PBAC rejections, and the lack of available appeal mechanisms, have been increasingly challenged in recent years. One route available is to pursue a legal challenge to the Federal Court of Australia for a review of the decision. In March 2000 the Federal Court rejected a pharmaceutical company's application to overturn the recommendation of the PBAC not to list a product on the scheme.

Following a recent review of the listing process, the opportunity for meetings between the PBAC and stakeholders has been established. These meetings are not intended as an appeals mechanism but as a "without prejudice", non-adversarial process to facilitate a resubmission by the sponsor. A stakeholder meeting may be sought where the drug is indicated for a serious or disabling or life-threatening condition for which there is no other realistic management option. The "Guidelines for Stakeholder Meetings" are available from the PBS website.

6.4.3 Pricing of products on the PBS

The PBPA makes recommendations to the Department of Health on the prices for new items that have been recommended for PBS listing by the PBAC. It also reviews the prices for all items listed on the Schedule of Pharmaceutical Benefits at least once per annum. The PBAC provides advice to the PBPA regarding comparison with other treatments and comparative cost-effectiveness.

The Commonwealth Government negotiates an agreed wholesale price with the pharmaceutical company sponsor, through a senior officer in the Pharmaceutical Benefits Branch. This process applies to all products subsidised as PBS-listed items under Section 85 of the National Health Act, including products that are priced below the general patient co-payment.

A wholesaler margin is then set on the supplier's price, a pharmacist margin is applied to the wholesaler's price, and a pharmacist dispensing fee is also added, determined by the Pharmaceutical Benefits Remuneration Tribunal. Patients pay the co-payment (and any premiums) to the pharmacist when the PBS-listed medicine is dispensed, with the balance of the cost of the product being paid to the pharmacist by the Government.

Consumers' contributions to the cost of their medicines are limited by safety net thresholds, which are adjusted annually in relation to the Consumer Price Index (CPI). Under the PBS the maximum cost for a listed item at 1 January 2002 was AUD$3·60 for concessional patients and AUD$22·40 for general patients, except where a brand premium, therapeutic group premium or special patient contribution applies. There are two safety net thresholds – one for general patients and one for concessional patients (pensioners, seniors, repatriation health beneficiaries). For general patients, once a patient has spent AUD\$686·40 on PBS medicines the patient co-payment decreases to the concessional level of AUD\$3·60 for the rest of the calendar year. For concessional patients the safety net threshold is AUD\$187·20. Once concessional patients reach this level they receive PBS items free of charge for the rest of the calendar year.

The Commonwealth Government has announced that it intends to increase patient co-payments for the PBS to AUD\$4·60 per item for concessional patients and AUD\$28·60 per item for general patients. In addition, from 1 January 2003, the level at which the co-payment safety nets will apply is to be increased to AUD\$239·20 (concessional) and AUD\$874·90 (general patients).

Determination of the agreed price for a product to be listed on the PBS is understandably one of the most contentious areas between the pharmaceutical industry and government. The pricing procedure and methods used by the PBPA in recommending prices for new items and in its annual review of prices of all items listed on the PBS, including Reference Pricing and Weighted Average Monthly Treatment Cost (WAMTC), are explained in a document that is available from the PBS website.

The PBPA sometimes recommends the use of price/volume arrangements, particularly where unit prices are reasonably high and there is the potential for significant volumes or where there is uncertainty about future volumes.

If the predicted annual cost to the government is greater than AUD\$5 million in one year, including consideration of the potential for prescribing outside of the agreed restrictions, the Department of Health must obtain the Department of Finance's agreement to the estimated costs. If the predicted annual cost to government is greater than AUD\$10 million, the listing must be approved by the Prime Minister and the Minister for Finance, in addition to the Minister for Health.

The PBAC and PBPA also consider the prices of pharmaceuticals listed under Section 100 of the National Health Act, which allows for an alternative means of providing an adequate pharmaceutical service in circumstances where pharmaceutical benefits cannot be conveniently and efficiently supplied in the usual manner under the PBS. Drugs in this category, such as medicines for HIV/AIDS, are reviewed by the Highly Specialised Drugs Working Party and are generally supplied through different dispensing arrangements in public hospitals under agreements with the States, and exclude wholesaler involvement.

6.4.4 Brand premiums

Where there are two or more brands of the same form and strength of a drug listed on the PBS that are bioequivalent and hence interchangeable, the PBPA recommends the benchmark price for that drug, being the price of the lowest priced brand. Sponsors of the other brands may charge a premium above the benchmark price. Brands that are considered interchangeable are indicated in the Schedule by alphabetic superscripts. The cost of the brand premium must be paid by the consumer in addition to any co-payment. A pharmacist may substitute brands to avoid a consumer paying a premium, provided the prescriber does not specifically prohibit this and the consumer agrees.

6.4.5 Special patient contribution arrangements

A sponsor may not seek to charge a product premium above the agreed listing price unless there is an alternative brand of the drug in the same form and strength listed on the PBS. If the sponsor and government cannot agree on a listing price for a new product, and there is no alternative listed on the PBS, the product cannot be listed with a brand premium. However, on rare occasions a special patient contribution can apply. Currently (2002) this applies to only one item on the PBS and has applied in only three instances in the past five years.

6.4.6 Reference pricing and Therapeutic Group Premiums

In 1997, the Commonwealth Government announced the introduction of Therapeutic Group Premiums (TGPs), a form of reference pricing, to certain therapeutic drug classes listed on the PBS, to take effect from 1998. Under this policy the Government agreed to subsidise all drug products in a therapeutic subgroup up to the price of the lowest priced product in the group, the benchmark. Different chemical entities in a therapeutic group were deemed to be equivalent for the purpose of pricing, including patented and out of patent products. If a sponsor chooses to charge a premium above the benchmark price, that premium must be paid by the consumer in addition to the co-payment. This premium does not count towards the PBS safety net threshold.

A prescriber may apply to the HIC for a TGP exemption for an individual patient for a particular product if adverse effects or reactions are expected to occur with all of the benchmark priced products, or the transfer to a benchmark priced product would cause patient confusion leading to problems with compliance. Pharmacists may not substitute between different chemical entities in a therapeutic group.

Six therapeutic groups were initially proposed – H_2 receptor antagonists, ACE inhibitors, HMG CoA reductase inhibitors (statins), calcium channel blockers, β-blockers, and SSRI antidepressants. SSRIs and β-blockers, were subsequently excluded from this measure as the chemical entities within these groups could not be considered therapeutically equivalent. When the policy was introduced it was thought that some sponsors would maintain significant premiums for their products over the benchmark price.

Table 6.1   Time frame for application for PBS listing

Action	Weeks prior to PBAC meeting
Cut off date for major submissions	11
Cut off date for minor submissions	6–7
ESC agenda sent to members	4
PES evaluation sent to sponsor	2·5–3
ESC meeting	2·5
PBAC agenda sent to members	2·5
Pre-PBAC comments provided by sponsor	1·5
ESC report and sponsor comments sent to PBAC	1
PBAC meeting	0

Action	Weeks post-PBAC meeting
Written advice of recommendation sent to sponsor	3
Unratified minutes sent to sponsor	4–5
PBPA meeting	4–6
Approval by Minister for Health/ Parliamentary Secretary	10–12
Closing date to amend Schedule of Pharmaceutical Benefits	12
Listing in the Schedule of Pharmaceutical Benefits	20

However, over time, many have reduced their price to the benchmark price or charged a reduced premium compared with the price prior to introduction of the TGP policy. The premiums currently range from AUD$7·01 to AUD$1·40 in three of the four groups, with no premium charged on any of the HMG CoA reductase inhibitors.

6.4.7   Time frames

It takes a minimum of 32 weeks from submission of an application for PBS listing to the time it may be prescribed as a PBS item if the application is successful the first time it is considered, although some of this process may overlap the final stages of registration approval. The time is set out in Table 6.1.

Before listing, the National Health Act also requires that a product must have been cleared with respect to chemistry and quality control matters. This is currently undertaken by the TGA Laboratories Branch. Products are frequently not launched in Australia until the outcome of the PBS listing application is known.

6.5 Access to medicines not registered or listed on the ARTG

Guidelines detailing the four avenues available for access to medicines not registered or listed on the ARTG are available through the following websites:

Clinical Trials: www.health.gov.au/tga/docs/html/clintrials.htm
Special Access Scheme: www.health.gov.au/tga/docs/html/sasinfo.htm
Authorised Prescriber: www.health.gov.au/tga/docs/html/authpres.htm
Personal Importation: www.health.gov.au/tga/docs/html/personalimp.htm

6.5.1 Clinical trials

There are two schemes under which clinical trials involving therapeutic goods may be conducted in Australia – the Clinical Trial Notification Scheme and the Clinical Trial Exemption Scheme. These schemes are used for clinical trials involving any product not entered on the ARTG, or use of a registered or listed product in a clinical trial beyond the conditions of its marketing approval.

Clinical trials in which registered or listed medicines (or medical devices) are used within the conditions of their marketing approval are not subject to CTN or CTX requirements but still need to be approved by a Human Research Ethics Committee (HREC) before the trial may commence.

All CTN and CTX trials must have an Australian sponsor. The sponsor is that person, body, organisation or institution which takes overall responsibility for the conduct of the trial. It need not be a pharmaceutical company. The sponsor usually initiates, organises, and supports a clinical study and carries the medicolegal responsibility associated with the conduct of the trial.

In 2000–01 there were 1989 CTN scheme notifications. It should be noted, however, that this does not indicate the number of different clinical trial protocols, which is approximately 400 per annum. This contrasts with four CTX applications in that period – three 50 working day and one 30 working day application.

6.5.1.1 The Clinical Trial Notification scheme

Under the CTN scheme the sponsor of the clinical trial provides detailed information about the proposed trial to the principal investigator who submits an application to conduct the clinical trial to the HREC at the institution or other site at which the trial is proposed to be conducted. The clinical trial application generally includes the protocol, the investigator's brochure, related patient information, supporting data, and the CTN form. HRECs usually have their own standard format for applications to conduct a CTN trial at their institution. The HREC evaluates the scientific and ethical validity of the proposed clinical trial and the safety and efficacy of the medicine in the context of its stage of development. The TGA does not evaluate any information about the clinical trial.

If the HREC approves the conduct of the clinical trial, the chairman of the HREC signs the CTN form. The institution or organisation at which the trial will be conducted, referred to as the Approving Authority, gives the final approval for the conduct of the trial at the site, having due regard to advice from the HREC, and also must sign the CTN form. In some cases the HREC can also be the approving authority for a particular trial site.

In signing the CTN form the signatories agree that they will comply with all legislative and regulatory requirements, that the trial will be conducted in accordance with Guidelines for Good Clinical Practice (GCP), and the National Health and Medical Research Council (NHMRC) National Statement on the Ethical Conduct of Research Involving Humans 1999 (National Statement), and that they will agree to release information to the TGA about the conduct of the trial in the event of an inquiry or audit of the trial.

The form is then submitted by the sponsor of the trial to the TGA, along with the appropriate notification fee. The 2001–02 notification fee is AUD$210 for each notification, which can comprise a single site conducting the same clinical trial, or multiple sites notified together. Once the CTN form has been submitted to the TGA along with the relevant fee, the clinical trial may commence. The TGA acknowledges receipt of the CTN form and fee, which takes two or three days. Some sponsors choose to wait for receipt of this acknowledgement before commencing a trial, although this is not strictly necessary.

There is one CTN form for each site conducting the same clinical trial, such as multicentre trials. In some cases a composite site can be notified where a single HREC and approving authority have responsibility for all sites conducting the trial, such as a general practice network.

To assist the TGA to maintain a record of each CTN trial, the sponsor must subsequently notify the TGA of the date the trial was completed, the reason the trial ceased (for example, concluded normally; insufficient recruits), and any changes to the trial in respect of information previously submitted.

6.5.1.2 The CTX scheme

Under the CTX scheme, a sponsor submits an application to conduct clinical trials to both the TGA and the HREC at each institution or site at which it is proposed to conduct the clinical trial. The TGA reviews the information about the product provided by the sponsor, including whether the medicine is under investigation or approved for marketing in other countries, proposed usage guidelines, a pharmaceutical data sheet, and a summary of the preclinical data and clinical data.

There are two levels of evaluation of applications for clinical trials of medicines under the CTX scheme. A 30 working day period for evaluation of a CTX application applies when the supporting data relate only to chemical, pharmaceutical, and biological issues. A 50 working day period applies for applications supported by chemical, pharmaceutical and biological, preclinical, and clinical data. These evaluation times commence from the date of acceptance of the application or receipt of the appropriate fee. The fee for a 30 day CTX application in 2001–02 is AUD\$1170 and for a 50 day application, AUD\$14 390.

If the TGA delegate raises an objection, trials may not proceed until the objection has been addressed to the delegate's satisfaction. Even if no objection is raised, the delegate usually provides comments on the accuracy or interpretation of the summary information supplied by the sponsor. The sponsor must forward these comments to the HREC(s) at sites at which the sponsor intends to conduct the trial.

As with the CTN scheme, the sponsor prepares information for submission by the principal investigator to the HREC at the institution or other site at which the trial is proposed to be conducted. The HREC in each host institution/organisation is responsible for approving the proposed trial protocol after reviewing the summary information received from the sponsor and any additional comments from the TGA delegate. The approving authority gives the final approval for the conduct of the trial at the site, having due regard to advice from the HREC.

A sponsor may not commence a CTX trial until written advice has been received from the TGA regarding the application, and approval has been obtained from the HREC and the institution at which the trial will be conducted.

There are two forms relating to the CTX scheme that must be submitted to the TGA by the sponsor. Part 1 is the formal CTX application and must be completed by the sponsor of the trial and submitted to the TGA with data for evaluation. Part 2 is used to notify the commencement of each new trial conducted under the CTX as well as new sites in ongoing CTX trials. It requires the signature of the chairman of the HREC, the responsible person from the approving authority, the principal investigator and the sponsor, and must be submitted within 28 days of the commencement of supply of goods under the CTX. There is no fee for notification of additional trials.

Applications can be lodged simultaneously with the TGA and the institution(s) at which studies are proposed to be conducted. However, if the application is lodged simultaneously with the TGA and HREC(s), the sponsor is required to convey any TGA comments or revisions on the application and/or objections to the HREC(s).

The sponsor may conduct any number of clinical trials under the CTX application without further assessment by the TGA, provided use of the product in the trials falls within the original approved usage guidelines.

174

However, HREC approval of each protocol and approval from the institution or organisation for the conduct of each trial are still required.

6.5.1.3 TGA investigation of clinical trials

In 2000 the Therapeutic Goods Regulations were amended to expand and strengthen the TGA's powers to require provision of information about the conduct of any clinical trial being conducted under the legislation, and to audit a clinical trial. These amendments were introduced following a review of the clinical trial legislation and regulation which indicated that the TGA's powers were inadequate to enable it to investigate complaints about clinical trials conducted under the Therapeutic Goods Act and Regulations.

New provisions allow an authorised person to enter a site at which a clinical trial is being conducted and examine anything at the site relating to the clinical trial, including any documents or records relating to the trial. The revised regulations also require the principal investigator to give assurances that the trial will be conducted in accordance with the guidelines on GCP, and will comply with an audit of the trial by an authorised person.

6.5.1.4 Reporting adverse events and adverse drug reactions during clinical trials

Australia has largely harmonised its reporting requirements for adverse events and adverse drug reactions occurring during clinical trials with international requirements and has adopted, in principle, the "Note for Guidance on Clinical Safety Data Management: Definitions and Standards for Expedited Reporting CPMP/ICH/377/95)" – in particular the definitions and reporting time frames.

Whilst the TGA has adopted these international requirements, the local interpretation of these guidelines in relation to reporting serious and unexpected adverse reactions must be adhered to. Sponsors of clinical trials are required to report to TGA single cases of serious and unexpected adverse reactions. Fatal or life-threatening ADRs should be reported within seven calendar days of the reaction first being notified to the sponsor. This should be followed by as complete a report as possible within eight additional calendar days. All other serious and unexpected ADRs should be reported to the TGA within 15 calendar days of first knowledge of the sponsor.

Information should be provided in the form of a detailed summary in the ADRAC "Blue Card" format. Even if initial information is scanty, these details should be forwarded to the TGA pending receipt and provision of further data. This procedure should be followed even when the medicine in question is the subject of an application for registration and is under evaluation by the TGA.

Sponsors are not required, as a matter of routine, to submit individual patient reports to the TGA of suspected adverse drug reactions occurring with use of the same product in another country, even if a trial is ongoing at Australian sites. However, the TGA requires that sponsors advise the Experimental Drugs Section of DSEB within 72 hours of any significant safety issue which has arisen from an analysis of overseas reports or action with respect to safety taken by another country's regulatory agency. This advice must include the basis for such action.

6.5.1.5 Good clinical practice and ethical conduct of clinical trials

The TGA's regulation of clinical trials involving new medicines requires adherence to international standards of ethical conduct and GCP.

In 2000 the TGA Guidelines on Good Clinical Research Practice 1991 were replaced by the CPMP/ICH "Note for Guidance on Good Clinical Practice (CPMP/ICH/135/95)", with some amendments to reflect Australian regulatory requirements.

Furthermore, Australia has a strong framework in place to support the ethical conduct of clinical trials, provided by the NHMRC, its principal committees, and HRECs. In 2000–01 there were 210 active HRECs in Australia – 99 hospital, 45 university, 35 government, and 31 associated with professional and other bodies.

The strategic intent of the NHMRC is to provide leadership and work with other relevant organisations to improve the health of all Australians by:

- fostering and supporting a high quality and internationally recognised research base
- providing evidence-based advice
- applying research evidence to health issues thus translating research into better health practice and outcomes
- promoting informed debate on health and medical research, health ethics and related issues.

A principal committee of the NHMRC, the Australian Health Ethics Committee (AHEC), provides guidance and support for HRECs in Australia, and is responsible for developing and publishing the National Statement on the Ethical Conduct of Research Involving Humans 1999, which replaced the previous NHMRC Statement on Human Experimentation and Supplementary Notes 1992.

Compliance with the National Statement is a requirement for all clinical trials conducted in Australia under the CTX and CTN Schemes. The chairman of the HREC certifies that the HREC is constituted in accordance with guidelines issued by the NHMRC, has registered with the AHEC, and has approved the clinical trial in accordance with the guidance provided by the National Statement.

The increased awareness of ethical issues relating to human research has led to the release in 2002 of the Human Research Ethics Handbook, including detailed commentary on the National Statement and discussion of ethical and legal issues, to further assist HRECs to assess and facilitate the ethical conduct of research involving human participants, and resolve the challenges encountered during this process.

Both the National Statement and the associated Handbook are available at www.health.gov.au/nhmrc (NHMRC website).

AHEC is currently working with HRECs around Australia to develop a nationally accepted clinical trial application format that will be acceptable to all HRECs. This will significantly benefit sponsors of clinical trials who currently have to prepare applications in different formats to meet individual HREC requirements, which delays submission of applications in Australia and adds to the workload.

6.5.1.6 Status of the Declaration of Helsinki

The clinical trial guidelines published by the TGA specify that all clinical trials must be conducted in accordance with the Declaration of Helsinki, October 1996. The World Medical Association (WMA) updated the Declaration of Helsinki in October 2000 but these changes were not adopted in Australia due to concerns in relation to the interpretation of two new clauses.

Clause 29 has been interpreted to mean that it prohibits use of a placebo where there is a current therapy available. Clause 30 has been considered unrealistic as few sponsors would be willing to guarantee ongoing access to an experimental therapy at the conclusion of a clinical trial.

The AHEC has advised HRECs to continue to regard the National Statement as the definitive guideline for the review and conduct of research in Australia. In October 2001 the WMA issued a note of clarification on the interpretation of its guideline on the ethical use of placebo-controlled trials. The note of clarification has reduced any differences between the National Statement and the Declaration of Helsinki, but AHEC has advised HRECs that wherever there is doubt regarding the interpretation and application of various ethical guidelines, the National Statement should always take precedence.

6.5.1.7 Clinical trial compensation guidelines and indemnity

In order to promote a uniform approach to offering compensation to subjects and indemnity to investigators and institutions conducting clinical trials, Medicines Australia (formerly the Australian Pharmaceutical Manufacturers Association) has published a "Form of Indemnity for Clinical Trials" and "Guidelines for Compensation for Injury Resulting from Participation in a Company-Sponsored Clinical Trial". These documents are based on those published by the Association of the British Pharmaceutical Industry and are available from www.medicinesaustralia. com.au (Medicines Australia website).

6.5.2 Special Access Scheme (SAS)

The Special Access Scheme (SAS) allows for the import and supply of an unapproved therapeutic good to an individual patient on a case by case basis. The scheme envisages two categories of patients – Category A patients, who are defined in the regulations as "persons who are seriously ill with a condition from which death is reasonably likely to occur within a matter of months, or from which premature death is reasonably likely to occur in the absence of early treatment", and Category B, all other patients. A medical practitioner can supply an unapproved product to a Category A patient without the approval of the TGA, but must inform the TGA within 4 weeks following supply. Thus, no prior approval is required from the TGA. For Category B patients, individual approval for each patient must be obtained from a TGA delegate or a delegate outside the TGA, referred to as an external delegate.

Classification of a patient as Category A or B lies with the medical practitioner. However, the TGA may review, seek clarification and request information regarding the classification of patients under Category A.

A medical practitioner can supply any unapproved medicine to a Category A patient, except medicines listed in Schedule 9 of the SUSDP, which are primarily drugs of abuse such as heroin or cannabis.

Adverse event and ADR reporting requirements are similar to those for clinical trials, with greater emphasis on the prescriber being responsible for reporting any ADR to the TGA, the sponsor, and HREC.

6.5.3 Authorised prescribers

Another avenue for limited access to an unapproved medicine is through the Authorised Prescriber provisions of the Act. The TGA grants certain medical practitioners authority to prescribe a specific unapproved therapeutic good or class of unapproved therapeutic goods to specified recipients or classes of recipients (identified by their medical condition) in their immediate care without further approval from the TGA. The authorised prescriber must also have the endorsement of an appropriate HREC to supply the product.

A pharmaceutical company is not obliged to supply an unapproved product under the authorised prescriber provisions. If it does supply the specified product, the company must provide six monthly reports of the amount of product supplied to authorised prescribers.

Adverse event and ADR reporting requirements are similar to those for clinical trials, with greater emphasis on the authorised prescriber being responsible for reporting any ADR to the TGA, the sponsor and HREC as the sponsor will not normally be actively monitoring the use of the product.

6.5.4 Personal importation

Individuals may personally import an unapproved therapeutic good by either bringing the goods with them as they enter Australia or arranging for someone outside Australia to send the goods to them. Personal importation may only be used for that person or their immediate family, i.e. the goods may not be given or sold to another person. Furthermore, the quantity that may be imported is restricted to 3 months' supply at one time and a total of 15 months' supply in a 12 month period at the manufacturer's recommended maximum dosage.

If a prescription medicine is to be imported in this way, the importer must have a prescription from a medical practitioner, unless the goods are being carried with the person.

Certain medicines may not be imported under the personal importation provisions, including drugs of abuse such as narcotics, amphetamines, psychotropic substances, anabolic substances, androgenic steroids, and treatments for alcohol and drug addiction. There are also controls over certain other medicines including erythropoietin, growth hormones, and gonadotrophins.

An individual cannot import injections that contain substances of human or animal origin (except insulin) without a SAS approval. The TGA considers that these injections represent a high risk from inadequately or improperly prepared materials (including a lack of sterility) and, therefore, approvals will only be granted to the supervising physician.

6.6   Presentation

Under the Therapeutic Goods Act, presentation means the way in which the goods are presented for supply, and includes matters relating to the name of the goods, the labelling and packaging of the goods, and any advertising or other informational material associated with the goods. The term label refers to the display of printed information on or supplied with the goods and their packaging, rather than the broader meaning applied in the USA, which includes approved uses of the product. Labels fall within the definition of advertising.

6.6.1   Standard for the Uniform Scheduling of Drugs and Poisons (SUSDP)

The SUSDP lists drugs and poisons according to the recommended restrictions on their availability to the public. The categories of the SUSDP most relevant to medicines on the ARTG are:

- Schedule 8 – controlled drugs (for example, strong analgesics such as morphine)
- Schedule 4 – prescription only medicines
- Schedule 3 – non-prescription medicines for supply by pharmacists only
- Schedule 2 – non-prescription medicines the safe use of which may require advice from a pharmacist.

Schedules 5 and 6 of the SUSDP also include some medicines, such as head lice preparations and some essential oils.

The National Drugs and Poisons Schedule Committee (NDPSC), established under the Therapeutic Goods Act, is responsible for the SUSDP, which includes requirements for signal headings, warning statements, and safety directions to be included on the labels of medicines containing scheduled substances, and exemptions from scheduling gained by placement of specified warnings on labels.

Access to the substances listed in the SUSDP is usually restricted for a number of reasons, including toxicity, safety, and the risks and benefits associated with the use of the product.

NDPSC decisions in relation to the SUSDP have no force in Commonwealth law. However, State legislation refers to or reflects the SUSDP (occasionally with some differences in some States) and may impose warning statements and other labelling and packaging requirements additional to those covered by Commonwealth legislation and associated Therapeutic Goods Orders (TGOs).

Medicines that are not scheduled in the SUSDP can be sold through any distribution outlet, such as a supermarket or health food store. Examples of medicines that are unscheduled include small packs of simple pain relievers, and most vitamins and minerals.

6.6.2 Labels and packaging

The labels of medicines are required to conform to TGO69: General Requirements for Labels for Medicines, except for goods solely for export or for use in clinical trials. The requirements include names and quantities of active ingredients, dosage form, batch number, expiry date, the registration or listing number (AUSTR or AUSTL number, respectively), identification of inactive ingredients, what labelling is adequate for special packs and small containers, and letter size and additional requirements in particular circumstances. TGO69 recently replaced TGO48, and there is a phase-in period of several years for existing products. In addition, labels for medicines must conform to requirements for labelling described in the SUSDP. TGO69 is available on the TGA website.

Certain medicines considered to have a high risk of poisoning children must be packaged in child-resistant packaging. The specified medicines and acceptable types of packaging are described in TGO33: Child Resistant Containers.

Evaluation areas within the TGA responsible for the different categories of registered medicines make recommendations on the labelling of individual products as part of the registration process. Listed medicines are entered into the ARTG with a declaration from the sponsor that they meet the relevant standards and advertising requirements, and have acceptable presentations. Labels are not examined at the time of listing, but may be assessed following listing either as a result of a random review or if a problem arises.

6.6.3 Country of origin

Country of origin is generally not indicated on the labels of therapeutic goods marketed in Australia.

As prescription medicines are prescribed by a medical practitioner rather than purchased "off the shelf" by the consumer, there is generally little incentive to convey country of origin information. Where manufacturers choose to do so, they must comply with State Fair Trading Acts, and the Commonwealth Trade Practices Act 1974.

Prior to December 1994, an "essential character" test, was used to determine the validity of country of origin claims, in the context of Sections 52 and 53 (eb) of the Trade Practices Act 1974 in relation to false or misleading statements. However, in 1994 the Federal Court handed down a decision that effectively rejected the essential character test and created uncertainty about outcomes of future cases in this area.

In 1998, the Trade Practices Amendment (Country of Origin Representations) Act 1998 came into force. Manufacturers making unqualified statements about country of origin, such as "Made in ..." must be able to demonstrate substantial transformation and exceed a 50% local production costs threshold. They therefore tend to use qualified claims, such as "Made in Australia from local and imported ingredients", to ensure that labels are not misleading or deceptive.

6.6.4 Advertising

The Therapeutic Goods Act and Regulations, Trade Practices Act, and State legislation all contain sections relating to the promotion of therapeutic goods. In particular, the Therapeutic Goods Act specifies that advertising of a therapeutic good can only refer to the approved indications for that good.

Prescription medicines may only be advertised to healthcare professionals – they may not be advertised to consumers. Advertisements of prescription medicines directed at healthcare professionals are regulated under a self-regulatory Code of Conduct administered by Medicines Australia. First published in 1960, it includes standards for appropriate advertising, the behaviour of medical representatives, and relationships with healthcare professionals, and is available from the Medicines Australia website.

The Therapeutic Goods Advertising Code forms the basis for determining the acceptability of advertisements directed to consumers. All advertisements for therapeutic goods directed to consumers, published or broadcast in mainstream (designated) media, must be approved before publication or broadcast. The Minister for Health has delegated this responsibility to the Australian Self-Medication Industry and the Complementary Healthcare Council.

6.7 Patents

The Patents Act 1990 conveys a 20 year standard term of patent protection. From July 1999, holders of patents for a pharmaceutical substance have been permitted to apply for an extension beyond the standard term, so long as the application is made within six months of the first marketing approval of a pharmaceutical product containing the substance. The extension granted may be for no more than 5 years and will permit a maximum of 15 years' protection after marketing approval. Sponsors of generic products containing that substance are permitted to undertake certain preparatory activities, known as "springboarding", from the date the extension is granted.

6.8 Non-prescription medicines and complementary medicines

Non-prescription or over the counter (OTC) medicines are considered to be "low risk" in comparison with prescription medicines. They are evaluated for quality, safety and efficacy by the TGA and the Medicines Evaluation Committee (MEC), in accordance with the "Australian Guidelines for the Registration of Drugs – Volume 2: Non-Prescription Drugs Registered via the Compliance Branch" (AGRD2) before they may be registered on the ARTG. Revision of the AGRD2 is currently under way, and the final document will be published on the TGA website in due course under the new title "Australian Guidelines for the Registration of Medicines" (AGRM).

Complementary medicines are most frequently listed rather than registered, but this depends on the ingredients and claims made. The document "Guidelines for Levels and Kinds of Evidence to Support Indications and Claims" was developed to assist sponsors in determining the appropriate evidence to support indications and claims made in relation to complementary medicines, sunscreens and other listable medicines, and is available from the TGA website. The Complementary Medicines Evaluation Committee (CMEC) provides scientific and policy advice relating to controls on the supply and use of complementary medicines, with particular reference to the quality and safety of products and, where appropriate, efficacy relating to the claims made.

A product's principal use and the claims made are also key determinants of whether it is deemed to be a medicine or a food, or a medicine or a cosmetic. Guidance on these distinctions are available from the TGA website.

6.9 Medical devices

The Therapeutic Device Program was established in 1984. In 1987 the Customs (Prohibited Imports) Regulations were amended to require the

Department of Health's approval before devices in five "designated" categories could be imported, and the Therapeutic Device Evaluation Committee (TDEC) was established.

The Commonwealth Government gradually introduced regulatory requirements for devices akin to those for medicines, especially where higher risks were associated to their use. These include formal guidelines for marketing and clinical trial applications, GMP requirements and an adverse event reporting scheme. However, TDEC is not as involved as ADEC in considering individual marketing applications.

When the Therapeutic Goods Act came into effect, most therapeutic devices were classified as listable goods. Registrable devices include implantable devices, biomaterials, intraocular lenses and fluids, intrauterine and other contraceptive devices, and drug infusion systems.

A Mutual Recognition Agreement (MRA) on standards and conformity assessment between Australia and the EC came into effect from 1999, covering eight industry sectors including GMP inspection and batch certification of medicinal products, and conformity assessment of medical devices.

The ECMRA applies to medical devices manufactured in the EC, Australia, and New Zealand. It recognises the competence of designated conformity assessment bodies (CABs) in the EC to undertake conformity assessment of medical devices to Australian regulatory requirements, and the competence of the TGA to undertake assessment of medical devices for compliance with the requirements for certification (CE Marking) for entry onto the EC market.

Devices incorporating animal-derived tissues, radioactive materials, in vitro diagnostics and devices manufactured in other countries such as the USA (even those devices that have CE marking) are excluded.

For registrable devices, the MRA included an 18 month transition period, to allow each party to gain confidence in the other's procedures and processes for pre-market assessment.

The Therapeutic Goods Amendment (Medical Devices) Bill 2002 and the Therapeutic Goods (Charges) Amendment Bill 2002 passed by Parliament in March 2002 provide for the introduction of an internationally harmonised framework for the regulation of medical devices in Australia. The new regulatory system for medical devices commenced on 4 October 2002. The Therapeutic Goods (Medical Devices) Regulations and associated guidelines further clarify the new arrangements. The Therapeutic Goods Amendment (Medical Devices) Act 2002 has made provision for a range of transition periods for certain therapeutic goods.

The TGA has also initiated development of a new regulatory framework for in vitro diagnostic devices (IVDs) that is to be harmonised with international best practice. The IVD framework will complement the new regulatory system for medical devices and it is expected that implementation will be phased in from late 2003.

Current details of the regulation of medical devices in Australia may be obtained through the TGA website.

References

1   Baume PE. *A question of balance: Report on the future of drug evaluation in Australia.* Canberra, AGPS, 1991.
2   Sloan C. *A history of the pharmaceutical benefits scheme, 1947–1992.* Canberra, AGPS, 1995.
3   Australian Institute of Health and Welfare. *Australia's health 2000: The seventh biennial health report of the Australian Institute of Health and Welfare.* Canberra, AIHW, 2000.

7: **Regulatory and clinical trial systems in Japan***

YUICHI KUBO, JOHN O'GRADY

7.1 Introduction

Japan, with its population exceeding 100 000 000, is the second largest country in the world in terms of pharmaceutical market. The importance of this market has long been recognised, but many pharmaceutical companies have excluded this particular area from their global development strategy. One reason for such omission is the unique marketing/distributing rules that handicap newcomers. Another reason was the unique clinical trial system, represented by the now abolished general guideline that required the primary endpoint of a clinical study to be categorised to FGIR (final global improvement rate), and by old Japanese good clinical practice (GCP) which did not require study site monitoring or auditing. The other obstacle was the notion of the Japanese themselves that they are unique and different in every respect from the rest of the world, and that therefore clinical data obtained in foreign countries are not applicable to the Japanese population.

Marketing/distributing rules in Japan have become almost identical to those in the western world, and GCP is updated in line with ICH GCP. ICH discussion on ethnic factors established a concept that foreign clinical data are acceptable for new drug applications if there are no concerns about ethnic differences in the effects or adverse effects of the product.

Because of these changes, many multinational pharmaceutical companies include Japan in their global development and marketing strategies. It is important to understand, however, that there are still many peculiarities for conducting clinical trials in Japan. Many of these are due to differences in medical practice and/or the attitude of Japanese people towards the effects and side effects of medicinal products, and may not harmonise with the west in a short period of time. Therefore, it is important to conduct a

---

*The views expressed in this chapter are those of the authors and not necessarily those of Daiichi Pharmaceutical Co. Ltd.

careful feasibility study before commencing clinical trials in Japan if global development is planned.

7.2 Regulatory systems

7.2.1 Introduction

The procedures described below are essentially those that apply to the approval of ethical pharmaceutical products containing new chemical entities. Approval procedures for drugs containing agents already listed in the Japanese Pharmacopoeia, or which are modifications of already approved drugs, or are *in vitro* diagnostic agents, are all subject to slightly different procedures. For a full description of these variations the reader is referred to *Drug Licensing and Approval Procedures in Japan*.[1]

In 1996 (effective from 1 April 1997), the Japanese government passed a bill that significantly amended the Pharmaceutical Affairs Law. These changes reflected recommendations made by the Ministry of Health and Welfare (MHW) Study Committee on Measures to Ensure Drug Safety, set up in 1993 following an unforeseen fatal drug interaction in which at least 15 people died. Major changes have been made to the regulatory review and clinical trial system. A revised GCP based on ICH has become a legal requirement, effective from 1 April 1997. A clinical trial review procedure has been instigated with a 30-day review period before trial initiation. Although clinical trial applications were previously sent to the MHW, the hospital and in-house Institutional Review Boards also undertook active review. Another significant change is that advice on clinical trials can be sought from the Organisation for Pharmaceutical Safety and Research (the Drug Organisation, also known as Kiko, an extra-government organisation).

Responsibility for regulatory review has passed to a Pharmaceutical and Medical Devices Evaluation Centre (Evaluation Centre) within the National Institute of Health Sciences (NIHS). The Drug Organisation now intensively checks applications for GCP compliance and reliability compliance. In an effort to minimise the review period, substantial review process re-engineering took place in the year 2000 to introduce intensive review within the Evaluation Centre and to abolish review by the Sub-Committees on New Drug Evaluation in the Pharmaceutical Affairs and Food Sanitation Council (PAFSC). From January 2001 the MHW merged with Ministry of Labour and became the Ministry of Health, Labour and Welfare (MHLW), but the basic structures of drug regulation have been preserved.

7.2.2 Type of approval

Under the Japanese system the MHLW grants approvals for new drugs. Approvals fall into three categories, namely manufacturing, import and foreign manufacturing. Manufacturing approvals cover those products that will be manufactured in Japan, whereas import approvals refer to products manufactured outside Japan that will be imported into the country. Foreign manufacturing approvals were introduced in 1983 with a change to the Pharmaceutical Affairs Law and permit foreign manufacturers to apply directly to the MHLW for approval of their product via use of an "in-country caretaker".

Criteria for the selection of the "in-country caretaker" are specified in Article 26–5 of the Enforcement Regulations of the Pharmaceutical Affairs Law. In essence, he or she must be resident in Japan and must be a pharmacist (or physician, microbiologist, etc. in the case of biological products), or must employ someone with this qualification. The designated person must take responsibility for the development, registration and post-marketing surveillance of the product on behalf of the foreign manufacturer in respect of ensuring compliance with the Pharmaceutical Affairs Law.

Once a drug is registered, any changes to items in a drug approval will require the filing of a partial change application.

7.2.3   Review process

The procedure by which applications for all new drugs are reviewed is described below, and for all new drugs is shown schematically in Figures 7.1 and 7.2.

Applications for approval to manufacture or import drugs must be made either via the Government of the Prefecture where the applicant is domiciled, where the head office is located in Japan, or where the factory that will manufacture the product is located. In foreign manufacturing approval applications are made via the Government of the Prefecture where the in-country caretaker is located.

The application then passes to the Evaluation Centre, where it divides into different routes, that is, GLP, GCP and reliability compliance check by the Drug Organisation, and application review by the Evaluation Centre.

First, the Drug Organisation will conduct a compliance review to ensure that the dossier meets the standards of GCP, GLP and reliability. The GCP compliance check is based on the inspection of both study sites and sponsor. For the submission of a new active substance four study sites are inspected. If the pivotal studies are conducted overseas, the inspection may be conducted by MHLW instead of the Drug Organisation.

As well as GCP site inspections an examination is undertaken of the raw or source data and records of Chemistry and Manufacturing Controls (CMC), non-clinical and clinical reports that are the basis of the application. This is to ensure that the application dossier accurately reflects the source data. The procedure issued by the Drug Organisation details that two lists of raw data and records must be provided: one is the "list of documents to be submitted" and the other is the "list of documents not to be submitted".

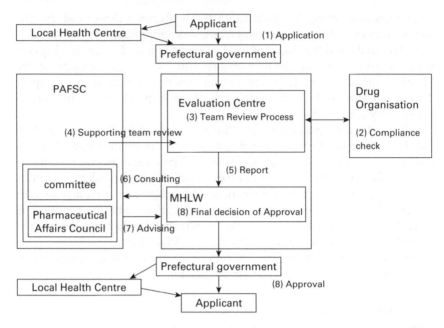

Figure 7.1 Japanese regulatory review process. Flow of new drug application submission, review and approval. PAFSC, Pharmaceutical Affairs and Food Sanitation Council; MHLW, Ministry of Health, Labour and Welfare.

The applicant is required to bring the data and records to the Drug Organisation on the specified days, and when the examination finishes they should be retrieved. Therefore, the raw data and records stored at overseas sites are usually categorised as "documents not to be submitted" and not subject to reliability review by the Drug Organisation. Instead, the MHLW may investigate the data from non-Japanese studies at the site of storage as submission of a photocopy of data is not permitted. The Drug Organisation sends a report of compliance to the Evaluation Centre.

Review of the submission dossier will begin simultaneously with the above-mentioned compliance check. Review is undertaken by one of the four Evaluation Centre teams, which comprise experts from medicine, pharmaceutical sciences, veterinary sciences and statistics. The team also includes experts from PAFSC. Evaluation meetings are held at which questions are raised by the reviewing team and the applicant has the opportunity to discuss issues with the reviewers. The Evaluation Centre will prepare a report of the application for the next stage of the regulatory review, undertaken by the First or Second Committee on New Drugs of PAFSC. If the drugs fall into the categories of applied recombinant DNA technology or gene therapy, there will be a review by an expert subcommittee before it goes to the Committee on Biotechnology.

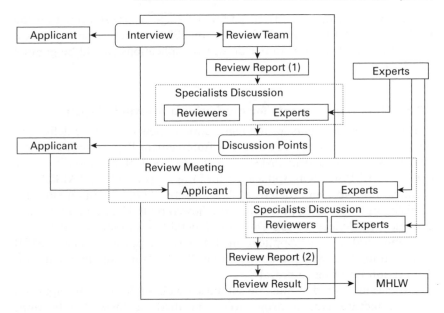

Figure 7.2 Review process at the Evaluation Centre. The new drug application dossier is reviewed at the Pharmaceutical and Medical Devices Evaluation Centre. The Centre organises a review team with scientific support from external experts. The applicant has two opportunities to meet the team during the review process.

The period required from receipt to approval of the application is treated as that for handling of the standard clerical service, except for that for replying to PAFSC inquiries and that for correcting incomplete applications. The period for handling the standard clerical service is 12 months, applicable to applications received on and after April 2000.

7.2.4 Priority review

An October 1993 amendment of the Pharmaceutical Affairs Law (Article 14–4) made provision for priority review for orphan drugs, orphan medical devices and "innovative drugs or medical devices that have been authorised to be highly necessary from a medical standpoint". The new ordinance sets out standards to define both orphan drugs and the criteria by which "innovative drugs" will be decided for priority review.

The priority review system, although having only a limited impact on the procedure for the majority of drugs, is being applied to a number of important drugs. The criteria for gaining priority status as an innovative drug requires that either the chemical structure or the pharmacological action of the agent is new and that the agent is for treating a severe disease, as designated in the categories for orphan drugs.

189

For orphan drugs there is an additional stage of pre-screening by the Evaluation and Licensing Division of the Pharmaceutical and Medical Safety Bureau of MHLW to decide which applications should be granted priority review.

7.2.5 Data requirements for marketing approval in Japan

The data requirements for the registration of new drugs were defined in the Pharmaceutical Affairs Law and its Enforcement Regulations. Practical guidelines were issued in PMSB Director-General Notification No. 481 dated 8 April 1999, "On Application for Drug Approval" and PMSB/ELD Notification No. 666 dated 8 April 1999, "On Requirements for Application for Drug Approval", then followed by ICH common technical document guidelines, PMSB Director-General Notification No. 481 dated 21 June 2001, "On Application for Drug Approval" and PMSB Notification No. 899 dated 21 June 2001, "On Requirements for Application for Drug Approval".

The various data that must be submitted with applications for approval to manufacture ethical drugs were specified in these Notifications (Tables 7.1 and 7.2).

The application in either conventional format or common technical document (CTD) format has been accepted since July 2001 but only CTD format will be accepted from July 2003. The regional specific requirements are in Modules 1 and 5 of CTD, which are described below.

7.2.5.1 Module 1

NDA application form (format based on Pharmaceutical Affairs Law Enforcement Regulations)

Certificates (including statement by a responsible person supervising the collection and preparation of application data, documents related to GLP and GCP, copy of a written contract of co-development)

Patent status information

Origin, background of the discovery and research and development history (formerly in the first part of GAIYO. This can be described in Module 2 instead of in Module 1)

Status of use in foreign countries

List of other pharmaceuticals with similar pharmacological effect(s) and/or indications(s)

Draft package insert (labelling)

Documentation of non-proprietary name

Format for designation of poisonous/deleterious pharmaceutical ingredients

Draft protocol for post-marketing surveillance (if necessary)

List of information/documents complied in the dossier

Table 7.1 Information required for new drug application in Japan

Type of drug	A* 1	2	3	B* 1	2	3	C* 1	2	3	D* 1	2	3	4	5	6	7	E* 1	2	3	F* 1	2	3	4	5	6	G* 1
Drug with new active ingredients	×	×	×	×	×	×	×	×	×	×	×	×	/	×	/	/	×	×	/	×	×	×	×	−	/	×
New combination prescription drugs	×	×	×	−	−	×	×	×	×	×	×	−	−	−	/	−	×	/	/	×	×	×	×	−	/	×
Drug with new route of administration	×	×	×	−	−	×	×	×	×	×	×	−	/	×	/	/	×	/	/	×	×	×	×	−	/	×
Drugs with new ingredients	×	×	×	−	−	−	−	−	−	−	−	−	−	−	−	−	×	−	−	/	/	/	/	−	/	×
Drugs with new dosage forms	×	×	×	−	−	×	×	×	×	−	−	−	−	−	−	−	−	−	−	×	×	×	×	−	/	×
Drugs with new doses	×	×	×	−	−	−	−	−	−	−	−	−	−	−	−	−	×	−	−	×	×	×	×	−	/	×

Type of drug is defined in the article 18–3, Paragraph 1, Item 1 of MHLW Ordinance
*Refer to Table 7.2
×: required
/: required case-by-case basis, depending on individual new drug application
−: not required in principle

Table 7.2   Key for Table 7.1

A. Data on the origin and background of the discovery and conditions of use in foreign countries, etc.	Data on: 1. origin and background of discovery 2. conditions of use in foreign countries 3. properties and comparative studies with other drugs
B. Data on physical and chemical properties, specifications, testing methods, etc.	Data on: 1. determination of structure 2. physical and chemical properties, etc. 3. specifications and testing methods
C. Data on stability	Data on: 1. long-term shelf life tests 2. stress tests 3. accelerated tests
D. Data on acute, subacute and chronic toxicity, teratogenicity and other types of toxicity	Data on: 1. single-dose toxicity 2. repeated-dose toxicity 3. genotoxicity 4. carcinogenicity 5. development and reproductive toxicity 6. local irritation 7. other types of toxicity
E. Data on pharmacological effects	Data on: 1. tests supporting the efficacy 2. general pharmacology
F. Data on absorption, distribution, metabolism and excretion	Data on: 1. absorption 2. distribution 3. metabolism 4. excretion 5. biological equivalence
G. Data on results of clinical studies	Clinical study results

In addition to the Section 5.3.7 of Module 5, "Case Report Forms and Individual Patients Listing", the following tabulations and charts are required.

The list of subjects in the pivotal studies of dose setting/efficacy clinical studies

The list of subjects with adverse reactions in all the submitted clinical studies

The list of subjects with serious adverse reactions in all the submitted clinical studies

The list of subjects with observed clinical data abnormal in all the submitted clinical studies

The charts that illustrate the progression of observed abnormal clinical test data.

If any consultation with the Drug Organisation took place, the official records should be incorporated into Module 5.4.

Module 2 will be termed GAIYO ("summary" in Japanese) as before and should be prepared in Japanese, except for the figures and tables if they are accompanied by translation of keywords. The original English reports will be accepted in Modules 3, 4 and 5 and a Japanese summary will no longer be required.

After the approval of the product, the sponsor is requested to disclose GAIYO to the public except for the parts containing trade secrets and private information. The electronic version of GAIYO for disclosure is obtainable from http://www.pharmasys.gr.jp. (NB: the home page is written in Japanese only.) The previous requirement to publish the result of pivotal clinical studies before submitting a new drug application is now abolished.

7.2.6 Clinical trial consultation

The Drug Organisation consults with sponsors on the protocol and the issues relating to drug development. There are four types of consultation for drug development stages, namely, "clinical trial consultation before initial protocol notification", "clinical trial consultation on completion of Phase II studies", "consultation prior to approval application", and individual consultation. Any of these consultations should be based on the scientific knowledge of the product obtained by the time of consultation, and the clear queries of sponsors either on the design of the study protocol, concepts of development or rationale for submission. The consultations provide the merits of both FDA meetings and EMEA scientific advice. The consultation is chargeable and the fee is in the range of about £7,000–16,000, depending on the type of consultation. The Drug Organisation prepares the official records of the consultation, which is attached to the new drug application and will be considered by the reviewers.

7.3 Clinical trial systems

7.3.1 Introduction

Based on Step 4 of the ICH Good Clinical Practice (GCP) guideline of May 1996, the Japanese Ministry of Health and Welfare (MHW) prepared an amendment to the previous GCP guideline and on 27 March 1997 this was issued as "MHW Ordinance of the Standards for Good Clinical Practice". This new GCP became effective as of 1 April 1997 with some moratoria (preparation of standard operating procedures (SOP) at medical institutes, source data verification, etc.), and full implementation was from 1 April 1998. Unlike the previous GCP guidelines, the new GCP is based on the revised Pharmaceutical Affairs Law of June 1996, which requires

---

Box 7.1 Responsibilities of the chief investigator

- Judge whether the clinical trial request is appropriate
- Develop the protocol
- Confirm whether the clinical trial is appropriately carried out according to the protocol
- Modify the protocol, if necessary
- Supervise the clinical trial and, if necessary, direct the physicians in charge
- Convey the information and data obtained from the sponsor to the physicians in charge and other clinical research staff participating in the clinical trial
- Discuss the protocol with the sponsor
- Confirm the completion of the clinical trial
- Keep records of the above tasks
- Prepare the final report and submit it to the sponsor
- Check the case report forms prepared by the physicians in charge and submit them to the sponsor

---

that the data for new drug applications are obtained at the standard set by the Ministry, and therefore it is legally obligatory to respect the new GCP in conducting clinical trials in Japan.

The new GCP follows the ICH GCP guideline but there are some unique aspects added in order to cope with Japanese medical and clinical practice. Although such modifications have been made, the concept of the ICH guidelines is maintained, and this led to significant changes in clinical trial practice in Japan. The main points of the changes in clinical trial practice between the old and new GCP, as well as unique aspects of Japanese GCP and clinical trial practice, are explained below.

7.3.2 Chief investigator

The old GCP was characterised by a dominant role of the chief investigator. This system has now been abolished, but it is of some benefit to explain the role of the chief investigator so as to understand the previous study reports and the influence of the old system on the new one.

It was the usual practice that medical decision-making and responsibility were given to an eminent specialist, who became the chief investigator. The chief investigator then appointed the other investigators, formed them into committees and arranged the protocol. Thus the company in Japan was rather more distant from the medical practice of the trial than is usual outside Japan, and hence the more frequent references in the old GCP guidelines to external people and functions concerned with this aspect of trial organisation and operation. The old GCP guidelines outlined the duties of the chief investigator; and, as Box 7.1 indicates, this individual had significant responsibility. It should be noted that some of the monitor's duties in Europe and the United States were previously defined as duties of the chief investigator in Japan.

Because the chief investigator had to play a leading role in the clinical trial, the person appointed by the sponsor was usually a physician or professor who was an authority on the subject of the clinical trial. In practice, however, such people were generally too busy to perform the duties mentioned here, and the sponsor wrote a draft protocol and a draft of the explanatory note used when obtaining informed consent from subjects. In addition, the sponsor's monitor conveyed data and information to the physician in charge, as well as collecting and checking the case report forms (CRFs).

7.3.3 Sponsor

The new GCP requires the sponsor to be fully responsible for all aspects of the clinical trial. This responsibility includes preparation of the study protocol, selection of investigators and study centres, monitoring and auditing, and writing the clinical reports. Under the old GCP system most of the responsibility for conduct of the clinical trial fell upon the chief investigator and, in a sense, the sponsoring company was immune from such responsibility. This mechanism deprived Japanese pharmaceutical companies of the incentive to build medical and other expertise within the company. As many Japanese pharmaceutical companies have little or no expertise in the clinical area, the new GCP guidelines require the sponsor to organise a study team consisting of specialists in a variety of aspects.

7.3.4 Medical adviser

It is not yet common for most Japanese pharmaceutical companies to have a medically qualified person in-house. The new GCP requires sponsoring companies to either employ or contract medical professionals in order to obtain medical advice on preparing protocols and conducting clinical trials.

7.3.5 Other specialists

Other specialists include biostatisticians, regulatory affairs personnel, pharmacokineticists and so on, but the new GCP does not specify these. If the sponsoring company does not possess such expertise they can contract it in.

7.3.6 In-house study review board

The Government had required that the sponsors should have their own in-house study review board to review the ethical aspects of clinical trial protocols. Such a requirement was based on the former Japanese GCP, which stipulates that the company should organise an internal formal body or mechanism to review and authorise its planned studies before submitting them to either study centres or the MHW for clinical trial plan notification. The new Japanese GCP no longer contains a clause to this effect, but it seems that the authorities expect the sponsor to maintain the procedures for an in-house study review board and to determine the appropriateness of the planned studies.

7.3.7 Contract research organisations

For the first time, contract research organisations (CROs) have been formally recognised. Previous legislation described as an "in-country caretaker" someone who operates as a CRO for foreign pharmaceutical companies aiming to obtain Japanese product approval without establishing a formal entity within Japan. Such activity was not open to Japanese pharmaceutical companies, as they were expected to have the full capacity to conduct clinical trials in Japan.

The new Japanese GCP explicitly stipulates that the sponsor may contract all or some parts of clinical trial activity to contract bodies, and in such a case the contract between the sponsor and the study site should be executed between the sponsor, the study site and the CRO.

7.3.8 Protocol development

The former requirement of a categorised result of efficacy, called final global improvement rate (FGIR), or utility, called global utility rate (GUR), is no longer required. For the confirmation studies, a single objective, clinically meaningful endpoint should be identified. Where an objective endpoint is not available, subjective endpoints can be used instead. If the endpoint is not well established or subjective, it must be validated. Study investigators or others who are involved in evaluation should be well trained, and their variation of evaluation results should be within an acceptable range.

Surrogate endpoints, if they are required, should be carefully chosen. Some surrogate endpoints, such as peak flow in asthma or haemoglobin A1c in diabetes mellitus, are well established and can be used in confirmation studies. Conducting a true endpoint study is difficult if it is not incorporated into a global study because patient recruitment is still slow in Japan, and hence relatively small numbers of study participants will be achieved in a reasonable time frame.

7.3.9 Study guidelines

It is always advisable to check whether there is a specific guideline for evaluating a given medicinal product in the area of interest. Some guidelines have not been updated for some time, and caution should be exercised to confirm that their contents are still valid.

The agency had requested sponsors to adhere strictly to the guidelines, but now it explicitly warns sponsors that the guidelines are those at the time of their issue and that the latest scientific standard will be applied when the agency reviews a new drug application.

7.3.10 Study design

A double-blind randomised study is recommended for the confirmation study unless there are substantial scientific reasons not to do so. In many cases an active comparator is preferred to inactive placebo, as evidence of similar efficacy to the premium-priced product will be advantageous for obtaining a favourable reimbursement price. Nevertheless, the use of placebo to demonstrate the absolute efficacy of the drug is increasing, and has been accepted by many study sites. However, there are still doubts about the use of inactive placebos in clinical trials, and the recent revision of the Declaration of Helsinki may strengthen this argument.

If multinational studies are being conducted in Japan, choice of active comparator may be a difficult issue. Many products are not available, or their indication, dose and dosage or conditions of use are different from those in other countries.

7.3.11 Selection of study centres and investigators

7.3.11.1 Study site

The new GCP requires that clinical study sites must have enough facilities to conduct clinical trials and be able to cope in case of emergency. There should also be adequately trained staff available. The sites must prepare standard operating procedures (SOPs) for accepting, reviewing and operating clinical trials. Additional SOPs are required for the operation of an Institutional Review Board (IRB). A clinical trial office and an office for IRB operation must be established in the study site. These requirements have been interpreted that any clinical trial should be conducted in hospitals with ample resources to manage many SOPs and office staff for clinical trials and IRB. Currently the requirements are so interpreted that the trial-related offices can be established among a collection of study sites if these are those of general practitioners or small clinics.

7.3.11.2 Number of study sites and number of patients at each site

It was customary for Phase III studies that study centres were chosen on marketing grounds as well as from the scientific aspect. Because many similar products were developed and launched, hospitals decided to list in their formularies only those drugs in whose development they had participated. A vital issue for sponsoring companies is that their product be listed in the formularies of major hospitals, such as university hospitals or main regional hospitals. Therefore, the Phase III clinical study sites tend to

197

spread all over Japan and favour at least one hospital in each prefecture. Although the number of participating hospitals is large, the number of patients involved in Phase III was rather limited, and therefore many studies were conducted with only a few patients per centre.

If the number of patients at each centre is small, doctors cannot gain experience in the study and they cannot compare the responses of patients to the study medications. Study monitors have to cover a wide geographic area and large number of study-related personnel in order to monitor relatively small numbers of patients. This old practice might be expected to reduce the quality and credibility of the study.

Currently the agency recommends sponsors to recruit more than ten patients at each centre, and most of the study centres are able to accommodate this number. Overall, the number of clinical trials has itself declined because of new GCP and unfavourable pricing rules for the new products with limited advantages over existing products.

7.3.11.3 Institutional Review Board (IRB)

The new GCP has expanded the IRB constitution and its role in the clinical trial. The IRB must consist of more than five members and must include non-medical personnel and a person who does not relate to the study centre. There are no requirements regarding the balance of gender. The head of the institute can attend the IRB meetings but cannot be a member, nor discuss or vote at the meeting.

The IRB is responsible for judging all studies to be conducted at the centre concerned by reviewing protocols, the informed consent sheet, the investigator's brochure and other materials relating to the conduct of clinical trials. The IRB is also responsible for monitoring whether the clinical trials are conducted in compliance with both GCP and IRB requirements, if any. When the study period of a clinical trial exceeds one year the IRB should review the study every year. As the new GCP allows the study sponsor to pay a reasonable amount of money to the subjects, the IRB is expected to review whether the amount and method of payment is reasonable and does not infringe the ethical aspects of the study. Also, the advertisement of a trial for patient recruitment is allowed, but the IRB's approval to implement this at the study centre is required.

The new GCP stipulates that many study centres may share an IRB, or an IRB may be established by academic organisations from which medical centres can seek advice on the studies. As the maintenance and operation of full IRBs may be a burden to some medical institutes, it is likely that such "public" IRBs will become a practical option.

7.3.11.4 Investigators

The new GCP clarifies the role of the investigators, who are expected to take an active part in the study from the planning stage. Previously, the number of patients and the study protocols were allotted to each centre by the chief investigator, but now it is the responsibility of investigators to decide whether they accept the protocol and the number of patients to be recruited and then take part in the study.

Preparation of the patient informed consent sheet is the responsibility of each investigator, although support of the sponsor is requested.

The investigator can nominate sub-investigators and other support staff for the study and establish a study team. The member list of the study team should be submitted to and confirmed by the head of the institute.

The investigator should endorse the study protocol and the study contract, and must comply with them. Any deviations from the protocol should be recorded and reported to both the head of institute and the sponsor.

The selection of study investigators is difficult and involves many factors, among which possible patient recruitment is the most important. It is not easy to predict patient recruitment at the time of protocol discussion, because the attitude of patients towards clinical trials is not entirely in favour of participation. Whether the study site is acceptable in the light of GCP is another important issue for the choice of investigators. Although many centres are "GCP compliant", close monitoring is required to confirm that such status is maintained during the conduct of clinical trials. The GCP system in hospitals is maintained by a small number of competent staff, mostly pharmacy staff, and therefore the retirement or movement of main staff may change the situation.

7.3.11.5 *Controller*

In Japanese clinical trials, a controller is often appointed. This is usually an academic expert (for example a professor of clinical pharmacology or biostatistics) who should be independent of both the sponsoring company and the investigators. His role is "to ensure that the study is performed safely, and without bias, and that the published results are accurate". Therefore, his function includes, for example, randomisation, confirmation of the double-blindness of the study medications, and confirmation of code envelope integrity at the end of the study.

7.3.12 Clinical trial plan notification

An outline of the data from non-clinical studies must be submitted to the MHLW with the protocol for the proposed clinical study before the trial begins. A notification is required for each protocol. The list of items required for clinical trial plan notification is shown in Box 7.2. Furthermore, supplementary data must be added on entry to subsequent clinical phases, that is, general clinical trials and comparative trials. Such data are reviewed by the MHLW, and for this purpose the sponsor must wait 30 days after submitting the initial notification before

---

Box 7.2 List of items required for "clinical trial plan notification"

- Description of trial drug
- Manufacturing method
- Anticipated indications, dose and dosage
- Purpose of trial
- Trial details including study period
- Name and address of each study centre
- Names of all investigators
- Amount of clinical supply for each centre
- Reasons if the supply is free of charge
- (Name and address of local CT manager)

---

executing a contract with the medical institute. For a subsequent notification the review period is reduced to 14 days. The notification also requires the names of all investigators, whether investigators or sub-investigators, and this list must be kept updated throughout the study period.

7.3.13 Contracts and funding

7.3.13.1 Head of study centre

Japanese GCP requires that the head of the medical institute and the sponsor must execute a study contract, and does not allow the investigator to contract directly with the sponsor. Historically, a clinical trial is considered an activity of the hospital as a whole, not of an individual investigator. The reason behind this is that the investigator cannot conduct any study without the full support of hospital staff and access to hospital facilities. The head of the medical institute is responsible for organising an IRB in-house, or to make it available outside the hospital organisation if the hospital is not large enough to maintain an IRB. Once the sponsoring company submits the clinical study plan to the hospital, the head of the medical institute should submit the study document to the IRB for their opinion. The head cannot be a member of the IRB, is not allowed to discuss or vote on the clinical trial, but nevertheless attendance to the IRB is not prohibited.

After receiving a favourable opinion from the IRB the head of the medical institute should sign the study contract. The head cannot accept the study if the IRB decision is not favourable. GCP stipulates essential clauses of the contract (Box 7.3).

In addition to IRB members, the head of the institute must appoint a study drug manager, a document archiving manager, and administration

---

Box 7.3 Essential clauses of the contract between study sponsor and medical institution

- Date of contract
- Name and address of person sponsoring clinical trial
- In cases where part of the work is entrusted to a CRO, name and address of CRO and range of the work entrusted
- Name and address of medical institution
- Name and title of persons responsible for contract
- Names and titles of investigators and others
- Period of clinical trial
- Target number of subjects
- Matters related to control of clinical trial drugs
- Matters related to preservation of records (including data)
- Matters related to report by sponsor and persons engaged at medical institution pursuant to the GCP
- Matters related to conservation of subjects' privacy
- Matters related to costs of clinical trials
- Statement that medical institution will conduct the clinical trial in conformity with the protocol
- Statement that medical institution will allow access to records (including documents) specified by GCP at request of sponsor
- Where it is evident that medical institution adversely interfered with the proper conduct of the clinical trial by violating GCP, protocol or the contract, the sponsor can cancel the contract
- Matters related to compensation for subjects for damage to health
- Other matters necessary for ensuring that the clinical trial can be conducted properly

---

staff for both clinical trials and the IRB. In order to handle clinical trials in such a complex structure, SOPs for conducting clinical trials must be prepared at the hospital.

All serious adverse events, deviations from the protocol, extensions of the study period or increases in patient numbers should be reported to the head of the institute by the investigator.

7.3.13.2 Clinical trial funding

The regulations on clinical trial funding differ between hospitals, based on their background. For example, in national university hospitals there is a standard table that categorises clinical trial activities. To calculate the study budget, the activities are added up for each protocol and some hospital overheads, which cover general management costs, are also added. The entire study points are then multiplied by the index to change the points into actual currency. This index is set as ¥ 6000 (about £35). Private university hospitals set a similar rule but with greater overheads.

The costs calculated at the beginning of the study should include all the activities of the trial. Therefore, the investigators expect no additional payment. For example, the fund should include travel and accommodation costs if investigator meetings are planned during the trial.

Although the new rules make clinical trial funding transparent, they may cause other confusions. First, it is not clear how investigators receive benefit from the fund. The clinical trial is now considered an official activity of the hospital and the fund may be allocated purely to the personnel cost. If investigators do not obtain any benefit from conducting a clinical trial, they may not find it attractive in their busy clinical environment.

Second, many public hospitals run a yearly budget system. This system requires that all income and spending must balance within each fiscal year (from April to March the following year). It is often the case that the hospital refuses to refund study cost even if the recruitment rate of the hospital is very low at the end of each fiscal year. The sponsors have accepted this, as the required number of patients at each centre was low. However, the new calculation system doubled or tripled the study costs and, with an increased number of patients to be recruited at each centre, this yearly budget system became a major concern to the sponsors.

7.3.14 Ethical issues

7.3.14.1 Informed consent

The patient's informed consent was required by the old GCP, with a wording of "in writing as a rule". A survey performed in the early 1990s showed that a limited number of informed consents were obtained in writing and the rest were in the form of verbal agreements without witnesses. There was concern about whether patients understood the nature of clinical trials because the informed consent sheet was rarely provided to the patient and, even if it was, the explanation might be too difficult for a layperson to understand.

Based on the ICH guidelines full written informed consent is now required for all participating patients. If the patient cannot consent because of his/her health condition, a responsible caretaker is allowed to give consent in lieu of the patient.

The investigator should prepare an informed consent form for every study to be performed at the institute and should obtain an approval from the IRB that covers the institute. GCP listed a dozen points to be covered by the informed consent form (IC) (see Box 7.4). The new GCP allows a reasonable amount of payment to the patient, such as transport costs.

Box 7.4 Items required in the informed consent form

- The fact that the clinical trial is conducted as a test
- Purpose of the clinical trial
- Name and title of the investigator and contact site
- Methods of the clinical trial
- Anticipated efficacy of the clinical trial drugs and anticipated disadvantage to the subject
- Matters on other therapeutic methods
- Duration of participation in the clinical trial
- The fact that agreement to participate in the clinical trial can be withdrawn at any time
- The fact that the subject is never placed at any disadvantage by refusing to participate or withdrawal of participation
- The fact that monitor, auditor, and the institutional review board can have access to source data on condition that the subjects' anonymity is maintained
- Contact site of the medical institution in case of damage to health
- Matters regarding compensation for damage to study subjects' health
- Other necessary matters related to the clinical trial

Patients should allow clinical trial monitors, auditors, IRB members, and inspectors from the regulatory authority to verify the source documents. This new requirement of obligatory written informed consent is regarded as a major challenge for the conduct of clinical trials in Japan. In Japan, patients are usually not informed about their medications and are unaware of possible outcomes or side effects. As this is normal practice in Japan, patients do not expect any detailed explanation of their condition, nor to participate in decision-making regarding treatment choices. Also, it must be borne in mind that in Japan verbal agreements or contracts are widely accepted, not only in the clinical setting but also in society in general. It is easily imaginable in such an environment that patients may be frightened by very detailed explanations of disease, possible treatment options, including the study drug, possible side-effects (sometimes including death) and compensation policy.

Informed consent has recently become much more popular, not only for clinical studies but also for daily medical practice, and patients are now much more accustomed to giving their consent. Clinical studies become more visible to the general public and the media reports studies with potential therapeutic benefit in a favourable manner. This is a significant change from the past, when most media coverage of clinical studies was scandalous or sensational without sound scientific reason.

7.3.14.2 Patient recruitment

Recent changes in the operation of the Pharmaceutical Affairs Law and Medical Practice Law provided options for patient recruitment for both sponsors and hospitals. Pharmaceutical Affairs Law prohibits the advertisement of non-approved drugs, that is, clinical study drugs, but if the study drug is not identified the sponsor can advertise the clinical trial itself in order to recruit patients.

Similarly, hospitals were not able to advertise their involvement in clinical studies. There are detailed regulations about what hospitals can advertise, and they were amended in April 2001 so that hospitals can now recruit patients through the mass media. Before the introduction of such advertising only posters were allowed in hospitals.

7.3.14.3 Payment to participating patients

Participation in a clinical study should be voluntary and there will be no payment unless the study provides no therapeutic benefit, such as pharmacokinetic studies in healthy volunteers. When the new GCP were introduced there was substantial discussion about whether, if patients were required to visit study sites more often than usual, for example to attend additional examinations or treatments, it would be fair to place the whole financial burden on them.

In Japan, when patients receive medical services they need to pay 10–30% of actual medical costs, depending upon the type of insurance. The insurer pays the rest. There are ceilings for patient payment if it exceeds predefined monthly limits, or the patient fall into a certain category, such as the elderly or those suffering from diseases designated by the government as difficult to treat. The body of insurers and sponsoring companies agreed that the sponsoring company of the trial must pay (1) all laboratory costs, including radiological imaging during the study period, and (2) concomitant medication costs if such medication is used for the disease of concern in the study. For this purpose the study period is defined as "between the first day of dosing and the last day of dosing".

In addition, many study sites rule that patients should be paid for their attendance at clinical examination or treatment during the study. This is roughly considered as the reimbursement of travel costs. There are no statistics on the amounts of these payments, but the majority of hospitals set a standard of about £40 for each visit, based on the protocol requirements.

7.3.15 Monitoring

The old GCP did not contain the word "monitoring". The lack of monitoring was based on the general view at the time of legislation that "the culprits are pharmaceutical companies". The new GCP requires monitoring and on-site audit, including source data verification (SDV) as in the ICH GCP guidelines. The difficulty in circumventing violation of privacy laws (medical law, criminal law and other related regulations) was resolved by obtaining an informed consent from the patient that allows sponsors' monitors, auditors, IRB members and inspectors from regulatory authorities to access the source record provided that the subjects' privacy is respected.

The monitors place much emphasis on source data verification, as it is a new concept in Japanese clinical trials. The way case record forms (CRFs) are prepared causes difficulties in monitoring. Most CRFs used in Japan are in the form of 8–12 page booklets. Investigators fill them in after the completion of each case, or sometimes after completion of all cases. Therefore, there was a vague understanding that SDV is a post-hoc confirmation of the CRF against the source data. This view is changing, and more emphasis is being placed on the initiation of and ongoing monitoring to confirm that investigators adhere to the study protocol. Visit-type CRFs are being introduced in this context, and this becomes possible as sponsors reinforce their data management capabilities and study sites/investigators introduce clinical study coordinators.

Once many sponsors started monitoring based on the new GCP, they found that they were heavily understaffed. In previous times, a monitor was able to take care of 15–20 centres all over Japan. Now most sponsoring companies consider the appropriate number of centres per monitor to be around five. This reflects not only the workload of study site monitoring, but also complicated study initiation procedures required by the new GCP and serious adverse reaction reporting procedures, as some major hospitals require the personal presence of the monitor to report such events. The sponsors are also aware there is a mismatch of monitors' qualifications, as most monitors in major pharmaceutical companies are graduates, postgraduates or sometimes doctors in pharmaceutical/biosciences but are not trained in the bedside setting. Their responsibilities are not limited to monitoring but include study planning, administration and medical writing, to mention but a few. Sponsors recognise this is not an ideal situation, and they are introducing more medically trained monitors and separate other activities from them.

7.3.15.1 Clinical research co-ordinator (CRC)

It is agreed in Japan that the key person for the successful conduct of clinical trials is the clinical research co-ordinator (CRC). It is now common to refer to the study nurse or study co-ordinator as the CRC, although such a concept is rather new in Japan. It may take some time to introduce the

CRC to hospitals, as there is no history of such a role and the rather rigid labour environment of Japan makes it difficult to establish a new activity in hospitals.

The possible role of the CRC will be identical to that of their European or American counterparts, or may be more complex because of the complicated Japanese GCP and medical system. It is considered that successful implementation of Japanese GCP relies on the successful introduction of the CRC in major hospitals. Many professional bodies, some backed up by regulatory bodies and academia, have started training courses for CRCs. Although the numbers of courses and trainees are still limited, the activities of graduates have enhanced the quality and productivity of clinical trials in Japan.

7.3.15.2   Audit

In the previous GCP guidelines, the auditor's activity was confined to the company. The auditor used the CRF as a source document and checked the clinical database and final report against it.

The new GCP requires that: "sponsors shall compile plan and operating procedures on auditing and implement auditing in conformity with the plan and the procedures", thus expanding the scope of audit toward the clinical site.

7.3.16   Safety issues

7.3.16.1   Serious adverse event (SAE) reporting

All unexpected, serious and drug-related adverse events should be reported to MHLW, the investigators and study sites. The requirement to report to the MHLW is identical to ICH guidelines, with an additional definition that adverse events include any suspicious infection related to a study drug. This addition reflects bitter experience of the spread of AIDS among haemophilia patients due to HIV-contaminated non-heat treated human plasma products.

The agency rigorously reinforces the SAE reporting system during clinical studies, and this is reiterated at the time of GCP inspection. Some hospitals require the chief investigator to acknowledge the report before the sponsor submits it to the hospital study office. As the number of study centres for each protocol is rather large in Japan, such requirements are resource consuming for sponsoring companies.

Study suspension or the obtaining of additional written informed consent from participating patients based on new serious adverse experience varies from one ethics committee to another. There is no clear rule for this, and the decision of sponsors as to whether they would suspend an entire study or not may differ. It is worth noting that not only is the serious adverse event described here life-threatening or potentially harmful to the entire study population, but that moderate or sometime mild adverse conditions may nevertheless fall within the definition of serious.

7.3.17 Safety concerns

Concerns about the safety of the study drug may characterise the Japanese clinical trial. In a Phase I study, the dose escalation stops at the level of expected therapeutic dose or double it, and is never escalated to identify any toxicity (except for anticancer drugs). If toxicity is observed in a Phase I study, even if it is at the highest dose or under experimental conditions, further study will be difficult. Everyone in the clinical trial is used to handling study drugs with no safety problems and there is the general concept that the drug must be "safe".

This concept becomes an absolute requirement of drug development, with Japanese companies developing many compounds that are an improvement over established products. Under such circumstances the effect of the study drug is guaranteed and the major point of characterisation of the product is "enhanced safety". Sponsoring companies have tried to establish the therapeutic dose as low as possible so as to give a larger safety margin and a lower incidence of side effects. This attitude has led to lower dosage levels of drugs in Japan than in the USA or Europe.

This situation will change as a simultaneous development of a product between Europe, Japan and the USA becomes popular, and the same level of side-effects at the same dose and dosage conditions is expected.

7.4 Conclusion

The introduction of the new GCP and other study practices is aimed at bringing Japanese clinical studies to be accepted by regulatory bodies worldwide. Hospitals, regulatory authorities and pharmaceutical industries have worked to change many aspects of clinical studies, and although it is difficult they are establishing the new clinical study system. There have been dramatic improvements in the quality and reliability of clinical trials, and the objectives of the new GCP are being achieved in many ways. As the differences in medical practice and ethnic factors will nevertheless remain, sponsors should consider incorporating such differences into their global development plans and conduct.

References

1 Drug Approval and Licensing Procedures in Japan 2000, Jiho Co. Ltd, Tokyo ICH guidelines implemented in Japan is obtainable in: Japan's and ICH Guidelines for New Drug Registration, Supplement 2000, Yakuji Nippo Ltd, Tokyo.

THE REGULATION OF MEDICAL PRODUCTS

More information on regulatory procedures relating to the Japanese pharmaceutical industry can be found at the following websites:
http://www.kiko.go.jp/English/E_Top.html
http://www.nihs.go.jp/index.html
http://www.nihs.go.jp/pmdec/outline.htm
http://www.mhlw.go.jp/english/index.html

8: The regulation of drug products by the United States Food and Drug Administration

PETER BARTON HUTT

8.1 Introduction

The regulation of drug products by the Food and Drug Administration (FDA) in the United States is extraordinarily detailed and complex, and has enormous public costs as well as public benefits.[1] This chapter provides only a broad overview of this subject. Entire books,[2] and thousands of articles, have been devoted both to a comprehensive review of the area and to specific aspects. Anyone who wishes to understand it in greater detail must consult the governing statutes, regulations and guidance, as well as the experience of experts who have spent their entire careers working in the field. This chapter therefore presents a bare outline, permitting a glimpse into this extremely important and fascinating area but not a definitive analysis of any of its myriad aspects.

8.2 Regulatory framework

8.2.1 Federal regulatory requirements

In the United States, regulatory policies are established by statutes enacted by Congress and signed by the President. These laws govern all regulatory requirements imposed by FDA upon drug products. No additional or different requirements can be imposed by any administrative official, but the statutory requirements are continually subject to reinterpretation and thus expansion as they are implemented by administrative action.

Laws are usually written by Congress in relatively general terms. They are intended to be implemented and enforced by administrative officials, in this instance located in FDA. Under the Federal Food, Drug, and Cosmetic Act (FD&C Act) of 1938,[3] FDA is empowered to promulgate regulations implementing the statute, in accordance with the procedural requirements established by the Administrative Procedure Act.[4] These procedural requirements require that most regulations initially be published as proposals in the Federal Register, accompanied by a lengthy preamble explaining the purpose and meaning of the proposed regulations.[5] Time is then given for public comment. After all public comment has been received, FDA reviews the comment, makes a final decision on the regulations and promulgates the final regulations, together with a preamble explaining the decision with respect to each comment received and the reasons for the final version of the regulation. The regulations are then codified in the Code of Federal Regulations, without the explanatory preambles.

Following the promulgation of a federal regulation, any interested person may challenge the legality of the regulation in the courts.[6] The primary grounds for any such legal challenge are that the regulation exceeds the FDA statutory authority or that it is arbitrary or capricious. Any person who challenges an FDA regulation in this way has a heavy burden to demonstrate that the regulation is illegal, and in most instances the FDA regulations are upheld by the courts.

Even though the FDA regulations are more detailed than the governing statute, they are nonetheless still often worded in general terms, and thus it becomes important to have more specific and detailed documents to guide daily decision-making in the agency. Such detailed policy comes in many forms, including the preambles to the regulations, written guidance, letters, speeches, and a host of other documents, as well as unwritten tradition and practice. It is this area that largely governs daily FDA action. Because the vast bulk of FDA policy is not set forth either in the statute or in the regulations, it is uniquely a field where experience and judgement play a very large role.

8.2.2 State regulatory requirements

Decades ago, the individual states played an important part in the regulation of pharmaceutical products. As pharmaceutical science has become more complex and as the FDA regulation of the pharmaceutical industry has become more intense and pervasive, however, the states have shifted their traditional regulatory responsibilities to concentrate more heavily on food products and other items that are more appropriate for local control. Thus, state regulation of drug products is a relatively insignificant aspect of drug regulation in the United States today.

The individual states have retained their statutes governing both non-prescription and prescription drugs, however, and on occasion will exercise their authority to regulate in these areas. In recent years, this regulation has largely been limited to non-prescription drugs. For example, California has guidelines for slack fill in the packaging of non-prescription drugs.[7] On occasion, states have also switched a non-prescription drug to prescription status in order to address a local abuse problem – usually only for a short duration. State regulation of drugs is not considered further in this chapter.

8.2.3 Product liability

The one aspect of state "regulation" of pharmaceutical products that has increased is that of product liability. Drawing upon common law precedent extending back to medieval English origins, an individual harmed by a pharmaceutical product may bring a civil tort action under state law against the manufacturer or distributor of the drug for damages sustained. This can be a potent form of regulation. If a pharmaceutical product causes widespread damage to patients, the resulting tort liability could endanger the future of the manufacturer. One example is the Dalkon Shield, the damage actions from which resulted in the bankruptcy of AH Robbins. Further discussion of the field of product liability is beyond the scope of this chapter.

8.3   FDA history[8]

The United States Patent Office began its interest in agricultural matters in the 1830s. Eventually, an Agricultural Division was established in the Patent Office, and a chemical laboratory was funded in that Division.

When Congress created the United States Department of Agriculture (USDA) by statute in 1862,[9] the Agricultural Division of the Patent Office, and its chemical laboratory, were transferred to form the nucleus of the new Department. A Chemical Division was immediately formed within USDA. This became the Division of Chemistry in 1890,[10] the Bureau of Chemistry in 1901,[11] the Food, Drug, and Insecticide Administration in 1927,[12] and the FDA in 1930.[13]

FDA remained a part of USDA until it was transferred to the new Federal Security Agency in 1940.[14] When the Department of Health, Education and Welfare (HEW) was established in 1953, as a successor to the Federal Security Agency, FDA became a part of HEW.[15] HEW was renamed the Department of Health and Human Services (HHS) in 1979.[16]

Throughout this entire period, FDA (and its predecessor agencies) were created by administrative action, not by Congress. The governing statutes were all officially delegated for implementation and enforcement to the Secretary of Agriculture/HEW/HHS, not to the Commissioner of Food and Drugs. It was not until the Food and Drug Administration Act of 1988[17] that Congress officially established FDA as a government agency. To this day, however, the governing statutes delegate responsibility for implementation and enforcement to the Secretary of HHS.

Throughout this history, the Commissioner of Food and Drugs and his predecessors have also occupied a position that was created solely by administrative action, not by Congress. The Food and Drug Administration Act of 1988 also officially created the position of the Commissioner of Food and Drugs, and required that the Commissioner be appointed by the President by and with the advice and consent of the Senate.

The Secretary of HHS is a Cabinet position, appointed by the President with the advice and consent of the Senate. The Commissioner of Food and Drugs reports to the Secretary of HHS.

Within FDA, there is an Office of the Commissioner and five product-oriented centres (for food, drugs, biologics, medical devices and veterinary medicine) located in the Washington DC area.[18] The Center for Drug Evaluation and Research and the Center for Biologics Evaluation and Research are responsible for regulation of drug products. Outside Washington DC, FDA has an extensive field force located in regions and districts throughout the United States, where FDA employees inspect drug establishments and conduct enforcement activities. The FDA field force is also responsible for the inspection of foreign drug establishments located throughout the world.

8.4 Historical overview of drug regulation statutes

Government concern about the adulteration and misbranding of pharmaceutical products extends back to ancient times.[19] Pliny the Elder, for example, in the first century AD, criticised "the fashionable druggists' shops which spoil everything with fraudulent adulterations".[20] As a result, various forms of government control to prevent the adulteration and misbranding of food and drugs can be found in virtually every recorded civilisation. These regulatory controls were brought to the American colonies by early settlers, were enacted into state law following the American Revolution, and eventually were adopted by Congress as nationwide requirements in a series of federal statutes.

During most of the 19th century regulation of food and drug products was thought to be a matter of state and local concern, not appropriate for federal legislation, under the United States Constitution. During this period, most federal laws governing food and drugs therefore related to foreign commerce rather than to domestic commerce. It is only since 1900 that regulation of food and drugs in the United States has been concluded to be a matter of national concern that justifies the enactment of federal statutes. The following paragraphs present a brief chronology of the major federal regulatory statutes governing non-prescription and prescription drug products in the United States.

8.4.1 The Vaccine Act of 1813[21]

Following Edward Jenner's discovery of a smallpox vaccine in 1798, and the demonstration by Benjamin Waterhouse in the United States in 1800 that the vaccine was effective, fraudulent versions of the vaccine were marketed throughout the country. A Baltimore physician, John Smith, initially convinced the Maryland legislature to enact a statute designed to ensure the availability of an effective smallpox vaccine supply, and then persuaded Congress to enact the Vaccine Act of 1813 for the same purpose. This statute authorised the President to appoint a federal agent to "preserve the genuine vaccine matter and to furnish the same to any citizen" who requested it.

The President promptly appointed Dr Smith as the first and, as it turned out, only federal vaccine agent. Following an outbreak of smallpox in North Carolina in 1821 that was thought to be caused by a contaminated lot of vaccine supplied by Dr Smith under the 1813 statute, the matter was investigated by two committees of the House of Representatives. The second committee concluded that regulation of smallpox vaccine should be undertaken by state and local officials rather than by the federal government, and as a result the 1813 Act was repealed in 1822.[22] As will be discussed below, 80 years later another drug tragedy led to the enactment of a new statute in 1902 under which vaccines are currently regulated by FDA.

8.4.2 The Import Drug Act of 1848[23]

A congressional investigation in 1848 discovered that a wide variety of drugs imported into the United States for use by American troops in Mexico were adulterated. Congress therefore enacted a statute dealing solely with imported drugs. The 1848 Act required that all imported drugs be labelled with the name of the manufacturer and the place of preparation, and be examined and appraised by the United States Customs Service for "quality, purity, and fitness for medical purposes". The Customs Service was directed to deny entry into the United States of any drug determined to be so adulterated or deteriorated as to be "improper, unsafe, or dangerous to be used for medical purposes". This law remained in effect until it was replaced by another statute in 1922.[24]

8.4.3 The Biologics Act of 1902[25]

As the result of a series of problems with biological drugs during the late 1890s, culminating in the death of several children in St Louis from a tetanus-infected diphtheria antitoxin, Congress enacted the Biologics Act of 1902. This statute is the first known regulatory law in any country that required premarket approval. It required approval of both a product licence application (PLA) and an establishment licence application (ELA) before any biological product could be marketed in interstate commerce.

Although it was recodified in 1944[26] and 1997,[27] it has remained in effect without significant change since 1902. It was initially implemented by the Public Health Service, but was transferred to FDA in 1972.[28] Today it is implemented by the Center for Biologics Evaluation and Review (CBER) within FDA, which is located in buildings on the campus of the National Institutes of Health, where it had been located prior to the 1972 transfer to FDA.

8.4.4 The Federal Food and Drugs Act of 1906[29]

The first legislation to establish comprehensive nationwide regulation of all food and drugs was introduced in Congress in 1879. Largely because regulation of food and drugs was at that time thought to be a matter for state and local control, Congress debated this legislation for 27 years, ultimately enacting the Federal Food and Drugs Act in 1906. This law broadly prohibited any adulteration or misbranding of drugs marketed in interstate commerce. Although it was quite short, and very broad and general in nature, it was extremely progressive for its time and included sufficient authority to permit FDA to take strong enforcement action against the unsafe, ineffective and mislabelled products that flooded the United States market in the late 1800s. Unlike the Biologics Act of 1902, however, it contained no provisions requiring pre-market testing or approval for new drug products. An attempt by FDA to obtain this type of authority in 1912 was unsuccessful. Thus, Congress initially provided pre-market approval authority for biological drugs but not for other drugs.

8.4.5 The Federal Food, Drug, and Cosmetic Act of 1938[30]

Shortly after President Franklin D Roosevelt took office in 1933, the Commissioner of Food and Drugs persuaded the new administration to propose legislation to modernise the Federal Food and Drugs Act of 1906. The legislation introduced in 1933, and ultimately enacted as the Federal Food, Drug, and Cosmetic Act of 1938 (the FD&C Act), was debated by Congress for five years. Initially, it was intended primarily to add cosmetics and medical devices to the 1906 Act and to require additional affirmative labelling for food and drug products. In September 1937, however, more than 100 people died of diethylene glycol poisoning following use of Elixir Sulfanilamide, which used this chemical as the solvent without any form of safety testing. As a result, Congress added a pre-market notification requirement for new drugs to the pending legislation and enacted the new law in June 1938. Under this statute, a "new drug" was defined as a drug that was not generally recognised as safe for its intended use. Before a new drug could be marketed, it was required to be tested on humans in accordance with investigational new drug (IND) regulations promulgated by FDA. When sufficient data were obtained under the IND to demonstrate the safety of the drug, the manufacturer was required to submit a new drug application (NDA) for the drug to FDA. If FDA did not disapprove the NDA within 60 days after filing, the NDA became effective and the drug could be marketed. The FD&C Act has been amended more than 100 times since 1938, and is now a very lengthy, detailed and complex law. The more important amendments relating to drugs are summarised below.

8.4.6 The Insulin and Antibiotics Amendments[31]

Following enactment of the FD&C Act in 1938, insulin, penicillin and other antibiotic drugs were developed and marketed. Because of the unique production processes for these new pharmaceutical products, Congress enacted special provisions in the law requiring both that FDA approve each of them as safe and that FDA have the authority to require that each batch be certified by FDA as conforming to standards established for them by the Agency. Thus, insulin and antibiotics were regulated by FDA under provisions that were similar to, but nonetheless different from, those established both for biologics and for chemical drugs.

8.4.7 The Durham–Humphrey Amendments of 1951[32]

The FD&C Act made no distinction between non-prescription and prescription drugs. A company could label a drug either way, depending upon marketing strategy. In 1939, however, FDA promulgated regulations declaring that any drug for which adequate directions for lay use could not be prepared must be sold only on prescription, thereby for the first time creating a mandatory prescription class of drugs. In order to make certain that the same drug, at the same dosage and for the same indication, could not be marketed both as a non-prescription and a prescription drug, in 1951 Congress codified the FDA regulations into law by enacting the Durham–Humphrey Amendments.

8.4.8 The Drug Amendments of 1962[33]

Although thalidomide was marketed throughout Europe, the NDA for this drug did not become effective in the United States. When it was learned in mid-1962 that thalidomide was a potent human teratogen, Congress immediately enacted the Drug Amendments of 1962 to strengthen the new drug regulatory system to make certain that FDA had adequate statutory authority to ensure that no such drug could be marketed in the future. The 1962 Amendments made a number of important changes. First, and most important, the amended law requires FDA explicitly to approve an NDA, rather than simply allowing the NDA to become effective through FDA inaction. Thus, the new drug provisions of the law were converted in 1962 from pre-market notification to pre-market approval, making them parallel with the Biologics Act of 1902.

Second, a new drug was required to be shown to be effective as well as safe. Third, FDA was given additional authority to require compliance with current good manufacturing practices (GMP), to control the advertising of prescription drugs, to register drug establishments, and to implement other regulatory requirements. Finally, FDA was required to review all NDAs that had become effective during 1938–1962, to determine whether these drugs were effective as well as safe.

8.4.9 The Controlled Substances Act of 1970[34]

Beginning in the early 1900s, Congress enacted a series of laws to control narcotic drugs and other drugs subject to abuse. All of these laws were repealed in 1970 and replaced by the Controlled Substances Act. Responsibility for enforcement rests with the Drug Enforcement Administration (DEA) of the Department of Justice. FDA may approve an NDA for any controlled substance that has a legitimate medical use, but DEA may impose upon any new drug that is also a controlled substance additional regulatory requirements to prevent abuse and misuse by classifying it into one of four categories: schedules II (most restrictive) to V (least restrictive).

8.4.10 The Poison Prevention Packaging Act of 1970[35]

In response to concern about household poisoning of children with hazardous household products, Congress enacted the Poison Prevention Packaging Act to require the use of special child-resistant packaging. In accordance with regulations established by the Consumer Product Safety Commission, this type of packaging is now common for virtually all prescription drugs and for most non-prescription drugs.[36]

8.4.11 The Drug Listing Act of 1972[37]

The Drug Amendments of 1962 included a requirement that every owner of a United States drug establishment register that establishment with FDA. Congress enacted the Drug Listing Act of 1972 to add the requirement that every person who registers an establishment shall include a list of all drugs manufactured at that establishment.

8.4.12 The Orphan Drug Act of 1983[38]

An orphan drug is one that is intended for use for rare diseases and thus for which there is not a sufficient market to justify the investment needed to demonstrate safety and effectiveness in order to obtain approval of an NDA. For more than 20 years FDA had permitted orphan drugs to be distributed through a permanent IND, with little or no thought that it would ever progress to an approved NDA. In 1983, Congress enacted the Orphan Drug Act to provide economic incentives for industry to make the investment necessary to develop this category of drugs. When that proved

216

insufficient, the Act was amended in 1984 to expand its coverage substantially, by providing that any drug with a use that has a target patient population of fewer than 200 000 people is automatically classified as an orphan drug.[39] Although the Orphan Drug Act does not provide for any different regulatory requirements from those applied to non-orphan drugs, the tax incentives and, in particular, a seven-year period of market exclusivity during which no competing NDA may be approved by FDA, combined with the extraordinary expansion in 1984 of the number of drugs covered by this statute, has had a major impact on drug development in the United States.

8.4.13 The Drug Price Competition and Patent Term Restoration Act of 1984[40]

Under the new drug provisions as initially enacted in 1938 and as amended in 1962, all information in an IND and NDA was regarded as confidential proprietary business information that could not be revealed by FDA to the public or any competitor, and could not be used as the basis for any subsequent approval of a generic version of the pioneer new drug. Even after the patent for a pioneer new drug expired, competitors were unable to obtain an approved NDA for a generic version without duplicating all the animal and human testing needed to demonstrate safety and effectiveness. Congress therefore enacted the Drug Price Competition and Patent Term Restoration Act of 1984, which authorised FDA to approve an abbreviated NDA for a generic version of a pioneer new drug after the patent and the statutory period of market exclusivity for the pioneer drug had expired. The result has been a substantial increase in the number of generic drugs available in the United States.

At the same time, Congress recognised that the effective patent term of pioneer drugs was dramatically reduced because of the time required for drug development by the FDA IND/NDA requirements prior to marketing. On average, the effective patent life for a pioneer drug was less than half the 17-year period then specified by Congress under the patent law, as of the time of NDA approval. For some drugs, no patent could be obtained. As part of the 1984 legislation, Congress therefore directed the Patent Office to extend the patent for a pioneer drug for up to five years in order to compensate for the lost patent life resulting from FDA regulatory review requirements. Congress also specified a minimum period of three or five years of market exclusivity during which no generic version could be approved by FDA even if there were no patent protection.

8.4.14 The Drug Export Amendments Act of 1986[41]

Under the FD&C Act as enacted in 1938, adulterated and misbranded drugs may lawfully be exported but an unapproved new drug could not. This was a drafting error, but it was nonetheless enforced by FDA.

Congress therefore enacted the Drug Export Amendments Act of 1986, which authorised the limited export of unapproved new human drugs and biological products after FDA had approved an export application. An export application could be approved only if there was an active IND; approval of an NDA was actively being pursued in the United States; the product was for export to one or more of 21 listed countries with sophisticated regulatory systems; the product was currently approved and marketed in the receiving country; FDA had not disapproved the product; the product was manufactured in conformity with GMP and was not adulterated; the product's labelling listed the countries to which FDA permitted it to be exported; FDA had not determined that domestic manufacture of the drug for export was contrary to the public health and safety of the United States; and the product was properly labelled for export. Not surprisingly, these restrictions were so tight that most United States companies preferred to move their manufacturing facilities overseas, and thus to source the drug from abroad, rather than to make it in the United States and attempt to obtain FDA approval for an export application. As a result, in 1996 the 1986 Amendments were repealed and replaced with substantially more flexible provisions.[42]

8.4.15 The Prescription Drug Marketing Act of 1987[43]

Congressional investigations in the mid-1980s demonstrated that pharmaceutical products were being exported from the United States and later imported back into the country without adequate assurance that they had not become adulterated or misbranded while abroad. Congress responded by enacting the Prescription Drug Marketing Act of 1987, which makes the importation of United States drugs by anyone other than the manufacturer illegal. It also prohibits the sale of drug samples and the resale of drug products initially sold to healthcare institutions. Distribution of drug samples by pharmaceutical manufacturers is permitted only in response to a written request, for which a receipt is obtained. The provisions requiring state licensure of wholesale distributors of prescription drugs were subsequently clarified in the Prescription Drug Amendments of 1992.[44]

8.4.16 The Generic Drug Enforcement Act of 1992[45]

Following enactment of the Drug Price Competition and Patent Term Restoration Act of 1984, FDA embarked upon a major campaign to expedite approval of abbreviated NDAs for generic versions of important pioneer drugs for which the patents had expired. Because of the enormous economic profit that could be made by the generic drug company that marketed the first generic version of an important pioneer drug, a number of generic drug manufacturers submitted fraudulent data to FDA as part of abbreviated NDAs, and even paid illegal bribes to FDA officials in an attempt to obtain preferential handling of their applications. When this scandal came to light, in addition to the criminal prosecution of the individuals and companies involved, Congress enacted the Generic Drug Enforcement Act of 1992 to increase the penalties for such illegal behaviour. These new penalties include mandatory and permissive debarment of corporations and individuals, suspension and withdrawal of approval of abbreviated NDAs, and civil money penalties. Although the 1992 Act applies primarily to generic drugs, it also provides mandatory and permissive debarment for individuals who engage in wrongdoing with respect to any drug, whether generic or pioneer. All of the provisions of the Act apply to both non-prescription and prescription drugs.

8.4.17   The Prescription Drug User Fee Act of 1992[46]

Following enactment of the Drug Amendments of 1962, the time needed to develop the data and information to demonstrate the safety and effectiveness of a new drug, and to obtain FDA approval of an NDA, escalated. As a result, a "drug lag" developed between the pharmaceutical products available in the rest of the world and those available in the United States. FDA on many occasions pointed out that the time needed for FDA review of an IND or a NDA was at least in part a function of the resources available to the agency. Although both FDA and the pharmaceutical industry initially opposed the imposition on the industry of "user fees" that would generate additional revenue to permit FDA to hire additional people to review INDs and NDAs, both abruptly reversed their earlier positions and agreed to enactment of the Prescription Drug User Fee Act of 1992. Under this statute, FDA was authorised to collect user fees for five years based on annual fees levied for each pioneer prescription drug and each pioneer prescription drug establishment, as well as a one-time fee for each NDA for a pioneer new drug. The fees do not apply to generic or pioneer drugs after they become subject to generic competition. All of the revenue from these user fees is required to be in addition to the existing FDA budget and must be used solely for the IND/NDA review system. User fees were extended for another five years under the Food and Drug Modernization Act of 1997.[47]

8.4.18   The FDA Export Reform and Enhancement Act of 1996[48]

Following the November 1994 elections, in which the Republican Party won control of both the House of Representatives and the Senate for the first time in 40 years, Congress began to consider statutory reform of FDA in earnest. When the reform legislation became stalled in 1996, the provisions dealing with the export requirements of the FD&C Act were separated out and enacted. The 1996 Act repealed the Drug Export Amendments Act of 1986[49] and adopted a much more liberal and expansive approach. A drug that is not approved in the United States may now be exported to any country in the world if it complies with the laws of that country and has valid marketing authorisation by the appropriate authority in any country included in a new list of 25 countries with sophisticated regulatory systems. A drug that is not approved in the United States may be exported for investigational use in any listed country. FDA approval of the export of a drug that is not approved in the United States is required only if it is exported for investigational use in a non-listed country. Although the 1996 Act is a major improvement over the 1986 Act, the export provisions of the FD&C Act continue to be the most stringent in the world, and thus many United States companies continue to manufacture products abroad in order to avoid its cumbersome requirements.

8.4.19   The Food and Drug Administration Modernization Act of 1997[50]

One year after the drug export provisions of the FD&C Act were reformed, Congress enacted the remainder of the reform legislation that it had been considering. The Food and Drug Administration Modernization Act of 1997 is a lengthy, comprehensive and complex statute. Although the impact of this statute has been modest at best, it is the first since the FD&C Act was enacted in 1938 that has attempted significant reform. The following brief summary of the major provisions in the 1997 Act is sufficient to convey the broad scope of this legislation.

- Reauthorises prescription drug user fees for another five years.
- Establishes an additional six months of market exclusivity for paediatric studies of new drugs.
- Establishes a fast-track system for the study and approval of new drugs that address unmet medical needs related to serious or life-threatening conditions.
- Establishes a data bank in NIH to provide information on research relating to new drugs for serious or life-threatening diseases, for use by the general public.
- Establishes new criteria for permitting healthcare economic information relating to new drugs in labelling and advertising.
- Clarifies the requirements for NDA approval to say that data from one adequate and well-controlled study, together with confirmatory evidence, may, in the discretion of FDA, constitute substantial evidence of effectiveness of a new drug.
- Requires FDA to consult with NIH and representatives of the pharmaceutical industry to review and develop guidance on the inclusion of women and minorities in clinical trials.
- Adds a provision that is intended to reduce the number of post-market manufacturing changes requiring FDA approval and otherwise to make it easier to implement manufacturing changes for approved new drugs.

- Reduces the amount of information required to be submitted to FDA as part of an IND application.
- Clarifies the power of FDA to prevent or halt a clinical investigation of a new drug through use of a clinical hold.
- Requires FDA to issue guidance describing when abbreviated reports may be submitted in lieu of full reports for clinical and non-clinical studies required to be included in an NDA.
- Requires FDA to issue guidance for NDA reviewers relating to promptness in conducting the review, technical excellence, lack of bias and conflict of interest, and knowledge of regulatory and scientific standards.
- Requires FDA to meet with a sponsor upon reasonable written request for the purpose of reaching agreement on the design of pivotal trials, and provides that, after testing begins, the agreement cannot be changed unilaterally by FDA unless the director of the reviewing division issues a written decision that the change must be made because of a safety or effectiveness issue identified after the testing has begun.
- Provides that a decision by the reviewing division is binding on the FDA field and compliance personnel unless the reviewing division agrees to change its decision.
- States that no action of the reviewing division may be delayed based on a delay in action by field personnel.
- Provides for the use of scientific advisory committees to provide expert advice and recommendations to FDA regarding clinical investigation and approval of new drugs.
- Requires FDA to promulgate separate regulations governing the approval of radiopharmaceuticals.
- Amends the Public Health Service Act to eliminate the requirement of separate product and establishment licences and directs FDA to harmonise the review and approval requirements for biological products and new drugs to the extent possible.
- Provides that a drug manufactured in a pilot or other small-scale facility can be used to establish safety and effectiveness and to obtain marketing approval prior to scale-up unless FDA determines that a full-scale facility is necessary to ensure safety or effectiveness.
- Eliminates the separate regulatory requirements for insulin and antibiotics, and makes these drugs subject to the IND and NDA requirements.
- For prescription drugs, replaces the old label statement "Caution: Federal Law prohibits dispensing without a prescription" with a new "Rx Only" designation.
- Deletes the obsolete statutory provisions relating to labelling of 17 listed "habit-forming" drugs.
- Establishes an entire new programme to control pharmacy compounding.
- Reauthorises a clinical pharmacology programme in FDA.

221

- Establishes new requirements for phase IV studies which the manufacturer has agreed to conduct as a condition for NDA approval.
- Requires notice to FDA from the sole manufacturer of a life-supporting product six months before the manufacturer discontinues production.
- Establishes national uniformity in the regulation of non-prescription drugs.
- Requires the label of a non-prescription drug to bear the quantity or the proportion of each active ingredient.
- Requires the label of a non-prescription drug to bear the name of each inactive ingredient, listed in alphabetical order.
- Authorises manufacturers of new drugs to disseminate information on unapproved (off-label) uses of approved products under very limited conditions.
- Authorises expanded access to drugs that are still undergoing investigation for serious diseases and conditions.
- Attempts to reduce the disincentives to the submission of supplemental NDAs by reducing the cost and increasing the efficiency of handling them within FDA.
- Establishes dispute resolution mechanisms for the resolution of scientific controversies relating to new drugs.
- Requires FDA to promulgate a regulation regarding the development, issuance and use of guidance documents, and requires FDA to ensure that employees do not deviate from guidance without appropriate justification and supervisory concurrence.
- Establishes a statutory mission statement for FDA, which includes both the promotion of public health by taking appropriate action on the marketing of regulated products in a timely manner and the protection of public health by ensuring that regulated products are safe, effective and properly labelled.
- Requires FDA to publish a plan to bring the agency into compliance with each of the obligations established under the FD&C Act, and to review and revise the plan biennially.
- Requires FDA to publish an annual report in the Federal Register on its performance under the agency plan.
- Requires FDA to establish an information system regarding all submissions to the agency requesting agency action.
- Requires FDA to provide training and education programmes for employees relating to their regulatory responsibilities.
- Requires FDA to support the office of the United States Trade Representative to reduce the burden of regulation and harmonise international regulatory requirements consistent with the purposes of the FD&C Act.
- Requires FDA support of efforts to move toward the acceptance of mutual recognition agreements between the European Union and the United States.

- Requires FDA to participate in meetings with foreign governments to discuss and reach agreement on methods and approaches to harmonise regulatory requirements.
- Provides that an environmental impact statement prepared in accordance with the FDA regulations shall be considered to meet the requirements of the National Environmental Policy Act, notwithstanding any other provision of law.
- Requires FDA to implement programmes and policies that will foster collaboration between FDA, NIH and other science-based federal agencies in order to enhance the scientific and technical expertise available to FDA in discharging its duties with respect to regulating drugs.
- Authorises FDA to enter into contracts with any organisation or individual with relevant expertise to review and evaluate any application or submission for the approval or classification of an article, for the purpose of making recommendations to the agency on the matter.
- Provides that a person who submits an application or other submission under the FD&C Act may ask FDA for a determination respecting the proper regulatory classification of the product and the organisation within FDA that will regulate the product.
- Requires registration of foreign drug establishments.
- Establishes a rebuttable presumption of interstate commerce for drugs.
- Provides that any report or information relating to the safety of a drug that is submitted to FDA shall not be construed to reflect necessarily a conclusion that the report constitutes an admission that the product caused or contributed to an adverse experience.
- Repeals the former provision in the FD&C Act that prohibited any representation in labelling or advertising that FDA had approved an application for a new drug.

Only some of these provisions have been implemented by FDA, and the full impact of most of them remains to be determined.

8.5 Other pharmaceutical products

In addition to biological and chemical drugs, two other categories of pharmaceutical product deserve brief mention: animal drugs and human medical devices. Both are beyond the scope of the present chapter.

8.5.1 Animal drugs

Under the Federal Food and Drugs Act of 1906 and the FD&C Act of 1938 animal feed and drugs were regulated under the same provisions as human food and drugs. A separate statute, the Animal Virus, Serum, and Toxin Act of 1913,[51] was enacted by Congress to authorise USDA to regulate biological drugs intended for use in animals, and USDA retains jurisdiction over that statute to this day. To simplify FDA regulation of animal feed and drugs, Congress enacted the Animal Drug Amendments of 1968.[52] Following the approach of the 1984 statute authorising FDA approval of generic versions of human new drugs, Congress also enacted the Generic Animal Drug and Patent Term Restoration Act of 1988.[53]

8.5.2 Medical devices

Medical devices were first made subject to FDA regulation under the FD&C Act of 1938. At that time, the statute included no requirement for pre-market testing or approval. Congress enacted the Medical Device Amendments of 1976[54] to require pre-market notification for all medical devices, and pre-market approval for some old and new devices for which there is no adequate assurance of safety and effectiveness. The 1976 Amendments established a broad new array of statutory requirements and enforcement provisions. This new regulatory approach was supplemented by the Safe Medical Devices Act of 1990[55] and further refined by the Medical Device Amendments of 1992[56] and the Food and Drug Administration Modernization Act of 1997.[57]

8.6   Two classes of drug products

There are two classes of drug under the FD&C Act in the United States: non-prescription and prescription. Neither the Federal Food and Drugs Act of 1906 nor the FD&C Act of 1938 distinguished between non-prescription and prescription drugs or established a class of mandatory prescription drugs. Shortly after the FD&C Act was enacted in 1938, however, FDA promulgated regulations establishing criteria for a class of drugs that could only lawfully be sold by prescription.[58] Those regulations were later codified into law by Congress in the Durham–Humphrey Amendments of 1951.[59] Under this statute, prescription status is mandatory for drugs that are not safe for use except under a practitioner's supervision, and drugs limited to prescription sale under an NDA. The statutory criteria for determining prescription status are toxicity, other potential for harmful effect, and the method of use and collateral measures necessary to use the drug. In all instances today, the prescription or non-prescription status of a new drug is determined by the NDA.

A drug may be switched from prescription to non-prescription status.[60] Prior to 1970 this was most often accomplished by FDA promulgation of a regulation. During 1970–1990, a switch from prescription to non-prescription was most frequently accomplished as part of the FDA OTC Drug Review, discussed in detail below. Now that the OTC Drug Review is substantially complete, and with the availability of market exclusivity under the Drug Price Competition and Patent Term Restoration Act of 1984, a switch from prescription to non-prescription status is accomplished primarily through a supplemental NDA.

Non-prescription drugs may be sold at any kind of retail store in the United States, ranging from a pharmacy to a grocery store to a gasoline filling station. There are no criteria or limitations on their method of distribution and sale. Pharmacy groups have contended that FDA should establish a "third class" of drugs that would be available only through a pharmacy, and have used as one example of the need for such a new class those prescription drugs that are in the process of being switched to non-prescription status. FDA has declined to establish such a third class, on both policy and legal grounds.[61] First, FDA has stated that any drug switched by the agency from prescription to non-prescription status is sufficiently safe for sale in any retail establishment, and that a requirement limiting sale to a pharmacy would provide an unjustified monopoly to pharmacists. Second, FDA has stated that the FD&C Act provides no authority for FDA to restrict distribution of a non-prescription drug to pharmacies.

8.7   Regulation of non-prescription drugs

8.7.1   Adulteration and misbranding

Since 1906, the adulteration or misbranding of a non-prescription drug has been illegal in the United States.[62] Both "adulteration" and "misbranding" are terms of art, defined in the FD&C Act. Adulteration includes such acts as the failure to comply with good manufacturing practices; the use of a container that may render the contents injurious to health; the use of an illegal colour additive; failure to comply with *United States Pharmacopeia* requirements; failure to meet labelled strength or purity; and related prohibited acts. Misbranding includes such labelling violations as any false or misleading labelling; the failure to contain mandatory information relating to the name and address of the manufacturer and the net quantity of contents; the failure to bear adequate directions for use and warnings against unsafe use; the failure to meet packaging and labelling requirements established by the *United States Pharmacopeia*; the failure to use packaging and labelling to reduce product deterioration; danger to health when used as recommended in the labelling; the failure to obtain batch certification for an antibiotic for which such certification is required; and the failure to comply with a large number of other statutory requirements, including drug establishment registration and product listing, and poison prevention and tamper-resistant packaging. The adulteration and misbranding provisions of the statute itself are continually expanded by FDA regulations that impose additional requirements either for all non-prescription drugs or for specific categories. Accordingly, current requirements can be determined only by consulting FDA regulations and other policy statements, as well as the statute itself.

225

8.7.2 The IND/NDA system

Since 1938, non-prescription drugs have been subject to the new drug provisions of the Act as well as the adulteration and misbranding provisions. As a practical matter, however, the new drug provisions cover only those non-prescription drugs that have been switched from prescription status through a supplemental NDA. Almost all new chemical entity drugs are initially restricted by FDA to prescription status. Only a handful of new chemical entity drugs that require an NDA – perhaps one per decade – are marketed initially with non-prescription status. For those non-prescription drugs that do go through the IND/NDA system, the requirements are no different than for a prescription drug. These requirements are discussed in detail below.

8.7.3 The OTC drug review

During the period beginning with enactment of the new drug provisions in the FD&C Act in 1938 and ending with enactment of the Drug Amendments of 1962, there were approximately 420 NDAs for non-prescription drugs. Many of these NDAs were for long-established ingredients for which no NDA was actually required, but it was so simple to obtain an effective NDA during that time that many were submitted simply to obtain a perceived marketing advantage. As part of the Drug Amendments of 1962, FDA was required to review these 420 NDAs and to determine whether the drugs were effective as well as safe. Rather than limit its inquiry to these 420 specific non-prescription drug products, FDA decided instead to broaden the scope of its review to all active ingredients used in all non-prescription drugs on the market at that time. The agency also decided to review the safety and labelling as well as the effectiveness of the active ingredients in these products.

In 1972, FDA announced the beginning of its massive Over-the-Counter (OTC) Drug Review – the largest and most extensive review of the safety, effectiveness and labelling of non-prescription drugs ever undertaken.[63] FDA established panels of experts to review individual categories of non-prescription drugs and to prepare reports on their conclusions and recommendations. Those reports were published as proposed monographs establishing the conditions for safe, effective and properly labelled non-prescription drugs within each category. Following public comment, FDA published a tentative final monograph. Following additional public comment and a public hearing before the Commissioner, FDA established the final monograph. The documents that comprise these public proceedings represent an extremely important record of the status of non-prescription drug active ingredients and finished products in the United States.

By the early 1980s, all of the FDA panels had completed their deliberations and issued their reports. Because the industry largely followed the conclusions and recommendations of these reports, most of the impact of the OTC Drug Review has already been reflected in the marketplace. Nonetheless, a number of monographs remain to be completed and it will be some years before the OTC Drug Review is fully finished.

An OTC drug monograph establishes those conditions under which a non-prescription drug is generally recognised as safe and effective and properly labelled, and thus may be lawfully marketed in the United States without the need for an NDA or any other type of FDA approval. Any person may market a non-prescription drug in the United States today in compliance with one of these monographs (or, where no final monograph has been issued, in accordance with a tentative final monograph). One of the major purposes behind the OTC Drug Review was to establish, by regulations, the criteria under which an NDA is not required. Where a product is marketed with any deviation from an OTC drug monograph, however, some form of NDA is required in order to justify that deviation before marketing will be permitted.[64] In short, complete compliance with an OTC drug monograph guarantees immediate marketing without any form of pre-market approval. Of course, all non-prescription drugs must comply with the general adulteration and misbranding provisions of the law, including good manufacturing practices (GMP), establishment registration, and drug listing.

8.7.4 Tamper-resistant packaging

In September 1982 it was discovered that several people living in Chicago had died from cyanide poisoning after taking Extra-Strength Tylenol capsules. FDA promptly promulgated regulations requiring tamper-resistant packaging for most non-prescription drug products.[65] Congress followed by enacting the Federal Anti-Tampering Act of 1983,[66] which makes it a crime to tamper with a consumer product with reckless disregard for the risk of persons or with intent to cause injury to a business. A number of individuals have in fact been prosecuted for illegal tampering under this statute.

8.7.5 Non-prescription drug labelling

Based on an extensive rulemaking, FDA promulgated regulations in March 1999 establishing completely new labelling requirements for all non-prescription drug products.[67] The new regulations require the use of a "drug facts" box using a standardised format and type size. The new labelling requirements are being phased in, in coordination with the development of final monographs for non-prescription drugs. Industry has petitioned FDA for modification of some of the new requirements, and changes may be adopted through revision of the new labelling regulations, revisions of individual monographs, or the issuance of guidance.

8.7.6 Non-prescription drug advertising

In 1914, Congress enacted a statute to prohibit unfair methods of competition and created the Federal Trade Commission to implement this new law.[68] The FTC and the courts interpreted unfair methods of competition to include false or misleading labelling and advertising of non-prescription drugs and other consumer products. In 1933, when the legislation that became the FD&C Act was first introduced, it proposed to transfer the jurisdiction over food and drug advertising from the FTC to FDA. Not surprisingly, the FTC objected. Congress ultimately resolved this controversy in 1938, by enacting both the Wheeler–Lea Amendments to the FTC Act[69] and the FD&C Act. Congress gave the FTC jurisdiction over advertising and FDA jurisdiction over labelling. Because the FTC was also given jurisdiction over all unfair or deceptive acts or practices, however, it has jurisdiction over labelling as well as advertising. And because the courts have agreed with FDA that the agency may refer to advertising to determine the proper regulatory classification and requirements for a product under the FD&C Act, FDA to some extent indirectly regulates advertising. To clarify the situation, in September 1971 the FTC and FDA entered into a Memorandum of Understanding.[70] Under this agreement, the FTC has primary jurisdiction over advertising and FDA has primary jurisdiction over labelling of non-prescription drugs and other FDA-regulated products.

8.7.7 Industry self regulation

The Consumer Healthcare Products Association (CHPA), the United States trade association representing the non-prescription drug industry, has established a number of voluntary codes and guidelines to supplement FDA regulation of non-prescription drugs. Among these are recommended package sizes for non-prescription drug categories, label "flags" to bring the attention of consumers to significant product changes, bulk mail sampling of non-prescription drugs, expiry dating of non-prescription drugs, product identification of solid dosage non-prescription drugs, and label readability for non-prescription drugs. Although these are not legal requirements, they are widely followed in the non-prescription drug industry.

8.8 Regulation of prescription drugs

It is particularly difficult to summarise FDA regulation of prescription drugs. The statutory provisions are long and complex, the regulations consume hundreds of pages in the Code of Federal Regulations, the preambles cover thousands of pages in the Federal Register, and the guidelines and policy directives are numerous and diverse. The discussion will therefore begin with an historical overview of the development of FDA regulation of prescription drugs. This is followed by a brief analysis of how the current system works.

This section is limited to drugs regulated under the FD&C Act. Biological drugs are considered in the next section.

8.8.1   Historical overview[71]

As enacted in 1938, the FD&C Act defined a "new drug" as any drug that was not generally recognised as safe.[72] Section 505 of the 1938 Act provided that an NDA must be submitted for every new drug, and authorised FDA to permit an NDA to become effective or to disapprove it, but not affirmatively to approve an NDA. If FDA took no action within 60 days after the filing of an NDA, the NDA automatically became effective and the drug could lawfully be marketed.

During the first few years after 1938 the pharmaceutical industry submitted thousands of NDAs. Because FDA was unprepared to deal with this large number, it advised drug manufacturers that NDAs were not required for "old drugs" that were generally recognised as safe (GRAS), and in fact refused to accept NDAs for these drugs. This substantially reduced the numbers of NDAs that were submitted to and accepted by FDA. For example, more than 4000 NDAs had been submitted by 1941 but by 1962 NDAs for only 9457 individual drug products had become effective. Most prescription drugs were marketed on the conclusion of FDA or the manufacturer that they were GRAS, and hence old drugs that did not require an NDA.

Following enactment of the Drug Amendments of 1962, FDA immediately encountered two problems. First, the pharmaceutical industry submitted a substantially increased number of INDs and NDAs, which again overwhelmed the resources of FDA to deal with them. Second, the 1962 Amendments required FDA to review all of the NDAs that had become effective between 1938 and 1962 on the basis of a demonstration of safety, and to determine whether these drugs were also effective. Because of the overwhelming number of current INDs and NDAs for new products, FDA had no resources to devote to this requirement. Accordingly, in June 1966 FDA contracted with the National Academy of Sciences (NAS) to conduct the review of 1938–1962 NDAs.

The NAS review was conducted by panels of experts in specific drug categories. Drugs were rated in one or other of the following six categories: (1) effective, (2) probably effective, (3) possibly effective, (4) ineffective, (5) effective but other drugs are preferable, or (6) ineffective as a fixed combination. Because roughly half of the drugs were no longer marketed, the NAS ultimately reviewed approximately 4000 different drug formulations. Brief reports, many consisting only of a single sentence, were transmitted to FDA by the NAS in 1967–1968. FDA then undertook to implement these reports in the form of notices published in the Federal Register as part of what the agency called the Drug Efficacy Study Implementation (DESI) programme.

In order to implement the NAS reports, FDA found that it must first address a number of important policy issues. First, FDA was required to determine whether the NAS findings would apply only to the pioneer drug for which the NDA was submitted or would also apply to all subsequently marketed generic versions of the drug. FDA determined that the latter approach was required, which led to extensive litigation. The FDA policy on this matter was ultimately upheld by the Supreme Court in June 1973.[73]

Second, FDA had to confront the fact that prior to the 1962 Amendments it had issued hundreds of "old drug" opinion letters for generic versions of pioneer new drugs. It therefore issued a statement of policy in May 1968 revoking all of those opinions.[74]

Third, FDA was confronted with potentially thousands of requests for formal trial-type administrative hearings before it could remove from the market pre-1962 new drugs that were found to be less than effective. The requirement of formal administrative hearings would have effectively precluded implementation of the 1962 Amendments. FDA resolved this by publishing in the Federal Register regulations defining the new statutory requirement of adequate and well controlled clinical investigations,[75] and issuing summary judgement notices withdrawing approval of new drugs that failed to submit clinical studies which seemingly met the requirements of the new regulations. The regulations defining adequate and well controlled clinical investigations were upheld in the courts, and the summary judgement procedure was also upheld.[76] Thus, the number of drugs for which formal administrative hearings were required was substantially reduced.

Fourth, FDA established a new procedure for regulating generic versions of pre-1962 pioneer drugs that were found under the DESI programme to be safe and effective. FDA established the "abbreviated" NDA, which required the submission of information to FDA on bioequivalence and manufacturing controls only, and not on basic safety and effectiveness.[77] Any manufacturer who wished to market a generic version of a pre-1962 pioneer drug found to be safe and effective under the NAS review could obtain FDA approval through an abbreviated NDA.

In 1972, 10 years after the 1962 Amendments were enacted, three lower court rulings threatened to destroy the FDA approach to these matters. The agency successfully took all three cases, as well as a fourth in which FDA had prevailed, to the United States Supreme Court, and in June 1973 the Supreme Court sustained FDA on all of the legal issues involved.[78] From then on, the basic approach to FDA implementation of the 1962 Amendments was established and strengthened.

The FDA pace of implementation of the 1962 Amendments was, however, necessarily slow. The American Public Health Association therefore brought a lawsuit to require FDA to complete its DESI programme for pre-1962 new drugs, and the federal district court entered an order requiring completion within four years.[79] Although FDA to this day has still not completed this programme, the court order did impose a greater sense of urgency and led FDA to devote greater resources to the matter.

Throughout this time, FDA was groping for a consistent approach to the handling of generic drugs. Initially, it revoked all "old drug" opinion letters. Later, it proposed a procedure for determining old drug status for products.[80] Following that, it concluded that an abbreviated NDA should be submitted for all generic versions of pre-1962 new drugs.[81] In 1975, it again reversed itself and decided to develop old drug monographs, similar to the non-prescription drug monographs, for which an NDA would not be required.[82] Still later, it abandoned that approach and again stated that an abbreviated NDA would be required for all generic versions of pre-1962 new drugs.[83] That position was challenged in the courts, but was upheld by the Supreme Court.[84]

An attempt was made during 1977–1980 to resolve all of these issues through a comprehensive revision of the new drug provisions of the FD&C Act. The legislation passed the Senate in 1979[85] but did not reach the floor of the House and, because the legislation was so detailed and complex, it was never again seriously considered.

By 1980, a new problem had emerged. FDA had administratively created the concept of an abbreviated NDA to handle generic versions of pre-1962 pioneer new drugs, but there was no similar mechanism for the approval of generic versions of post-1962 new drugs. As time went by, more and more post-1962 pioneer new drugs lost patent protection, but retained an equivalent protection under the FD&C Act because FDA had no authority to approve any form of an abbreviated NDA for generic versions of these drugs. FDA therefore began to search for a solution to this problem. In 1978, FDA announced it would approve a "paper" NDA for a generic copy of a post-1962 pioneer new drug based on the published scientific data for the drug. This policy was upheld in the courts,[86] but it had relatively little impact because there were insufficient published animal and human data to approve generic versions of most post-1962 new drugs. Thus, relatively few paper NDAs were approved by FDA.

Another drug tragedy in early 1984 focused FDA on yet another aspect of regulating prescription new drugs. An intravenous vitamin E product marketed without an NDA produced serious adverse reactions that required a nationwide recall.[87] FDA concluded that there were approximately 5000 prescription drugs marketed without an approved NDA of any kind. Some 1800 would eventually be subject to the requirement for an abbreviated NDA when the DESI programme was fully implemented, but another 2400 were never subject to the NAS review because they were on the market prior to the FD&C Act of 1938, or were otherwise grandfathered. FDA was forced to concede that these products could remain on the market until the agency could find the resources to review them and consider appropriate regulation.[88] Indeed, new versions of these products can still be marketed as long as they are identical to the previously marketed versions. FDA did promulgate a regulation requiring adverse drug reaction reports for all prescription drugs marketed without an approved NDA, in order to track any potential public health problem.[89]

In the past two decades, FDA has proceeded slowly but surely with the DESI programme implementing the NAS review of pre-1962 new drugs.

Where drugs have been found ineffective, most have been taken off the market using the summary judgement procedure. A few manufacturers have succeeded in requiring an administrative hearing, but none has prevailed before an administrative law judge, the Commissioner, or the courts.

In a surprisingly large number of instances, manufacturers decided to market new drugs without any NDA, and outside the 1984 FDA policy that permits such products if they are identical to old products that never had an NDA, solely on the basis that they were old drugs because they were generally recognised as safe and effective (GRAS and GRAE) and therefore did not require an approved NDA. FDA brought enforcement actions against dozens of these products, and because the agency prevailed in every case, this approach is rarely tried today.

As indicated above, the status of generic versions of both pre-1962 and post-1962 new drugs was settled by Congress in the Drug Price Competition and Patent Term Restoration Act of 1984.[90] That statute will be discussed in greater detail below.

Accordingly, the large conceptual issues that confronted FDA following enactment of the Drug Amendments of 1962 have now been resolved, and most (but not all) of the large categories of DESI prescription drug products on the market have been brought under regulatory control. The major category of products that remains without any form of NDA approval are the approximately 2400 pre-1962 new drugs that were never the subject of an NDA and for which FDA has not yet conducted some form of regulatory review.

8.8.2 Regulatory categories of prescription drugs

There are two primary categories of prescription drug: those not currently subject to any form of NDA approval, and those subject to some form of NDA approval.

8.8.2.1 No NDA

Those not subject to any form of NDA approval consist largely of products for which an NDA has never been required or obtained, and which thus were not subject to the NAS review of 1938–1962 new drugs. This is a limited category.

In its 1984 policy statement[91] FDA stated that until some form of regulatory control was instituted new versions of these drugs could be marketed only if the new version was in all significant respects identical to the old version. The life of one of these products is, of course, uncertain. FDA could at any time decide to regulate any or all of these products in a more comprehensive way. The precise status of any of these drugs can be determined only by a detailed review of all of the facts available for the specific product involved.

8.8.2.2   Three forms of NDA

The vast bulk of prescription drugs on the market today are subject to the requirement for some form of an approved NDA. Following enactment of the Drug Price Competition and Patent Term Restoration Act of 1984, there are now three clearly established types of NDA: a full NDA, a paper NDA (now called a Section 505(b)(2) NDA, after the provision in the FD&C Act that created it), and an abbreviated NDA. Each of these is discussed in the sections that follow.

8.8.2.2.1   The full NDA   For any new chemical entity drug, whether or not it has been first marketed abroad, and whether or not it is chemically related to some other approved new drug, FDA requires compliance with the full IND/NDA process.

8.8.2.2.1.1   The IND[92]   Before submitting an NDA to FDA, the sponsor of a drug must conduct, or arrange to be conducted, various types of non-clinical (in vitro and animal) tests and clinical (human) studies designed to demonstrate that the drug is safe and effective for its intended use.

For non-human studies no IND is required. Companies may perform in vitro testing for example to obtain chemical information necessary to set exact specifications for the active ingredient or to obtain stability data. The company may also conduct animal toxicology tests to establish an adequate margin of human safety. Animal toxicology testing must be conducted in accordance with the FDA good laboratory practice (GLP) regulations,[93] but no IND or any other type of notice to FDA is required for any type of non-human studies. FDA also has both formal and informal guidelines to govern animal toxicity testing.

After adequate preclinical testing has been completed, an IND must be submitted to FDA to justify clinical investigation in humans. The content and format of an IND are set out in detail in the FDA regulations, and therefore need not be repeated here. The IND must contain all relevant information about the safety and effectiveness of the new drug, the protocols intended to be used in the investigations, the chemistry, manufacturing and control information, pharmacology and toxicology information, previous human experience, and other pertinent information. In all respects, the FDA IND regulations must be followed in detail.

After submission, FDA has 30 days within which to evaluate the IND. By the end of 30 days, one of several things will have occurred. First, FDA may approve the IND, in which case testing can begin. Second, FDA may place the IND on formal clinical hold, in which case testing cannot begin.[94] Third, FDA may say nothing, or may raise questions, or may offer suggestions, or may say virtually anything in response to the IND. The sponsor must then determine whether to proceed in light of these developments, or to delay testing until the matter is clarified. Many sponsors conclude that the only reasonable thing to do is to delay testing until all issues are fully resolved, but others proceed in the face of open questions.

Once the initial 30-day period has expired, the IND may be amended and updated periodically. For example, additional protocols may be added. There is no 30-day delay for any subsequent amendment. Once again, however, sponsors must determine whether to delay testing until FDA is consulted and any issues are fully resolved.

An essential element of the IND is approval of the investigation by an institutional review board (IRB), either constituted by the institution in which the drug will be tested or established as a for-profit private IRB.[95] The IRB is charged with reviewing the ethical and moral dimensions of the study as well as the scientific merit. IRB approval does not guarantee FDA approval, nor does FDA approval guarantee IRB approval. They are separate and independent requirements, and both must be fulfilled before testing may begin under an IND.

Adherence to the IND by the sponsor is essential: deviations from any aspect of it are not permitted. Before there can be any change in any aspect of the IND – including the specifications of the drug, the nature of the manufacturing process, the protocol for the investigation and the identity of the investigators, to name just a few – the IND must be amended.

No investigational new drug may be promoted or otherwise commercialised. No charge may be made for an investigational new drug without the prior approval of FDA.

The FDA IND regulations contain requirements for various types of records and reports, which must be adhered to without exception.[96] Immediate reports to FDA are required for any serious and unexpected adverse experience associated with the drug. Annual reports are required for every IND. Records must be kept to document all aspects of the IND.

Clinical testing under an IND is usually regarded as proceeding through three phases. Phase I includes the initial introduction of an investigational new drug into humans under closely monitored conditions, usually in a teaching hospital. This phase involves a relatively small number of subjects and is intended to obtain basic information on the pharmacology of the drug. Phase II includes controlled clinical studies conducted to evaluate the effectiveness and optimum dosage of the drug, and to determine common side effects and other risks. It involves a greater number of subjects, but is not a large-scale trial. Phase III involves expanded controlled and uncontrolled trials to gather additional information about safety and effectiveness that is needed to evaluate the overall benefit–risk relationship, and may involve up to several thousand subjects. In recent years, these three phases have tended to overlap substantially, and approval has been obtained on the basis of Phase II or Phase II/III studies for a number of important drugs.

Three types of unusual IND situations deserve special mention. First, the regulations contain a provision governing emergency use of an investigational new drug, where FDA will permit such use by telephone or other rapid communication means.[97] In these situations, the IND must subsequently be amended to reflect the new situation. Second, FDA will approve specific treatment protocols for compassionate use of an investigational new drug where the drug is intended to treat a serious or immediately life-threatening disease, there is no satisfactory alternative, the drug is under clinical investigation pursuant to an IND, and marketing approval is actively being pursued with due diligence.[98] After a treatment IND has been approved, the sponsor may provide the drug to any patient who meets the criteria in the treatment IND, and may charge in order to recoup the cost of the drug. Third, FDA will approve "parallel track" protocols for AIDS where there is no therapeutic alternative and individuals cannot participate in the controlled clinical trials, in order to assure widespread use of the most promising drugs at the earliest possible stage.[99] As a practical matter, it is difficult, if not impossible, to distinguish between a parallel track IND and a treatment IND.

Compassionate use of investigational new drugs has been permitted by FDA since the 1950s in order to assure that individual patients who have no other alternative are not denied any promising treatment. The more recent terminology of "treatment IND" and "parallel track" is therefore simply a continuation of this long-standing policy, with no significant substantive change. In addition to these new forms of compassionate-use INDs, the pharmaceutical industry continues to use the traditional form of compassionate-use protocol as well.

8.8.2.2.1.2 The NDA[100] After the sponsor has completed all non-clinical and clinical testing necessary to demonstrate the safety and effectiveness of the drug, the test results must be compiled in an NDA for submission to FDA. As with the IND, the content and format of the NDA are set forth in the FDA regulations and must be followed in detail. The NDA must begin with a summary, to be followed by technical sections relating to (1) chemistry, manufacturing and controls, (2) non-clinical pharmacology and toxicology, (3) human pharmacokinetics and bioavailability, (4) microbiology, (5) clinical data, and (6) statistics. Proposed labelling must also be included. The typical NDA comprises tens of thousands or even hundreds of thousands of pages.

The statute requires that a new drug be shown to be both safe and effective. Because no drug has ever been shown to be completely safe or effective, in all cases this has been interpreted to mean that the benefits of the drug outweigh its risks under the labelled conditions of use for a significant identified patient population. The statute is very broadly worded with respect to the required proof for safety and effectiveness, and FDA has exercised substantial discretion in applying these requirements. New drugs have been approved on the basis of only one study, on the basis of Phase II studies that have never progressed to Phase III, on the basis of foreign studies alone, and with results that could not be regarded as definitive from a scientific standpoint.

In most instances, FDA requires more than one adequate and well controlled clinical trial. In the FDA Modernization Act of 1997, however, Congress clarified the law by providing that FDA may base the approval of an NDA on data from one adequate and well controlled clinical investigation and confirmatory evidence.[101]

Under the FD&C Act, FDA has always been required to evaluate the NDA and approve or disapprove it within 180 days. Until 1992, this almost never occurred. The average time for approval of an NDA was between two and three years. This time remained largely unchanged for the years between 1962 and 1994, in spite of repeated promises and attempts by FDA to speed up the process. FDA was able to avoid the 180-day statutory time deadline in several ways. First, the agency started the clock when it accepted the NDA for filing, not when it was submitted. Second, FDA stopped the clock, and restarted it, whenever new submissions were made. Third, FDA requested an extension of time from the applicant, who had no choice but to agree. Fourth, FDA simply ignored the 180-day deadline, and there was nothing that the applicant could do about it anyway.

For many years it was proposed that user fees should be assessed on NDAs and that the proceeds should be used to hire sufficient FDA personnel to process applications more expeditiously. In 1992 the regulated industry and FDA finally agreed on this approach, and Congress enacted the Prescription Drug User Fee Act (PDUFA) of 1992.[102] PDUFA was initially authorised for five years, and was reauthorised for another five years under the FDA Modernization Act of 1997.[103] The legislation provides for three types of user fee: drug applications, drug products and drug establishments. These fees have allowed FDA to more than double the number of personnel reviewing NDAs. As a result, the time for NDA approval was initially halved. In 1999 and 2000, however, this trend has reversed and the time for approval has begun to increase significantly. PDUFA expires again in late 2002, and it is uncertain whether the statute will simply be extended or will be further revised in light of these recent developments. Reflecting this increase in approval time, FDA has begun to issue "approvable" letters within the user fee time guidelines, and then to take a substantial additional period to negotiate remaining issues (often including labelling) before a final approval letter is sent.

In response to criticism that the agency was not moving quickly enough to approve new drugs for AIDS and other serious or life-threatening illnesses, in 1992 FDA established regulations to establish an accelerated approval process.[104] This is commonly referred to as the subpart H process, after the designation in the FDA regulations. The regulations describe two subpart H procedures. Under the first, FDA is authorised to approve a new drug based on surrogate endpoint data if the sponsor agrees to conduct and submit data from post-marketing studies. Under the second procedure, FDA may grant accelerated approval to beneficial but highly toxic drugs if the sponsor agrees to post-approval distribution restrictions. Under the regulations, both of these procedures are voluntary. FDA has no legal authority to impose either procedure on an NDA sponsor.

Subsequent to the establishment of subpart H, Congress enacted separate "fast-track" procedures for new drugs to treat a serious or life-threatening condition that had the potential to address unmet medical needs under the FDA Modernization Act of 1997.[105] FDA is required to respond to requests for designation of new drugs as fast-track products within 60 days, and must expedite the development and review of a fast-track NDA. Approval may be based on a determination that the product has an effect on a clinical endpoint or on a surrogate endpoint. If it is based on a surrogate endpoint, post-approval studies can be required to confirm the effect on the clinical endpoint. The NDA sponsor must submit copies of all promotional materials prior to NDA approval and subsequently. Approval of a fast-track product may be withdrawn using expedited procedures. FDA has issued a guidance, but no regulations, to implement this provision.

Following market withdrawal of several new drugs because of toxicity that had not been uncovered in the non-clinical or IND studies, in 1998 FDA established a Task Force on Risk Management to evaluate the FDA system for managing the risks of FDA-approved medical products. The Task Force concluded that the rates of drug withdrawals and adverse events remain low, but recommended a new risk management approach in order better to identify and control these risks as early as possible in the NDA process.[106] Implementation of this report has had a substantial impact on the IND/NDA process. FDA reviewers are requiring more patients in clinical trials, longer follow-up and more trials. A number of NDAs that had been expected to obtain FDA approval were disapproved and will require additional evidence of safety and effectiveness. As already noted, the time for NDA approval has increased significantly following the release of the report. The release in late 1999 of the widely publicised Institute of Medicine report on the number of deaths caused by medication errors undoubtedly contributed to the new FDA wave of conservatism.[107] Patients have complained that their interests are not being considered, as drugs have been withdrawn or withheld because of concern about toxicity to a few individuals, and the benefits to large numbers of patients are not being taken into account.

During the NDA evaluation there are no guidelines or rules that require open communication between FDA and the applicant. It is impossible to generalise about the relationship between drug applicants and FDA reviewers. The Center for Drugs Evaluation and Research (CDER) review

237

divisions have quite varied reputations for openness, promptness and cordiality. Thus, discussion between an FDA review division and the applicant varies all the way from virtually no communication to constant discussion. Relations range from friendliness to near hostility. The NDA review process is, in short, entirely an ad hoc and informal process of negotiation that may go very well or very poorly, and over which the applicant has virtually no control. Attempts to obtain resolution of disputes through the FDA ombudsman or by appealing issues to higher officials are almost never successful, and often worsen relations with the NDA reviewers. Pharmaceutical companies uniformly fear retaliation unless they cooperate fully with every request from the NDA reviewers.

For every NDA, some clinical study is almost certain to remain in progress at the time when the NDA is submitted. Safety update reports are therefore required to be submitted to FDA by the applicant while the NDA is pending, and particularly following receipt of an approvable letter.[108] Detailed systems and procedures are required to ensure that the data in the NDA and the safety updates are accurate and complete, and failure to meet these requirements is regarded by FDA as a serious deficiency.

It is customary for FDA to submit one or more letters of disapproval as part of the NDA review process. These frequently lead to the submission of new information, a revision of labelling and further negotiation. In a relatively small number of cases, FDA will issue a definitive disapproval letter determining that there is no additional information on the basis of which the drug could be approved. There are then various administrative and judicial appeals that the applicant can make. In no instance since 1938, however, has any applicant successfully challenged FDA denial of approval of an NDA.[109] For this reason, it is generally understood that there is no practical way to challenge whatever FDA requires during the NDA process, and that the only realistic alternative is to negotiate the best possible approach with FDA in a cooperative spirit.

8.8.2.2.1.3 Confidentiality of information Under the Freedom of Information Act, all information in government files is subject to public disclosure unless it falls within a specified exemption.[110] Both the FD&C Act[111] and the Federal Trade Secrets Act[112] prohibit the public disclosure of confidential commercial information and trade secrets. FDA has promulgated detailed regulations governing the status of general categories of data and information in its files,[113] and particularly data and information submitted as part of an IND or NDA.[114] In general, no data or information submitted to FDA as part of an IND or NDA will be made public prior to FDA approval or disapproval of the NDA. Even the existence of an IND or NDA will be kept confidential by FDA if it has not been disclosed by the sponsor. Upon approval, FDA issues a summary of the basis for the agency approval of the product, which describes the safety and effectiveness data on which the agency relied.[115] Whether FDA will also release the reports and data relating to the testing for safety and effectiveness will depend upon whether the company can convince the agency that these data retain value as "confidential commercial information".[116] In general, FDA will release the full data and information on safety and effectiveness after a drug becomes subject to generic competition, but not before. Agency regulations spell out FDA's confidentiality policies in great detail, but there still are often disputes about their application to any particular set of facts.

8.8.2.2.1.4 Advisory committees There is no statutory requirement that FDA review the approval of an NDA with an advisory committee before final action is taken. Since the 1970s, however, this has been the customary practice, particularly with important new drugs. This prompted Congress to enact a specific provision dealing with the establishment of drug advisory committees under the FDA Modernization Act of 1997.[117]

The review of an NDA by an advisory committee is an extremely important step in the approval process. It represents the best opportunity that the applicant has to address the agency and the public about the evidence of safety and effectiveness and the importance of the drug to public health. In the vast majority of cases FDA accepts the recommendation of the advisory committee for approval, further testing, or outright disapproval. Where the advisory committee recommends approval and FDA disagrees, however, the agency will almost always take a long time to implement the advisory committee recommendations, or may even add additional testing requirements before approval is eventually obtained. The importance of advisory committee review is widely recognised in the pharmaceutical industry, and it is common for a company to engage in extensive preparation for the company presentation and to seek supportive statements from independent outside experts and patients as well.

8.8.2.2.1.5 Post-approval requirements Following approval of an NDA, FDA requires the submission of three different types of reports by the owner of the NDA.[118] First, serious and unexpected adverse drug experiences must be immediately reported to FDA regardless of whether or not the company believes they are causally related to the drug. Second, all adverse drug experiences, as well as other safety and effectiveness information, must be reported periodically to FDA, at intervals specified in the FDA regulations. Third, information relating to all other aspects of the drug must be reported immediately to FDA if they represent a potential problem, but otherwise may be included in an annual report. Foreign as well as domestic adverse experiences and other information must be included in these reports.

8.8.2.2.1.6 Changes in the NDA after approval Any significant change from the detailed terms and conditions specified in the approved NDA must be the subject of a supplemental NDA and cannot be put into effect until the supplemental NDA has been approved by FDA.[119] The only changes in an approved NDA that may be made without approval of a supplemental NDA are set forth in the FDA regulations, and those exceptions must be reflected in the annual report submitted to FDA. Where FDA finds that changes have been made from an approved NDA, beyond those permitted without a supplemental NDA, very stringent regulatory action can be taken, including recall of the product and the inability to manufacture any more product until the unapproved changes are eliminated or approved. Accordingly, it is essential that all aspects of an approved NDA be followed in detail unless a clear exception is created in the FDA regulations. In close cases, FDA should be consulted.

8.8.2.2.1.7 Summary suspension of approval The statute provides that the Secretary of HHS may summarily suspend approval of an NDA upon a finding that the drug represents an imminent hazard to the public health.[120] This authority is delegated to the Secretary of HHS alone, and cannot be exercised by FDA or anyone else. It has been used only once, and its use was upheld in the courts.[121]

8.8.2.2.1.8 Antibiotic drugs New antibiotic drugs are subject to the same IND and NDA requirements contained in the FDA regulations as other new drugs. Although the FD&C Act initially provided that FDA could require batch certification for antibiotics, in 1982 FDA exempted all classes of antibiotic drugs from this requirement because of the high level of manufacturer compliance with antibiotic standards. Because the FDA Modernization Act of 1997 repealed the old antibiotic provisions of the FD&C Act,[122] antibiotics today are regulated in basically the same way as all other new drugs.

8.8.2.2.1.9 User fees Under the Prescription Drug User Fee Act of 1992, as extended five more years by the FDA Modernization Act of 1997, FDA has authority to collect user fees for pioneering drugs until such time as generic competition is approved.[123] The fees include (1) a one-time NDA fee, (2) an annual product fee, and (3) an annual establishment fee. The precise amount of each fee escalates each year and is subject to modification according to detailed provisions in the statute. The funds obtained from these fees must be in addition to the existing congressionally appropriated resources for the IND/NDA system as adjusted for cost-of-living increases, and must be used solely for the IND/NDA process. In return for receiving user fees, FDA has committed to specific goals for improving the drug review process, by reducing the backlog of applications, meeting specified time deadlines, and making improvements in the process. The extent to which these commitments can be kept will become apparent only in the coming years.

8.8.2.2.2   The paper NDA   When Congress enacted the Drug Price Competition and Patent Term Restoration Act of 1984, it included a provision based on the concept of a paper NDA but which in fact expanded that concept significantly. The former paper NDA is therefore now called a Section 505(b)(2) NDA, after the statutory provision that creates it.[124] It applies to those situations where a pioneer drug is no longer protected by patents or market exclusivity but where an applicant is unable to submit an abbreviated NDA because the modified drug differs in some substantial way from the pioneer drug. A Section 505(b)(2) NDA relies upon the pioneer NDA for all information except the data needed to support the element of substantial difference. Thus, the Section 505(b)(2) NDA need not include any data relating to the basic safety and effectiveness of the drug, except insofar as the difference between the pioneer drug and the applicant's modification of that drug bears upon safety or effectiveness.

As will be discussed below, minor differences between a pioneer drug and a generic version of that drug may be approved by FDA as appropriate for an abbreviated NDA pursuant to a "suitability petition". Where those differences become substantial, however, FDA will deny the suitability petition and will require the approval of a more complete NDA. In these circumstances the Section 505(b)(2) paper NDA will be sufficient, and a full NDA will not be required. Thus, the Section 505(b)(2) NDA is midway between a full NDA and an abbreviated NDA. The same regulations and requirements apply to a Section 505(b)(2) paper NDA under the 1984 Act as apply to a full NDA.

8.8.2.2.3   The abbreviated NDA   All of the regulations and requirements for an abbreviated NDA developed by FDA in the late 1960s as part of the implementation of the Drug Amendments of 1962, and all of the proposed changes that FDA considered to adapt those requirements to post-1962 new drugs, were eliminated when Congress enacted the Drug Price Competition and Patent Term Restoration Act of 1984. The 1984 Act established detailed requirements that supersede everything that went before.[125]

Under the 1984 Act, an abbreviated NDA may be approved by FDA for a generic version of a pioneer new drug after (1) all relevant product and use patents have expired for the pioneer drug, and (2) all relevant periods of market exclusivity for the pioneer drug have also expired. The statute contains detailed and complex rules for determining precisely how this system works. No attempt will be made here to discuss the specific provisions, but they are extremely important in determining the commercial value of a pioneer new drug because they govern when the drug will become subject to generic competition. Of particular importance, Congress expanded the length of protection granted under the 1984 Act in the FDA Modernization Act of 1997, by providing an extra six months of market exclusivity at the end of the extended patent term (or market exclusivity term, if the patent has already expired) when the sponsor conducts paediatric testing requested and approved by FDA.[126]

There are basically two types of situation where an abbreviated NDA may be submitted. The first situation is where the generic version is the same as the pioneer version in all material respects. Where this is true, the applicant for the generic product simply submits the abbreviated NDA and FDA may approve it without further consideration about the basic safety and effectiveness of the drug. The second circumstance is where the generic version is different from the pioneer drug in any significant respect (for example a different active ingredient, route of administration, dosage form or strength). In these circumstances, the generic applicant must first submit to FDA a "suitability petition" demonstrating that the difference between the drugs is not sufficient to preclude an abbreviated NDA, and that additional studies to show safety and effectiveness are not needed. If FDA grants the suitability petition, an abbreviated NDA may be submitted. If the suitability petition is denied, the applicant must submit either a Section 505(b)(2) paper NDA or a full NDA. In all other respects the regulations and requirements for an abbreviated NDA are the same as those for a full NDA.

8.8.3 The Applications Integrity (Fraud) Policy

As a result of the generic drug scandal described above, where generic drug manufacturers submitted fraudulent data and bribed FDA officials, in September 1991 FDA adopted a "fraud policy", later called the Applications Integrity Policy, to cover situations where FDA concluded that an applicant who had engaged in a wrongful act would need to take corrective action to establish the reliability of data submitted to FDA in support of pending applications and to support the integrity of products already on the market.[127] Under this policy, FDA issues a formal letter invoking the policy and requiring the applicant to cooperate fully with the FDA investigation. The applicant is required to identify all individuals associated with the wrongful act and to ensure that they are removed from any substantive authority on matters under FDA jurisdiction. A credible internal review must be conducted to identify all instances of wrongful acts, to supplement FDA's own investigation. The internal review should involve an outside consultant or team qualified by training and experience to conduct such a review. Finally, the applicant must commit in writing to developing and implementing a corrective action operating plan. Although this fraud policy was developed in response to the generic drug scandal, it also applies to pioneer drug companies and to data in full NDAs.

8.8.4 Labelling and advertising

The labelling for a new drug must be included as part of the NDA and must be explicitly approved by FDA. No significant change may be made in the labelling without prior FDA approval through a supplemental NDA. Because this rule is so clear and so stringent, the pharmaceutical industry seldom takes chances with deviations in product labelling that could result in FDA enforcement action.

The Drug Amendments of 1962 gave FDA the authority to regulate advertising for prescription drugs, as well as labelling.[128] However, the FD&C Act was not amended to give FDA pre-market approval over advertising, similar to its pre-market approval over labelling. Accordingly, FDA must rely upon general policing of prescription drug advertising to determine whether it is false or misleading.

In accordance with its statutory authority, FDA has promulgated regulations that illustrate ways in which prescription drug advertising may be false, lacking in fair balance, or otherwise misleading.[129] As the pharmaceutical industry has expanded its promotional activities, FDA has also issued a variety of policy statements on various types of advertising practice that do not fall within the existing regulations. These policy statements deal with such issues as press conferences, medical seminars, journal supplements, TV and radio talk shows, and a wide variety of other means of communication.[130] It is essential that anyone engaging in prescription drug marketing be fully familiar with the latest FDA policy in these areas.

A recent innovation has been direct-to-consumer (DTC) prescription drug promotion in the broadcast media. Because FDA regulations require a summary of the entire approved package insert to appear with any prescription drug advertisement, it was extremely difficult to use radio or television advertising for this purpose. Most consumer advertising for prescription drugs was therefore limited to the print media. Beginning in July 1997, however, FDA has issued guidance that allows the package insert requirement to be satisfied with more flexible ways to provide the same information to consumers.[131] This has resulted in an explosion of DTC prescription drug advertising on television. FDA reviews these advertisements very carefully, and thus caution must be used in preparing them. It is sound practice to review proposed advertising of this type with FDA prior to its use.

8.8.5   Good manufacturing practices (GMP)

One of the most important parts of an NDA is the description of the chemistry, manufacturing and controls (CMC).[132] FDA has traditionally placed substantial reliance upon this part of the NDA in ensuring the safety and effectiveness of the drug. One study conducted a decade ago found that more questions were raised by FDA reviewers about this section of the NDA than about the safety and effectiveness of the drug itself.

Beginning in 1991, moreover, FDA announced a new enforcement technique designed to assure adequate GMP compliance before an NDA is approved.[133] Prior to FDA approval of the NDA, the FDA field force now conducts a pre-approval inspection (PAI) of the establishment where the new drug is to be manufactured. If the manufacturing facility deviates in any way from either the description in the NDA or the general requirements for GMP in the FDA regulations,[134] the NDA will be held hostage and will not be approved until full compliance is achieved. Pursuant to this policy, the approval of numerous NDAs has been substantially delayed. Compliance with GMP is therefore essential to any NDA approval. Because of widespread concern about this practice, Congress included in the FDA Modernization Act of 1997 a specific provision stating that an NDA approval may not be delayed because of unavailability of information from or action by the FDA field personnel unless the reviewing division determines that a delay is necessary to assure the marketing of a safe and effective drug.[135] In spite of this provision, FDA continues to hold drugs hostage as a result of a PAI without a finding that this is necessary to ensure the marketing of a safe and effective drug.

After approval of an NDA, FDA periodically inspects a drug establishment for two purposes. First, FDA determines whether any unapproved changes have been made in the manufacturing process from those set forth in the approved NDA. If any such changes are made beyond those permitted without a supplemental NDA, FDA may well bring stringent enforcement action. Second, FDA routinely inspects all establishments to determine compliance with GMP. Although FDA has not changed its GMP regulations, the interpretation and application of those regulations by FDA inspectors are thought by the pharmaceutical industry to have been substantially tightened and made more strict in the past few years.

Where FDA determines any deviation from GMP, the inspector leaves a Form FDA-483 specifying the manufacturing deficiencies. It is essential in these circumstances that the company immediately make all corrections and respond to FDA in writing about them. It can be expected that FDA will reinspect the establishment and look both for what has been done to correct the prior deficiencies and for any new deficiencies that can be found. The pharmaceutical industry believes that FDA often lists insignificant matters, that establishments which have passed without observed deficiencies in the past suddenly will be the subject of major deficiencies because of a change of inspectors or of interpretation, and that the requirements vary widely from individual inspector to individual inspector and from FDA district to FDA district. The industry has found, however, that its complaints fall on deaf ears, and thus that it must comply with whatever is required by the individual inspector or face the threat of serious regulatory action.

8.8.6 Distribution controls

On one occasion, FDA sought to limit the distribution of a new drug to hospital-based pharmacies and to prohibit it through community pharmacies. Upon challenge by the pharmacy profession, the courts ruled that this was an illegal restriction that was not authorised by the FD&C Act.[136] Since then, FDA has approved the labelling for new drugs under which the sponsor has voluntarily included restrictions on distribution, including under subpart H,[137] but the agency has not itself imposed distribution controls on any new drug.

8.8.7 Import and export

8.8.7.1 Import

In general, a prescription drug may lawfully be imported into the United States only in full compliance with all of the laws and regulations applicable to domestic drugs. There is, however, one exception. Since 1977, FDA has stated that the agency will not detain unapproved new drugs imported for personal use.[138] This became important when patients suffering from AIDS began to import drugs not available in the United States. Subsequently, AIDS organisations established buying clubs to import drugs for all of their members. FDA has not sought to prohibit this activity except where it is done for commercial profit or involves unsafe or fraudulent products for which the agency has issued an import alert (such as RU-486). Where FDA has considered cracking down on such imports, public pressure has forced the agency to back off from enforcement action.

8.8.7.2 Export

The FD&C Act of 1938, and even the Drug Export Amendments Act of 1986, placed such stringent limitations on the export of unapproved drugs from the United States that they raised enormous commercial potential for foreign countries. Many United States pharmaceutical companies reasonably anticipated that their drugs would receive approval for use outside the United States before they were approved by FDA, and could not take the risk that they would be able to obtain and maintain FDA approval of an export application. Under these circumstances, they had no option other than to build their manufacturing facilities abroad rather than in the United States. For that reason, foreign countries competed in attempting to attract these pharmaceutical factories.

The FDA Export Reform and Enhancement Act of 1996 eliminated many, but far from all, of the restrictions on FDA export of unapproved new drugs. For example, although unapproved new drugs may be exported to any of the 25 listed countries for investigational use, these drugs may not be shipped to any other country for the same purpose without FDA approval – which can take a year or more. No other country in the world controls exports in the same way as the United States, and thus a pharmaceutical establishment may be located anywhere other than the United States without fear of unreasonable limitations on international trade. Accordingly, it is essential for any United States or foreign company to be able to source its drugs abroad, rather than in the United States, if it is to be assured of the ability to investigate and market its new drugs throughout the world.

8.8.8 Orphan drugs

Under the Orphan Drug Act of 1983[139] and its numerous amendments, an orphan drug is eligible for two types of benefit. The first, which is often of minor significance, consists of tax credits. The second type, which has proved to be of enormous importance, is the market exclusivity provided by the prohibition against any form of FDA approval of the same drug for another company for seven years. The company that obtains FDA approval of an NDA for an orphan drug is thus assured of greater protection under the Orphan Drug Act than under any other statute, including the patent laws.

As enacted in 1983, the Orphan Drug Act had relatively little impact because the scope of the term "orphan drug" was considered by FDA to be relatively narrow. When Congress amended the law in 1984[140] to define an orphan drug as any drug, or any single indication for a drug, for a condition afflicting fewer than 200 000 patients in the United States, however, the impact of the law changed dramatically. Some orphan drugs are now blockbusters on which entire companies can be founded. Although Congress has considered legislation to cut back some of the provisions of the Orphan Drug Act, one such bill was vetoed by the President[141] and no other has since come close to enactment. Even if the benefits available from the Orphan Drug Act are changed, they are likely to remain important to drug companies for the foreseeable future.

8.8.9 Physician prescribing

The FD&C Act has been interpreted by FDA as applying only to the labelling, advertising and marketing of a new drug, not to the practice of medicine as reflected in the physician's prescription of the drug for a particular patient. In a policy first published in 1972[142] and reiterated many times,[143] FDA has stated that the physician may, within the practice of medicine, lawfully prescribe an approved drug for an unapproved use. Because the Drug Price Competition and Patent Term Restoration Act of 1984 provides no significant market protection for companies that obtain FDA approval of new uses for previously approved new drugs, companies rarely submit supplemental NDAs to request FDA approval of an unapproved use for an approved drug. As unapproved uses expand, the prescription drug package insert approved by FDA has become substantially outdated. In many areas, the unapproved uses of a new drug overwhelm the approved uses. Although FDA has deplored this fact, it has thus far done nothing to find an adequate resolution.

Although FDA has stated since 1938 that the agency has no authority to require an NDA sponsor to conduct testing for uses that the sponsor has not included in the proposed labelling, FDA nonetheless promulgated regulations in late 1998 to require paediatric testing of new drugs in most situations in order to reduce unapproved use of new drugs in infants and children.[144] The FDA regulation on paediatric testing is currently being contested in the courts. In the FDA Modernization Act of 1997, Congress included not only six months of marketing exclusivity for paediatric testing,[145] but also a provision to allow dissemination of information on unapproved uses of approved new drugs under specific limited conditions.[146]

While the 1997 Act was being considered by Congress, the FDA policy prohibiting dissemination of information on unapproved uses of approved new drugs was being challenged in the courts. The United States District Court held that the FDA policy violated the First Amendment to the United States Constitution, even taking into consideration the new statutory provision added by the 1997 Act, and issued an injunction that permitted a drug manufacturer to disseminate to physicians and other medical professionals information on unapproved uses of approved new drugs from a peer-reviewed professional journal or a reference textbook, or to suggest content or speakers to an independent programme adviser for a continuing medical education (CME) programme. The injunction permitted FDA to require the drug manufacturer to disclose the company's interest in the drug and the fact that the use of the drug had not been approved by FDA.[147] FDA then changed its legal position and argued on appeal that its policy merely constituted a "safe harbour", and that a violation would not necessarily bring an enforcement proceeding. As a result, the United States Court of Appeals reversed the District Court's decision on procedural grounds, without in any way disagreeing with it.[148] The District Court then revoked its injunction, although indicating that it had not changed its opinion on the matter.[149] FDA subsequently published a notice stating its continued intent to enforce its policy,[150] and the Washington Legal Foundation has returned to court on the matter. It is extremely unlikely that FDA will enforce its unapproved use policy under the circumstances permitted by the now-dissolved District Court injunction, regardless of the outcome of this case. Thus, the First Amendment right of free speech in the United States makes it even more difficult for FDA to attempt to force NDA sponsors to submit supplemental NDAs for unapproved uses, absent unequivocal statutory authority to require that drugs be tested for these uses, and that applications be submitted for including them in approved labelling. To the extent that a drug loses its patent status, of course, the problem of requiring the generic and the pioneer sponsors to conduct such testing is substantial.

8.8.10 Patient freedom of choice

Beginning with enactment of the Drug Amendments of 1962, organised patient groups have argued strenuously that they should have the freedom to purchase whatever drugs they may wish to use, regardless of their FDA status, particularly where individuals are suffering from life-threatening disease. Cancer patients argued for the use of Krebiozen and Laetrile, but FDA sought to prohibit those drugs by every means available, and the courts ultimately supported the agency.[151]

With the dramatic rise in AIDS, however, a larger, more vocal and more politically active interest group challenged the authority of FDA to deny experimental and unapproved drugs to any patient who wishes to use them. This time, the activists had a greater impact.[152] FDA has declined to take enforcement action in many instances where it would have done so in the past. The agency has also expedited the approval of AIDS drugs on the basis of scientific information that would not have been accepted as sufficient for any other disease area. Thus, FDA has bent its rules for putative AIDS treatments but has refused to expand its flexibility to include other disease areas as well. The result is an inconsistent series of decisions approving drugs for one disease on the basis of preliminary information and withholding approval of more extensively tested drugs for other diseases.

8.8.11   The costs and benefits of the IND/NDA system

There have been hundreds of investigations and reports on the IND/NDA system.[153] Numerous analyses have been done of the costs and benefits, and hundreds of recommendations have been made about ways to improve the system. Feelings run deep on these subjects, and the philosophical and emotional element often dwarfs the factual and analytical element.

A 1991 study demonstrated that the average NDA requires an investment of about $231 million.[154] In the last year of NDA approval, the average carrying cost (cost of capital) alone was $31 million. Today, these figures are about tripled to over $600 million.[155] Critics argue that this is largely the result of unrealistic regulatory requirements that cause higher drug prices, that the delay in drugs reaching the market substantially harms the public health, and that the high cost of drug development discourages drug research and development and directly hinders the development of life-saving drugs for the future. Supporters of the system point to drug tragedies of the past, argue that any relaxation of regulatory controls will dramatically increase drug risks and reduce drug effectiveness, and state that the only sound way to protect the public health is to continue and indeed to strengthen the present system. Supporters of biotechnology charge that the present system is destroying the opportunity presented by this new technology, and critics of biotechnology applaud that result.

8.9   Biological drugs

For a full century, biological drugs have been regulated under the Biologics Act of 1902, in accordance with statutory requirements that have not significantly changed.[156] When FDA was delegated the responsibility for regulating biologics in 1972, however, the agency promulgated regulations adding a number of the drug regulatory provisions under the FD&C Act to those already available under the Biologics Act. Current regulation of biologics therefore incorporates requirements from both statutes.

8.9.1 The Biologics Licence Application (BLA)

Prior to 1996, FDA required the submission and approval of both an establishment licence application (ELA) and a product licence application (PLA). This bifurcated submission and approval process was widely criticised as inefficient. Following the November 1994 elections and the realisation that FDA would be a major target for legislative reform, the agency revised its regulations to eliminate the requirement for a separate ELA and to substitute a single BLA for four categories of well-characterised biological products.[157] In the FDA Modernization Act of 1997, however, Congress eliminated the ELA and PLA for all biological products and substituted the single BLA.[158] Congress also ordered FDA to take measures to minimise differences in the review and approval of biological products under Section 351 of the Public Health Service Act and new drugs under Section 505(b)(1) of the FD&C Act. FDA promptly amended the regulations governing biologics licences to implement this requirement.[159]

Before a company may manufacture any biological product, a BLA must be submitted to and approved by FDA for the product involved. Under Section 351 of the Public Health Service Act as it is now revised, the product approval system for a biological drug is the same as for a new drug. Non-clinical studies may be conducted without FDA knowledge or approval. Clinical investigation in humans must be preceded by the submission of an IND, and all the IND regulations discussed above for chemical drugs apply equally to a biological drug. It is only the BLA that has a different name and a somewhat different focus.

A basic premise of the regulation of biological drugs is that, because they come from natural sources, they cannot adequately be characterised by chemical specifications and must instead be regulated very rigidly by rigorous adherence to detailed manufacturing procedures. For this reason, approval of a BLA depends upon the specific establishment specified and approved in that BLA. If the owner of an approved BLA wishes to manufacture all or part of the biological drug in a new establishment, it has long been standard policy under the Biologics Act to require not just that the new product be shown to be the same as the old, but also that new clinical studies independently demonstrate the safety and effectiveness of the new product as manufactured in the new establishment. This goes beyond the requirements that FDA has applied to new drugs.

With modern biotechnology, however, this rigid requirement by FDA is undergoing re-evaluation. Some biological products can be characterised by chemical or biological specifications as easily as chemical drugs. It is therefore likely that, in the future, FDA will adopt a more flexible policy on this matter.

With the advent of biotechnology, the work in the Center for Biologics Evaluation and Research has changed dramatically. For decades, the only biological products regulated under the Biologics Act of 1902 were vaccines, blood, allergenic extracts, and other related products that did not pose the difficult problems of balancing benefits against risks that were daily faced by the Center for Drug Evaluation and Research. As a result, CBER was able to review and approve ELAs and PLAs rapidly, in a fraction of the time that it took CDER to do the same job. Now, the two are indistinguishable. In the past few years, the time required for review and approval of a BLA has become even longer than that for an NDA. The backlog at CBER has risen dramatically. Critics have suggested that review and approval of new pharmaceutical products by CBER is now slower and more difficult than by CDER.

8.9.2 The Biologics Review

When implementation of the Biologics Act was transferred to FDA in 1972, a process was just being formulated by the Division of Biologics Standards in NIH to review the safety, effectiveness and labelling of the biological products that had been licensed during the past 70 years under the 1902 Act. FDA promptly established written procedures and undertook the Biologics Review.[160] The Biologics Review was patterned after the OTC Drug Review and is similarly not yet completed.

8.10   Enforcement

FDA has available to it a wide variety of formal and informal enforcement authorities under the FD&C Act. They apply equally to all products regulated by FDA. For generic drugs, FDA also can rely upon the provisions of the Generic Drug Enforcement Act of 1992. The following sections summarise some of the more important enforcement provisions used by FDA to regulate all pharmaceutical products.

8.10.1 Formal enforcement authority

8.10.1.1   Factory inspection[161]

For purposes of enforcing the law, FDA inspectors may at any time inspect any non-prescription or prescription drug. For both, FDA inspectors may see all records and documents except those that relate to financial data, sales data other than shipment data, pricing data, personnel data and research data.[162] An FDA inspector may spend whatever amount of time is necessary to complete such an inspection – even weeks or months. Where significant enforcement issues have been found, FDA inspectors have been known to spend more than a year at a single establishment.

8.10.1.2   Seizure[163]

FDA has statutory authority to request the Department of Justice to "seize" any illegal product. If FDA asserts that the drug is dangerous to health or the labelling is fraudulent or misleading in a material respect, the statute authorises multiple seizures throughout the country. Prior to 1997, FDA was required to prove the requisite shipment in interstate commerce in order to establish the agency's jurisdiction. Under the FDA Modernization Act of 1997, Congress established a rebuttable presumption of interstate commerce for purposes of FDA enforcement jurisdiction, thereby making all FDA enforcement action substantially simpler.[164]

8.10.1.3   Injunction[165]

FDA also has statutory authority to request the Department of Justice to seek a court injunction against continued violations of the law by a prescription drug manufacturer or distributor. FDA has had mixed results in attempting to obtain injunctions from the courts, who realise that an injunction can shut down a company entirely or subject it to arbitrary demands by FDA. FDA has therefore sought to obtain the equivalent in the form of stipulated agreements with companies that are filed in court as consent decrees and thus are fully enforceable as a requirement of law.

8.10.1.4   Criminal penalties[166]

All violations of the FD&C Act are automatically criminal violations of law. On two occasions the United States Supreme Court has held that any person standing in a responsible relationship to a violation of the FD&C Act is criminally liable, regardless of the lack of knowledge or intent.[167] The nature of the offence is the failure of an individual to take action to prevent a violation and to ensure compliance with the law.

This is an extremely harsh statute. As a practical matter, FDA exercises its prosecutorial discretion only to bring cases for continuing violations of the law, violations of an obvious and flagrant nature, and intentionally false or fraudulent violations. Although there have been attempts to change the criminal liability standard under the FD&C Act by legislation, none has so far been successful.

8.10.1.5   Section 305 hearing[168]

The FD&C Act provides that, before any violation is reported by FDA for institution of a criminal proceeding, the person against whom the proceeding is contemplated shall be given appropriate notice and an opportunity to present views. In accordance with this provision, it is the custom of FDA to provide an informal hearing to individuals, to show cause why they should not be prosecuted. When a grand jury is convened, however, FDA usually does not provide this type of hearing. Where such a hearing is given, it is obviously important for the individual to demonstrate a good faith attempt to comply with the law and an intent to correct and prevent any deficiencies in the future.

8.10.1.6   Other criminal statutes

The United States Code contains a number of criminal provisions related to enforcement of the FD&C Act. These laws prohibit any criminal conspiracy,[169] false reports to the government,[170] mail fraud,[171] bribery,[172] perjury,[173] and other similar illegal activity. FDA has in fact used these provisions on a number of occasions to bring criminal prosecution against individuals and companies who have violated the FD&C Act.

8.10.1.7   Civil money penalties[174]

The Prescription Drug Marketing Act of 1987 includes civil penalties for violation of the drug sample provisions of the FD&C Act. The law provides that a manufacturer or distributor who violates these provisions is subject to a civil penalty of not more than $50 000 for each of the first two violations resulting in a conviction in any ten-year period, and for not more than $1 million for each violation resulting in a conviction after the second conviction in any ten-year period. These penalties may be imposed only by a Federal District Court. FDA has no administrative authority to impose any civil penalties under these provisions.

8.10.1.8   Restitution

One court has interpreted the FD&C Act as not authorising FDA to require restitution by a manufacturer to purchasers of a product that has been found to violate the FD&C Act,[175] but a more recent court decision has upheld restitution.[176] The Medical Device Amendments of 1976 explicitly provide such authority for medical devices.[177]

8.10.2   Informal enforcement authority

8.10.2.1   Recall

For decades, FDA has worked with product manufacturers to request, and to help carry out, the recall of illegal products from the market. Courts have disagreed on whether the FD&C Act authorises an injunction that includes a requirement for product recall.[178] As a practical matter, however, the precise legal authority of FDA on this matter is irrelevant. Manufacturers routinely co-operate with FDA on the recall of any dangerous product. FDA has established detailed administrative policy governing recall procedures.[179]

8.10.2.2   Warning letters

The FD&C Act authorises FDA to decline to institute formal enforcement proceedings for minor violations whenever FDA believes that the public interest will be adequately served by a suitable written notice or warning. In accordance with this provision, in the early 1970s FDA began to issue a "regulatory letter" in lieu of bringing formal court enforcement action. This permitted more rapid, less costly and more efficient enforcement of the law. In the early 1990s regulatory letters were renamed "warning letters", and have lost their impact because they are no longer approved by FDA top management and the Chief Counsel. Nonetheless, any warning letter must be given immediate attention in order to avoid more serious formal enforcement action in the courts.

8.10.2.3 *Publicity*

FDA has explicit statutory authority to issue information to the public.[180] The courts have upheld the right of FDA to publicise illegal activity and to issue publicity about products and practices that it concludes to be harmful to the public health.[181] This is regarded by many as the most potent enforcement tool available to FDA.

8.10.3 Enforcement statistics

In the first few decades of the 1900s FDA brought hundreds of seizure and criminal actions to enforce the FD&C Act. Beginning in the 1970s, the formal court enforcement actions have been replaced in two ways. First, FDA has promulgated hundreds of regulations that establish the precise requirements of the law, thus reducing the need for many court enforcement actions. Second, formal court enforcement actions have been replaced by informal administrative enforcement actions such as recalls and warning letters. FDA statistics demonstrate that the increase in administrative enforcement actions has been greater than the decrease in formal court enforcement actions, and thus that overall FDA enforcement activity has continued to increase.

8.11 Conclusion

This brief survey of the FDA regulation of pharmaceutical products demonstrates the breadth and depth of FDA activity in this field. Although there are repeated calls for reform of the IND/NDA system, it appears unlikely that any substantial change will occur in the near future. It is therefore important that any person who enters the prescription drug industry in the United States be fully informed about the requirements, understand the regulatory risks involved, and comply adequately with all of the FDA requirements.

Addendum

Following completion of this chapter, FDA, Congress, and the courts have taken additional action that bears upon some of the subjects described.

Paediatric drug testing. The paediatric drug testing provisions in the Food and Drug Administration Modernization Act of 1997 had an automatic five year sunset limitation. In January 2002, Congress enacted the Best Pharmaceuticals for Children Act reauthorising those provisions, with changes, for another five years. The 2002 Act, like the 1997 provisions, relies upon incentives for voluntary industry testing of drugs used for children. Following enactment of the 2002 Act, a federal district court ruled that the FDA regulations that purported to require industry to test drugs used for children is not authorised by the FD&C Act and therefore is unenforceable. FDA has concluded not to appeal that decision and instead to ask Congress to enact new legislation that will give the agency explicit statutory authority to require testing in children of any drug that has a significant use in the paediatric population.

Pharmacy compounding. The pharmacy compounding provisions contained in the Food and Drug Administration Modernization Act of 1997 required that, to take advantage of the authority to compound, a pharmacy would be precluded from advertising that specific compounded drugs were available from that pharmacy. The Supreme Court ruled that this restriction was unconstitutional, in violation of the right of free speech under the First Amendment to the United States Constitution. Because a lower court had ruled that the advertising restriction could not be separated from the other pharmacy compounding provisions, the result is that none of these provisions remains effective. Accordingly, pharmacy compounding is now back to where it was before the 1997 Act. FDA has reiterated its views regarding when pharmacy compounding becomes illegal manufacture.

User fees. Both the Prescription Drug User Fee Act of 1992 (PDUFA I) and the Prescription Drug User Fee Act of 1997 (PDUFA II) contained five year sunset limitations. Congress therefore enacted the Prescription Fee Act of 2002 (PDUFA III) to extend user fees for new drugs and biological products for an additional five years. User fees will be increased over these five years to approximately half a million dollars per application and will fund 800–1000 FDA employees to review these applications. Critics have argued that user fees have resulted in early approval of unsafe drugs, resulting in withdrawal of an unusually large number of products after they are marketed and found to be unsafe. FDA has reviewed the data and has concluded that there is no statistically significant difference between the number of drugs withdrawn since user fees have been implemented and during any comparable prior period. Congress also enacted the Medical Device User Fee and Modernization Act of 2000 in order to collect the same type of user fees to support premarket notification submissions and premarket approval applications for medical devices, although the user fees will be at a much lower level than those for new drugs and biological products.

Bioterrorism. Congress passed the Public Health Security and Bioterrorism Preparedness and Response Act of 2002 as part of the Homeland Security Act, in response to the terrorism attacks of September 11, 2001. The new law contains several provisions that are designed to strengthen

254

the public health system generally and the availability of drugs, biological products, and medical devices for countering bioterrorism in particular.

FDA reorganisation. FDA has announced that the handling of biological drugs will be transferred from the Center for Biologics Evaluation and Research (CBER) to the Center for Drug Evaluation and Research (CDER), but that regulation of traditional biological products such as vaccines and blood will remain in CBER. Approximately one-third of the CBER resources will be transferred to CDER as part of this reorganisation.

References

1 An earlier version of this chapter was published in Denis M. Burley et al., *Pharmaceutical Medicine* ch. 9 (2d ed. 1993).
2 For example, Peter Barton Hutt and Richard A. Merrill, *Food and Drug Law: Cases and Materials* (2d ed. 1991).
3 52 Stat. 1040 (1938), 21 U.S.C. 301, et seq. FDA's internet website contains a large amount of information about the agency, the statutes it implements, its regulations and guidances, and other pertinent documents: www.fda.gov.
4 5 U.S.C. 551 et seq.
5 21 C.F.R. 10.40.
6 21 C.F.R. 10.45.
7 Section 12606 of the California Business and Professions Code.
8 Peter Barton Hutt, *A Historical Introduction*, 45 Food Drug Cosmetic Law Journal 17 (January 1990); Peter Barton Hutt, *The Transformation of United States Food and Drug Law*, 60 Journal of the Association of Food and Drug Officials 1 (September 1996).
9 12 Stat. 387 (1862).
10 26 Stat. 282, 283 (1890).
11 31 Stat. 922, 930 (1901).
12 44 Stat. 976, 1002 (1927).
13 46 Stat. 392, 422 (1930).
14 54 Stat. 1234, 1237 (1940).
15 67 Stat. 631, 632 (1953).
16 93 Stat. 668, 695 (1979).
17 102 Stat. 3048, 3120 (1988).
18 21 C.F.R. 5.200.
19 Peter Barton Hutt and Peter Barton Hutt II, *A History of Government Regulation of Adulteration and Misbranding of Food*, 39 Food Drug Cosmetic Law Journal 2 (January 1984).
20 9 Pliny, *Natural History* 207 (H. Rackham ed. 1949).
21 2 Stat. 806 (1813).
22 3 Stat. 677 (1822).
23 9 Stat. 237 (1848).
24 42 Stat. 858, 989 (1922).
25 32 Stat. 728 (1902).
26 58 Stat 682, 702 (1944).
27 111 Stat 2296, 2323 (1997), 42 U.S.C. 262.
28 37 Fed. Reg. 12865 (June 29, 1972).
29 34 Stat. 768 (1906).
30 Note 3 supra.
31 55 Stat. 851 (1941); 59 Stat. 463 (1945); 61 Stat. 11 (1947); 63 Stat. 409 (1949).
32 65 Stat. 648 (1951).
33 76 Stat. 780 (1962).
34 84 Stat. 1236, 1242 (1970), 21 U.S.C. 801.
35 84 Stat. 1670 (1970).
36 16 C.F.R. part 1700.
37 86 Stat. 559 (1972).
38 96 Stat. 2049 (1983).
39 98 Stat. 2815, 2817 (1984), section 526 (a)(2) of the FD&C Act, 21 U.S.C. 360bb(a)(2).
40 98 Stat. 1585 (1984).

41 100 Stat. 3743 (1986).
42 110 Stat. 1321, 1321–313 (1996), as amended, 110 Stat. 1569, 1594 (1996), section 802 of the FD&C Act, 21 U.S.C. 382.
43 102 Stat. 95 (1988).
44 106 Stat. 941 (1992).
45 106 Stat. 149 (1992).
46 106 Stat. 4491 (1992); Bruce N. Kuhlik, *Industry Funding of Improvements in the FDA's New Drug Approval Process: The Prescription Drug User Fee Act of 1992*, 47 Food and Drug Law Journal 483 (September 1992).
47 111 Stat. 2296, 2298 (1997).
48 Note 42 supra; Peter Barton Hutt and Bruce N. Kuhlik, Export Expertise: Understanding Export Law for Drugs, Devices and Biologics (1998).
49 Note 41 supra.
50 111 Stat. 2296 (1997).
51 37 Stat. 822 (1913), 21 U.S.C. 151.
52 82 Stat. 342 (1968), section 512 of the FD&C Act, 21 U.S.C. 360b.
53 102 Stat. 3971 (1988).
54 90 Stat. 540 (1976); Peter Barton Hutt, *A History of Government Regulation of Adulteration and Misbranding of Medical Devices*, 44 Food Drug Cosmetic Law Journal 99 (March 1989).
55 104 Stat. 4511 (1990); Ellen J. Flannery, *The Safe Medical Devices Act of 1990: An Overview*, 46 Food Drug Cosmetic Law Journal 129 (March 1991).
56 106 Stat. 238 (1992).
57 Title III of 111 Stat. 2296, 2332 (1997).
58 Peter Barton Hutt, *A Legal Framework for Future Decisions on Transferring Drugs from Prescription to Non-prescription Status*, 37 Food Drug Cosmetic Law Journal 427 (October 1982).
59 Note 32 supra.
60 Note 58 supra.
61 For example, 39 Fed. Reg. 19880, 19881 (June 4, 1974).
62 Sections 7 and 8 of the 1906 Act, 34 Stat. 768, 769–771 (1906); sections 501 and 502 of the FD&C Act, 21 U.S.C. 351 and 352.
63 37 Fed. Reg. 85 (January 5, 1972); 37 Fed. Reg. 9464 (May 11, 1972); 21 C.F.R. part 330.
64 21 C.F.R. 330.11.
65 47 Fed. Reg. 50442 (November 5, 1982); 21 C.F.R. 211.132.
66 97 Stat. 831 (1983), 18 U.S.C. 1365.
67 62 Fed. Reg. 9024 (February 27, 1997); 64 Fed. Reg. 131254 (March 17, 1999); 21 C.F.R. 201.66.
68 38 Stat. 717 (1914).
69 52 Stat. 111 (1938), 15 U.S.C. 41 et seq.
70 36 Fed. Reg. 18539 (September 16, 1971).
71 Note 2 supra at 477–487.
72 52 Stat. 1040–1042 (1938).
73 *USV Pharmaceutical Corp.* v. *Weinberger*, 412 U.S. 655 (1973).
74 33 Fed. Reg. 7758 (May 28, 1968), 21 C.F.R. 310.100.
75 34 Fed. Reg. 14596 (September 19, 1969); 35 Fed. Reg. 3073 (February 17, 1970); 35 Fed. Reg. 7250 (May 8, 1970); 21 C.F.R. 314.126.
76 *Upjohn* v. *Finch*, 422 F. 2d 944 (6th Cir. 1970); *Pharmaceutical Manufacturers Ass'n v. Richardson*, 318 F. Supp. 301 (D. Del. 1970).
77 34 Fed. Reg. 2673 (February 27, 1969); 35 Fed. Reg. 6574 (April 24, 1970).
78 *USV Pharmaceutical Corp.* v. *Weinberger*, 412 U.S. 655 (1973); *Weinberger* v. *Bentex Pharmaceuticals, Inc.*, 412 U.S. 645 (1973); *Ciba Corp.* v. *Weinberger*, 412 U.S. 640 (1973); *Weinberger* v. *Hynson, Westcott & Dunning, Inc.*, 412 U.S. 609 (1973).
79 *American Public Health Ass'n* v. *Veneman*, 349 F. Supp. 1311 (D.D.C. 1972).
80 33 Fed. Reg. 7762 (May 28, 1968).
81 Note 77 supra.
82 40 Fed. Reg. 26142 (June 20, 1975).
83 41 Fed. Reg. 41770 (September 23, 1976); FDA Compliance Policy Guide 440.100.
84 *United States* v. *Generix Drug Corp.*, 460 U.S. 453 (1983).
85 S. Rep. No. 96–321, 95th Cong. 1st Sess. (1979); 125 Cong. Rec. 26244–26275 (September 26, 1979).

86   *Burroughs Wellcome Co.* v. *Schweiker*, 649 F. 2d 221 (4th Cir. 1981); *Upjohn Manufacturing Co.* v. *Schweiker*, 681 F. 2d 480 (6th Cir. 1982).

87   "Deficiencies in FDA's Regulation of the Marketing of Unapproved New Drugs: The Case of E-Ferol," H.R. Rep. No. 98–1168, 98th Cong., 2d Sess. (1984).

88   49 Fed. Reg. 38190 (September 27, 1984); FDA Compliance Policy Guide 440.100.

89   50 Fed. Reg. 11478 (March 21, 1985); 51 Fed. Reg. 24476 (July 3, 1986); 21 C.F.R. 310.305.

90   Note 40 supra.

91   Note 88 supra.

92   21 C.F.R. part 312.

93   21 C.F.R. part 58.

94   Section 505(i)(3) of the FD&C Act, 21 U.S.C. 355(i)(3).

95   21 C.F.R. parts 50 and 56.

96   21 C.F.R. 312.32 and 312.33.

97   21 C.F.R. 312.36.

98   21 C.F.R. 312.34 and 312.35.

99   55 Fed. Reg. 20856 (May 21, 1990).

100   21 C.F.R. part 314.

101   Section 505(d) of the FD&C Act, 21 U.S.C. 355(d).

102   Note 46 supra.

103   Note 50 supra.

104   57 Fed. Reg. 13234 (April 15, 1992); 57 Fed. Reg. 58942 (December 11, 1992); 21 C.F.R. part 314, subpart H.

105   Section 506 of the FD&C Act, 21 U.S.C. 356.

106   FDA, *Managing the Risks from Medical Product Use: Creating a Risk Management Framework* (May 1999).

107   Institute of Medicine, *To Err is Human: Building a Safer Health System* (1999).

108   21 C.F.R. 314.50(d)(5)(vi)(b).

109   For example, *Ubiotica* Corp. v. *FDA*, 427 F.2d 376 (6th Cir. 1970); *Edison Pharmaceutical Co., Inc.* v. *FDA*, 600 F.2d 831 (D.C. Cir. 1979).

110   80 Stat. 250 (1966), 5 U.S.C. 552.

111   Section 301(j) of the FD&C Act, 21 U.S.C. 331(j).

112   18 U.S.C. 1905.

113   37 Fed. Reg. 9128 (May 5, 1972); 39 Fed. Reg. 44602 (December 24, 1974); 21 C.F.R. part 20.

114   21 C.F.R. 312.130 and 314.430.

115   21 C.F.R. 314.430(e)(2)(i).

116   21 C.F.R. 314.430(f); 130 Cong. Rec. 24977–24978 (September 12, 1984).

117   Section 505(n) of the FD&C Act, 21 U.S.C. 355(n); 21 C.F.R. 14.160.

118   Section 505(k) of the FD&C Act, 21 U.S.C. 355(k); 21 C.F.R. 314.80 and 314.81.

119   21 C.F.R. 314.70.

120   Section 505(e) of the FD&C Act, 21 U.S.C. 355(e); 21 C.F.R. 2.5.

121   *Forsham* v. *Califano*, 442 F. Supp. 203 (D.D.C. 1977).

122   111 Stat. 2296, 2325 (1997).

123   Section 735 of the FD&C Act, 21 U.S.C. 379g.

124   Section 505(b)(2) of the FD&C Act, 21 U.S.C. 355(b)(2); 21 C.F.R. 314.50.

125   Section 505(j) of the FD&C Act, 21 U.S.C. 355(j); Ellen J. Flannery and Peter Barton Hutt, *Balancing Competition and Patent Protection in the Drug Industry*, 40 Food Drug Cosmetic Law Journal 269 (July 1985).

126   Section 505A of the FD&C Act, 21 U.S.C. 355a.

127   55 Fed. Reg. 52323 (December 21, 1990); 56 Fed. Reg. 46191 (September 10, 1991); FDA Compliance Policy Guide 120.100.

128   Section 502(n)(2) of the FD&C Act, 21 U.S.C. 352(n).

129   21 C.F.R. part 202.

130   62 Fed. Reg. 14912 (March 28, 1997).

131   FDA, *Guidance for Industry: Consumer-Directed Broadcast Advertisements* (Draft July 1997, Final August 1999).

132   Section 505(b)(1)(D) of the FD&C Act, 21 U.S.C. 355 (b)(1)(D); 21 C.F.R. 314.50(d)(1).

133   58 Fed. Reg. 47340 (January 28, 1991); 56 Fed. Reg. 3180 (September 8, 1993).

134   21 C.F.R. parts 210 and 211.

135 Section 505(b)(4)(F) of the FD&C Act, 21 U.S.C. 355(b)(4)(F).
136 *American Pharmaceutical Ass'n* v. *Weinberger*, 377 F. Supp. 824 (D.D.C. 1974), affirmed per curiam, 530 F.2d 1054 (D.C. Cir. 1976).
137 Note 104 supra.
138 Note 2 supra at 563–565.
139 Note 38 supra.
140 Note 39 supra.
141 26 Weekly Compilation of Presidential Documents 1796 (October 9, 1990).
142 37 Fed. Reg. 16503 (August 15, 1972).
143 For example, 21 C.F.R. 312.2(d).
144 62 Fed. Reg. 43900 (August 15, 1997); 63 Fed. Reg. 66632 (December 2, 1998); 21 C.F.R. 314.55.
145 Note 126 supra.
146 Section 551 of the FD&C Act, 21 U.S.C. 360aaa.
147 Washington Legal Foundation v. Friedman, 13 F. Supp 2d 51 (D.D.C. 1998), 36 F. Supp. 2d 16 (D.D.C. 1999), and 56 F. Supp. 2d 81 (D.D.C. 1999).
148 Washington Legal Foundation v. Henney, 202 F. 3d 331 (D.C. Cir. 2000).
149 Washington Legal Foundation v. Henney, 128 F. Supp 2d 11 (D.D.C. 2000).
150 65 Fed. Reg. 14286 (March 16, 2000).
151 *United States* v. *Rutherford*, 442 U.S. 544(1979); *Rutherford* v. *United States*, 806 F. 2d 1455 (10th Cir. 1986).
152 Note 2 supra at 552–566.
153 Peter Barton Hutt, *Investigation and Reports Respecting FDA Regulation of New Drugs* Parts I and II, 33 Clinical Pharmacology and Therapeutics 537 and 674 (April and May 1983).
154 Joseph A. DiMasi et al., *Cost of Innovation in the Pharmaceutical Industry*, 10 Journal of Health Economics, No. 2, at 107 (February 1991).
155 Parexel, Inc., *Pharmaceutical R&D Statistical Sourcebook 2001* 73 (2001).
156 Notes 25, 26, and 27 supra.
157 61 Fed. Reg. 2733 (January 29, 1996); 61 Fed. Reg. 24227 (May 14, 1996).
158 Section 123 of the FDA Modernization Act of 1997, 111 Stat. 2296, 2323 (1997), Section 351(a) of the Public Health Service Act, 42 U.S.C. 262(a).
159 63 Fed. Reg. 40858 (July 31, 1998); 64 Fed. Reg. 56441 (October 20, 1999); 21 C.F.R. 601.2.
160 37 Fed. Reg. 16679 (August 18, 1972); 38 Fed. Reg. 4319 (February 13, 1973); 21 C.F.R. 601.25.
161 Section 704 of the FD&C Act, 21 U.S.C. 374.
162 The non-prescription drug industry traded records inspection for national uniformity under the FDA Modernization Act of 1997, 111 Stat. 2296, 2374, 2375 (1997).
163 Section 304 of the FD&C Act, 21 U.S.C. 334.
164 Section 709 of the FD&C Act, 21 U.S.C. 379a.
165 Section 302 of the FD&C Act, 21 U.S.C. 332.
166 Section 303(a) of the FD&C Act, 21 U.S.C. 333(a).
167 *United States* v. *Dotterweich*, 320 U.S. 277 (1943); *United States* v. *Park*, 421 U.S. 658 (1975).
168 Section 305 of the FD&C Act, 21 U.S.C. 335.
169 18 U.S.C. 371.
170 18 U.S.C. 1001.
171 18 U.S.C. 1341.
172 21 U.S.C. 209.
173 21 U.S.C. 1623.
174 Section 303(b) of the FD&C Act, 21 U.S.C. 333(b).
175 *United States* v. *Parkinson*, 240 F. 2d 918 (9th Cir. 1956).
176 *United States* v. *Universal Management Systems, Inc.*, 191 F. 3d 750 (6th Cir. 1999).
177 Section 518 of the FD&C Act, 21 U.S.C. 360h.
178 For example, *United States* v. *Superpharm Corp.*, 530 F. Supp. 408 (E.D.N.Y. 1981); *United States* v. *Barr Laboratories, Inc.*, 812 F. Supp. 458 (D.N.J. 1993).
179 21 C.F. R. 7.40.
180 Section 705 of the FD&C Act, 21 U.S.C. 375.
181 *Horsey Cancer Clinic* v. *Folson*, 155 F. Supp. 376 (D.D.C. 1957); *Ajay Nutrition Foods, Inc.* v. *FDA*, 378 F. Supp. 210 (D.N.J. 1974), affirmed, 513 F. 2d 625 (3rd Cir. 1975).

9: The US FDA in the drug development, evaluation, and approval process

RICHARD N SPIVEY, LOUIS LASAGNA,
JUDITH K JONES, WILLIAM WARDELL

9.1 Introduction

9.1.1 Information sources

The Food and Drug Administration (FDA) is one of the largest and most complex agencies dealing with drug development, evaluation and approval. Separate centres handle drugs, biologics, devices and food. At the same time, personnel within the agency are accessible and a wealth of information is readily available to help guide novice and experienced pharmaceutical personnel alike through the process. The FDA has a website (http//:www.fda.gov) that gives ready access to food and drug law, official guidelines, and unofficial guidance documents for drugs, biologics, devices and foods. Also, one can find FDA press releases and "talk papers" on a variety of topics of current interest as well as information concerning the FDA Advisory Committees. Chapter 21 of the Code of Federal Regulations contains the official regulations for the Food and Drug Administration. A printed version is available through the US Superintendent of Documents. The Public Health Service Act governs biologics. Regulation of biologics and drug development has been largely harmonised, and the FDA Modernization Act of 1997 (FDAMA)[1] furthered this process.

The FDA, like all drug regulatory agencies worldwide, is in the midst of rapid change in response to the pressures of consumers and healthcare professionals for more rapid approval of life-saving drugs and from the push for international harmonisation of review and approval procedures. FDAMA represents congressional response to some of these pressures. These are the most extensive legislative changes made to the Food, Drug

259

and Cosmetic Act (FD&C Act) since the landmark 1962 Kefauver–Harris amendments. For the most part, however, the law merely codified current FDA practice rather than making substantial reforms. Specific references will be made to the new law in this chapter, but it is important always to check the implementing regulations.

9.1.2 Phases of drug development

Clinical drug development leading to product approval is often described in three phases. In the US regulations Phase I is described as the initial introduction into humans. Studies conducted in this phase of development are intended to determine the tolerance (dose range), metabolism and pharmacologic actions of the drug in humans and to characterise the adverse experiences associated with increasing doses. Studies in Phase I are usually well monitored and may be conducted in patients as well as normal subjects, depending on the nature of the drug as well as the type of information being sought.

In Phase II the studies are conducted to prove the therapeutic concept and evaluate efficacy. They are usually closely monitored and well controlled in small to moderate numbers of patients with the condition of interest. These studies may also give some idea of common adverse events following short-term therapy.

Phase III studies are usually large and may be either controlled or uncontrolled in design. They provide expanded information concerning the efficacy and safety of the drug in the intended patient population. For the FDA these studies have traditionally been to provide information on benefit versus risk, as well as prescribing information for physicians. Historically, two adequate and well-controlled studies (usually Phase III) were required for drug approval. For oncology and AIDS drugs Phase II studies have been accepted, and in some cases only a single adequate and well-controlled study was considered sufficient. To clarify the requirement for the number of studies, FDAMA specifically states that a single "adequate and well-controlled" study is sufficient provided that "confirmatory evidence" is obtained before or after the trial.

It is important to note that the phases described above are not mutually exclusive and are not necessarily performed in strict linear order. These definitions have become increasingly blurred with the accelerated development plans seen with drugs for the treatment of serious and life-threatening disorders. It is becoming more important to ask of each study what will be learned and what does the study contribute to proof of either efficacy or safety, or ultimately to the product label?

9.1.3 FDA meetings: general considerations

The FDA is open to communication. Meetings can be by teleconference, videoconference, or face-to-face. The FDA procedure refers to a "center

[FDA] component", which in most cases will be the FDA division responsible for the IND and eventually for the new drug application (NDA) (or in the case of biologics, the biologics licence application (BLA). The request must be in writing, usually preceded by a telephone call to the Consumer Safety Officer (CSO)/Project Manager responsible for the drug to discuss the need for the meeting and to make preliminary arrangements. The written request for the meeting should include a statement on the purpose of the meeting, a list of specific objectives that the sponsor has for the meeting, a proposed agenda, a list of sponsor attendees, a request for FDA attendees, and the timing of submission of a background document for the meeting.

The director of the FDA component, usually the Division Director, will determine whether the meeting is appropriate. Normally the background document must be sent to the FDA at least four weeks prior to the meeting. Once the Division Director has agreed to a meeting the reviewing division has 14 days to set a date with the sponsor (the earliest date when FDA participants can be available) within 30–75 days, depending on the meeting type.

The FDA is usually quite accommodating about meetings, but meetings should not be requested frivolously or prematurely. In preparing for an FDA meeting the sponsor should prepare and submit an agenda and background document to the FDA reviewing division. This should not be too lengthy. Large documents should be submitted as appendices to the background document. Any presentation should conform to the written material submitted. Presentations should be succinct and focused. It is rare to obtain more than one hour and time must be allotted for dialogue. Rehearsal is important to avoid unclear presentations. The agency may even decide to dispense with the formal presentation and go straight to their questions and discussion. When the FDA requests that presentations be omitted, the sponsor should follow the agency's lead and listen and respond to the comments. If, during the discussion, there are areas that require clarification, there may be parts of the planned presentation that can be used. The timing of the meeting may have some importance in terms of confidentiality: for example, there are regulations concerning the confidentiality of an existing IND which may not apply to a meeting held before an IND has been submitted.

It is very important for the sponsor and the FDA to keep complete and accurate minutes of official meetings. The FDA procedure for meetings outlines distribution within the agency. The minutes of the meeting should be exchanged between agency and sponsor to minimise misunderstandings. These minutes provide a record of agreements reached and they may be very important as development proceeds and at the time of NDA submission. For example, Section 119 of FDAMA provides for meetings and written agreements on the design of clinical trials that are binding on the agency, except in very unusual circumstances. Thus, the

261

internal review by the sponsor of the draft meeting minutes and approval of the final minutes is a very important task.

9.2 The investigational new drug application (IND)

9.2.1 General considerations

An IND is required before clinical testing of a new drug can be undertaken in the United States. The information requirements for the IND are found in Chapter 21, part 312 of the Code of Federal Regulations (21 CFR 312). The purpose of the IND is to provide a scientific rationale for studying the drug in humans and sufficient information from preclinical studies to warrant the risk of exposure in humans. Although the information to be submitted is specified in the regulations, there is flexibility as to the amount and type of information needed, based on the design of the first trials to be performed under the IND. For example, if all that is needed initially is to test the bioavailability of a drug in man, the requirements for data may be less than for a more extensive Phase I programme. Although there are exceptions, FDA generally wants a separate IND for each dosage form and research target (for example heart failure and asthma). Cross-referencing to information contained in an existing IND is permitted and reduces the need for duplicate paperwork.

In November 1995, the FDA clarified the minimum requirements for an IND submission (in three areas: chemistry, toxicology reports [draft] and size [9″ maximum]) in an attempt to relax current practices somewhat, to the level required by a UK clinical trial exemption (CTX). However, full reports are to be provided within a short time after the initial drafts.

An individual (rather than an industrial sponsor) may also file an IND for the purpose of conducting clinical investigations. Such an individual is referred to as an investigator–sponsor. If the investigator plans to study a drug already subject to an IND held by an industrial or other sponsor, he or she can request that the sponsor allow them to cross-reference the existing IND. A letter from the IND sponsor allowing cross-referencing by the sponsor–investigator is usually all that is needed. These situations usually occur when an investigator wishes to pursue a research target not of interest to the industrial sponsor. The request for cross-referencing may be denied if the planned investigation is felt not to be consonant with the development of the drug. An investigator–sponsor may, however, proceed if he supplies information independent of the industrial sponsor to support the investigator–sponsor application and thus meet FDA data requirements.

The question of the benefits and risks of investigator-sponsored INDs is often raised by small pharmaceutical companies, who are attracted to the independence, and often the lower initial cost, that this entails. Investigators are responsible for all the administrative support of their own

INDs and maintain responsibility for meeting all IND reporting and performance obligations. Usually the initial costs are indeed less to the small company, as the investigator is often willing to handle the IND requirement because he or she may have independent funding for the conduct of the study. The risk to the company is the lack of control over the study (and the drug) that this independence entails. The investigator may not perform the study to the standards needed, or may fail to report safety data in an appropriate and timely manner. Any of these failures could raise issues for the development of the drug and could have an adverse impact on the drug, the programme and the company.

Similar issues of control and development priorities are raised when studies are conducted under the auspices of any organisation not contractually bound to the company. Examples include National Institute of Health (NIH) entities such as the National Cancer Institute (NCI) or any of the cancer cooperative study groups, or the AIDS Cooperative Trials Group (ACTG). The company is at the mercy of the priorities, sense of urgency, objectives, standard operating procedures (SOPs), auditing standards, case report forms, dictionaries and databases of these groups when they are the sponsors independent of the company. At the same time, these groups may well be the most cost-efficient and expeditious way of developing a new drug, and they may control access to specialised resources (for example specialised clinical laboratories). These factors (in addition to ownership issues) must be carefully weighed before a decision is taken to rely on any outside sponsorship for drug development.

9.2.2 IND submission and review

An IND is submitted to the appropriate reviewing division in either the Center for Drug Evaluation and Research (CDER) or the Center for Biologics Evaluation and Research (CBER). If there is uncertainty as to the appropriate reviewing divisions, one should check with the division considered most likely and obtain guidance. For both drugs and biologics one may also consult the office of the Deputy Director. Once an IND is submitted the reviewing division will acknowledge receipt, and the date of receipt becomes the official date for review purposes. Once an IND is submitted, the FDA reviewing division has 30 days from the official submission date in the acknowledgement letter in which to evaluate the information contained in the IND and to decide whether the information supports going forward with the initial human study protocol. There is no official "approval" of an IND. If FDA raises no "hold" issues during the 30-day evaluation period the sponsor is free to proceed. However, it is generally good practice to contact the agency prior to study initiation to confirm that there are no concerns related to starting the planned study.

The FDA may respond to the IND with questions and concerns in writing. These may be requests for clarification or issues that need to be addressed during the drug development process. If the FDA feels that the planned study poses a significant safety risk to human subjects they may inform the sponsor that the study cannot proceed. This act is referred to as placing a "clinical hold" on the IND. A clinical hold may be complete or partial. In the latter case the FDA may place a hold on certain aspects of the planned development while permitting the sponsor to proceed with other aspects. For example, the planned study may be a dose-escalation trial and the FDA may only permit a single dose level based on the information provided in the IND. FDAMA has codified FDA obligations to a sponsor whose IND is placed on clinical hold (Section 117). The FDA is obliged to explain its concern and make clear to the sponsor what is needed to respond. Guidance documents adopted before the legislative changes require the reviewing division to communicate its concerns by telephone and with a written communication within five working days. The sponsor then responds and the FDA must reply within 30 days as to the adequacy of the response. If the hold is not lifted, formal appeal to the Office level may be needed to resolve differences of opinion.

9.2.3 IND meetings

9.2.3.1 Early IND meetings

One of the decisions that a sponsor should make regarding the time immediately before or after filing an IND is whether to request a meeting with the FDA to discuss the submission. The FDA has become more receptive in recent years to offering early advice and counsel. As a result, meetings during early development are much more common than they were a decade ago. Reasons for requesting a meeting in the early phases of an IND are varied. The sponsor may have concerns regarding some element of the IND – for example, they may wish to have as a first study relatively long exposure, and there may be problems with the adequacy of the animal toxicological data to support the exposure planned. The sponsor may wish to introduce the FDA to what they feel is a very interesting and promising development project. Another reason for requesting a meeting might be to determine whether the early development programme is adequate to achieve the stated objectives. If the latter is the primary purpose of the meeting, it is highly recommended that the sponsor present a plan to the FDA for comment and discussion, rather than asking the agency how to proceed. This latter approach can lead to less productive dialogue and perhaps a less than focused or commercially feasible development programme.

9.2.3.2 End of Phase II meeting

For most drugs, one of the most important meetings with the FDA in the new drug development process is the End of Phase II meeting. This was initially directed at drugs of specific interest because of either medical need

264

or possible toxicity. This meeting is now standard at the FDA for development planning. Its purpose is to present to FDA the results of studies conducted during Phase I and Phase II to gain the agency's concurrence that it is safe and reasonable to proceed into Phase III. More importantly, assuming there is concurrence to proceed, the meeting serves to review plans for Phase III development. Under FDAMA, written agreements on the adequacy of design of the key efficacy trials can be obtained (Section 119). Because Phase III can be very expensive for the sponsor and critical to the ultimate approval of the drug, it is critical to obtain FDA commitment at this juncture.

The timing of the End of Phase II meeting is important. The meeting should be scheduled when sufficient information from earlier phases of development is available, yet early enough to permit planning and preparation for Phase III. The information available must be in a condition to permit adequate summary and analysis. The background package of information presented to the FDA is critical to achieving the objectives of the meeting. At this stage one should have ready a "target package insert" with clearly stated desired claims and careful annotation showing the existing or planned studies that are intended to support these claims. A clinical development plan has little meaning unless related to the precise language of a package insert "Indications" section. Also, if any specific safety statements are desired or anticipated these should be highlighted and the data supporting them referenced in the background material. This meeting needs intense preparation. In order to achieve the objectives in the limited time available, any presentations must be concise and focused. If the FDA has reviewed the background material the agency may wish to omit the sponsor's presentations, but the sponsor must still be prepared.

9.2.3.3   IND amendments

The IND evolves with the development programme. It is amended with each new protocol and with each meaningful change in an existing protocol. It is particularly important to remember to amend a protocol when there is a change in design or in the scope of the study. The sponsor may begin a new study or implement a change in protocol when the protocol or protocol amendment has been submitted to the FDA for review and approval obtained from the institutional review board (IRB) responsible for the study.

There are also informational amendments submitted to the IND that incorporate new information concerning the drug under study. Examples include new toxicology data or new information concerning chemistry, manufacturing or controls of the drug. These amendments are essential to support new clinical protocols or amendments. There are proposals currently being discussed to determine the feasibility and desirability of submitting the original IND and subsequent amendments electronically. If this is done well, the body of information can be more accessible to the

FDA reviewers and lead to a more comprehensive knowledge base in anticipation of a future NDA submission. This concept has been referred to as a "cumulative" IND.

The IND safety report is another important type of IND amendment. Any serious, unexpected adverse experience associated with the use of the drug occurring in clinical trials *or in animal studies* must be submitted to the IND. The regulations define "serious" and "unexpected" (21 CFR 312.32). "Associated with" is somewhat more subjectively defined as an event for "which there is a reasonable possibility that the event might have been caused by the drug". The sponsor must report to the FDA and notify all participating investigators in writing within 15 calendar days following the initial receipt by the sponsor of the report. It does not matter whether or not the source of the event was a study conducted under the IND for it to be reportable. If the safety report concerns a fatal or life-threatening event of the type described, the FDA is to be notified by telephone within five calendar days. This is to be followed by the written report within 15 calendar days. It is critical that the regulations concerning IND safety reports be reviewed in detail as there are several nuances of interpretation, and strict compliance is essential.

9.2.3.4 IND annual reports

Within 60 days of the anniversary date on which the IND went into effect, the sponsor must submit an annual report. The Code of Federal Regulations (21 CFR 312.33) outlines the requirements for this report. It should include a brief summary of the status of each study completed or in progress. If a study is complete, a brief description of the findings should be presented, and if in progress any, interim results available should be summarised. A summary of all IND safety reports submitted during the year must be included, along with tabulations of the most frequent and serious adverse experiences observed. Listings of all patients who died or who discontinued the study because of adverse events (regardless of causality) must also be included. All preclinical studies completed or in progress during the year should be listed and any new findings summarised. New manufacturing information should also be presented. There is flexibility in the format of the report but it is important to submit it in a timely manner. Extensions may be granted upon request to the agency. The Code of Federal Regulations should be consulted for further details.

9.2.3.5 IND issues for drugs that treat serious or life-threatening conditions

FDAMA widens and codifies "fast-track" procedures that had previously been addressed in part by 21 CFR 312 Subpart E for drugs intended to treat "life-threatening and severely debilitating illnesses". The act refers to drugs "intended for the treatment of a serious or life-threatening condition and it demonstrates the potential to address unmet medical needs for such a condition" (Section 112). Sponsors apply for "fast-track" status and, if this is granted, receive expedited review of the application based on clinical or surrogate measures "reasonably likely to predict clinical benefit". The Act also codifies the process of a "rolling review", whereby an incomplete application can be reviewed while results from ongoing studies are added as the review progresses. Both the Act and existing Subpart E regulations place several conditions and limitations on drugs approved under "fast track". These include commitments to carry out definitive studies post-approval, preclearance of promotional material by the FDA, and a procedure for accelerated withdrawal of the drug from the market in cases where clinical benefit is not confirmed. Because development is accelerated under this procedure, sponsor and agency interactions are more frequent and intense than for other applications. For example, the enhanced interactions in this section allow for an End of Phase I meeting, where guidance might be offered that would allow an adequate and well-controlled Phase II study or studies to be used as the basis of approval.

Another set of regulations, 21 CFR 312.34, governs the availability of a treatment IND or protocol. A treatment IND protocol allows a drug to be made available to patients not otherwise eligible for the drug development programme. A treatment protocol may be filed when the drug provides a possible treatment for a serious or life-threatening disorder where no alternative therapy is available. A treatment protocol may be filed during Phase III, or when all clinical studies have been completed. When the drug is clearly valuable, a treatment IND can be filed as early as Phase II. The regulations spell out the information that must be provided when submitting a treatment protocol. The FDA must determine that there is sufficient information to suggest that the drug may offer the prospect of efficacy and that the risks for use are acceptable. The sponsor must also give assurances that they are continuing the development of a drug with due diligence. The sponsor should be aware that there is a risk that making the drug available under a treatment protocol may reduce the ability of the sponsor to recruit patients into the controlled trials, thereby delaying ultimate approval of the NDA.

9.3 The new drug application (NDA or BLA)

9.3.1 General considerations

The NDA is an organised presentation of all the information collected during the drug development process assembled into a form allowing FDA review. The regulations governing the NDA are found in 21 CFR 314. In addition, the FDA has issued detailed guidelines on the content and format of the NDA, which can be accessed on the FDA website. It is important to note, however, that the reviewing division may have specific format or organisational needs for the data to ensure speedy review (see pre-NDA meeting). Commonly, case report forms and data tabulations have been submitted in electronic portable document file (PDF) format, greatly reducing the volume of paper that needs to be submitted to FDA. It is now possible – and soon to be mandatory – that NDAs be submitted entirely in electronic form. Several guidelines have been issued which outline the requirements for such submissions, including the need for electronic signatures.

The NDA is a "layered" document. There are summary documents, individual study reports and actual data tabulations. It differs in two main ways from the dossier submitted in the European Union: (1) in the amount of raw data contained in the NDA submission, and (2) in the presence of expert reports in the European dossier, compared with well-defined integrated summaries in the NDA. This resulted from historical, cultural and structural differences between US and European regulatory bodies. In general, Europeans have relied more heavily on outside experts to review applications. The International Conferences on Harmonisation (ICH) have made considerable progress in harmonising the content of many sections of the US NDA and the EU dossier. ICH has now agreed on the common technical document (CTD) which will, as the name implies, be a common approach to dossiers in the three participating regions of the world, the US, the EU and Japan. In addition, work has begun on elaborating the requirements for the electronic version, the e-CTD.

9.3.2 The pre-NDA meeting

As preparations for the submission of an NDA begin, there needs to be a pre-NDA meeting with the FDA reviewing division. This meeting is important to eliminate delays that can occur when an NDA does not meet the specific needs of the assigned reviewers at the FDA (21 CFR 312.47). The sponsor should provide to the FDA an idea of the types and volume of information to he submitted, as well as the plan for data summary, presentation and analysis. The FDA should provide to the sponsor any specific requests for the display and analysis of data. Electronic formats and requests have become more routine, and a good understanding of what is planned and needed can help minimise later difficulties.

9.3.3 NDA submission

The sponsor submits the NDA along with an appropriate application fee, and the FDA reviews the application for completeness, that is to determine whether all parts of the NDA are present, and in particular the information critical for their review. If the NDA is complete enough for review it is "filed" by the FDA. The agency has 60 days in which to perform this "completeness" review. The completeness review is important under user fee legislation, as the review clock starts with FDA's acceptance of an NDA for review. If the FDA finds that some critical information is missing, the agency will notify the sponsor that the NDA is not filed (that is, not complete). In that case the agency must state the nature of the deficiency so the sponsor can resubmit with the needed information. The sponsor forfeits half of the application fee if the NDA is not accepted for filing. For drugs reviewed under fast-track procedures an incomplete NDA can be filed for review and additional data submitted during the review process (the "rolling review" referred to earlier).

The official filing date is 60 days after receipt of the submission if the 50-day review (45 for abbreviated NDAs) has found no deficiencies. FDA then has 180 days in which to review the content of the application for its acceptability for approval. This time frame was almost never met in the past, and until recently was usually much longer. The Prescription Drug User Fee Act of 1992 (PDUFA) set specific performance targets for the agency, listed below. Performance has improved considerably since the passage of this Act. There is a "sunset" clause in PDUFA which requires reapproval every five years. It was renewed in 1997, and is due for renewal by Congress again in 2002. Unless renewed, it will expire on 30 September 2002.

9.3.4 NDA classification

PDUFA provides for the classification of NDA submissions as being subject to either standard or priority review. Priority applications are targeted for, and tracked to, an action at six months. The standard applications are targeted for action at ten months. The sponsor may request the priority review status to be applied. This request is usually contained in the cover letter, along with the rationale for the request. Although there are general guidelines that address the basis for ascribing priority review status, decisions are not always clear-cut and arguments provided by the sponsor may help guide the agency.

9.3.5 Monitoring the review of the NDA

Once the NDA has been filed, the sponsor must monitor the progress of the NDA review in order to detect problems or concerns at the earliest possible moment. This monitoring or tracking must be carried out with great sensitivity. If contacts are too frequent or poorly timed they can quickly become an annoyance, which can hamper further communications. The Project Manager or Consumer Safety Officer is the usual point of contact. If there is difficulty with a particular review then the reviewer should be contacted (with consideration, obviously, for the reviewer's time).

One must consider the reviewer's style and preferred method of communication. Some reviewers prefer requests to go through the Project

Manager or CSO. One reviewer might be very responsive to e-mail, whereas another might prefer a telephone call. The contacts during an NDA review can be numerous – the exact number will vary with the application and the reviewing division. The purpose of contacts should not only be to track or monitor, but whenever possible to assist the reviewer in resolving quickly minor issues that can sometimes cause the reviewer to slow or even halt a review.

All substantial requests, whether received informally or through official notification, must be addressed as promptly and completely as possible. An attempt to gloss over an issue usually leads to further delay. Issues raised by the reviewer represent significant concerns and should be treated as such. The amount and type of any new information needed to answer a request must be carefully considered. Under user fee guidelines the FDA likes to keep the review moving without the need to review large amounts of new data which, if too large, may cause FDA to "reset the clock", that is, extend the review time frame. The effect of such a submission on the review should be discussed with the agency and balanced against the need for the information.

9.3.6 FDA actions

Until quite recently the actions of the FDA concerning an NDA were expressed in either an approval letter, an approvable letter or a non-approval letter. In the case of a non-approval letter the deficiencies were noted and were felt by the agency to require sufficient action by the sponsor that a positive action by the agency in the present review cycle was not possible. Where the issues could be solved promptly by the sponsor, a non-approval letter was not necessarily a bad result because it officially clarified the remaining issues.

An approvable letter usually stated some minor area of concern that needed to be resolved prior to final approval. The letter usually stated that if these concerns were resolved approval would be granted.

In contrast, an approval letter meant that the information provided justified approval. The only action usually requested for this type of letter was the submission of final printed labelling and advertising. In some cases an approval letter could spell out other conditions for approval, such as post-approval studies, or restrictions on distribution or promotion. These conditions were generally discussed with the sponsor and agreed to prior to receipt of the letter.

There is now a move to replace the non-approval and approvable letters with a "complete response letter", which lists all the deficiencies the sponsor will need to correct to obtain approval. If deficiencies are substantial the letter will read more like the old non-approval letter; if the deficiencies are minor, the letter would read more like an approvable letter. To date, the use of such letters has been random at best, and it is still most common to receive one of the three "action" letters noted above.

The sponsor will usually be made aware of the deficiencies prior to the action letter, and this allows a more rapid response. If post-approval studies are to be performed as a condition of approval, the agency now has clear authority to require the sponsor to report on those studies under Section 130 of FDAMA. Under the previous law FDA's authority in this regard was never clear, and post-approval studies had been conducted under a "gentleman's agreement" without a firm legal basis.

9.3.7 Post-approval reporting

Following the approval of an NDA, the sponsor has ongoing reporting responsibilities. The most important of these is the monitoring of clinical safety once the drug is on the market, to ensure that the product's benefits outweigh any risks identified when it is introduced to larger, more diverse populations. Clinical safety regulations for drugs are found at 21 CFR 314.80, and for biologics at 21 CFR 600.80. These regulations describe specific and rigidly enforced requirements as to the timing of submissions of individual spontaneous reports of suspected adverse events, determined by the type of report (for example, serious and unlabelled events are reported in 15 calendar days, whereas most other events are submitted in periodic reports). The information required is described on a standard form, the 3500A, which closely corresponds to the international CIOMS form for event reporting that is accepted in most countries.

In addition to the requirements for reporting individual adverse events, the FDA requires periodic safety reports at quarterly intervals for the first three years after a drug is marketed, and annually thereafter. The agency has the right to request that quarterly reporting continue if circumstances warrant. There are efforts under way through ICH to harmonise the individual and periodic reports that are required to be submitted to health authorities worldwide. The FDA has adopted some ICH recommendations, such as the timing of reports, and has taken the lead by adopting the Medical Dictionary for Regulatory Activities (MedDRA) terminology for coding of the events, and encouraging adoption of the ICH E2B standards for electronic submissions of spontaneous reports.

In the past decade there has been increased emphasis on drug safety, and more public visibility of safety problems. The volume of reports now exceeds 250 000 spontaneous reports per year, and adverse events have been highlighted in the medical sector and also in the media. In parallel, the FDA has focused more intently on this area in both NDA reviews and in the post-marketing period. This has accompanied withdrawals of a number of products, such as cisapride, phenylpropanolamine and terfenadine, and special scrutiny of products associated with particular adverse events, such as cardiac arrhythmias (*torsades de pointes*) and hepatic necrosis. The result has been an emphasis on the concept of risk management of a product. This concept, which is due to be described in forthcoming FDA recommendations, stresses the need to identify potential risks in the indication population and to make special efforts to prevent them in various ways. This area should be a focus for the agency in the near future, and definitive guidelines are awaited.

In addition to safety reporting there is a requirement for an NDA annual report that contains other information relevant to the NDA. Again, the requirements are detailed in the Code of Federal Regulations. Annual reports must contain a brief summary of new information which might bear on the safety, efficacy or labelling of the drug. This summary should also include any actions taken or planned as a result of the new information. The report also contains product distribution data, current labelling with any changes highlighted, as well as new information from preclinical and clinical studies. Updates are also needed for any ongoing studies. Some changes in chemistry, manufacturing or controls may be included in the annual report, whereas others must be submitted for approval prior to implementation. Copies of new promotional materials must be submitted at the time of their first use.

The NDA is a living document for as long as a drug is marketed. Supplements must be submitted for labelling modifications and for any change in the NDA that requires prior approval, including major manufacturing changes. Supplements may also be required for notification purposes.

The maintenance of an NDA is nearly as important as the approval, because any neglect in this activity can place the product in jeopardy.

9.4 The future of the FDA

9.4.1 Background

The FDA has undergone significant changes since the 1962 Kefauver–Harris Amendments to the FDC Act. Before that time, for example, regulatory decisions that required medical evaluation were made by just a handful of physicians. Today there are hundreds of reviewers in the agency, including physicians, pharmacists and PhD scientists.

Before Kefauver–Harris, the FDA was legally empowered to evaluate the evidence on safety of a proposed new pharmaceutical, but not the evidence on effectiveness. In practice, however, a decision to approve a drug for marketing had necessarily to involve both safety and efficacy, because the amount of risk allowable had to take into account the drug's efficacy; but legally this was not acknowledged.

Another important change after 1962 was the involvement of the agency in the drug development process upon submission of the IND; previously the FDA had played no role until an NDA was submitted. Now, as shown in this chapter, there is usually close involvement and expert guidance available from the agency.

There has been a tremendous increase over the years in the amount of knowledge available about a candidate drug at the time of NDA submission.

The size of NDAs has grown enormously, and it is not uncommon for them to contain data generated from scores of trials involving more than 10 000 patients, and sometimes several tens of thousands. Despite this, public debate about drug approval standards has increased, particularly when new adverse reactions occur with marketed drugs. For many years now, 2–3% of new drugs approved by the FDA in a given year (and UK data are similar) have been ultimately removed from the market, almost invariably because of rare serious side effects not apparent at the time of approval. This is understandable because, just as we do not know all the good a drug can do at NDA approval, current scientific understanding does not enable us to know all its potential harm either, no matter how large the number of patients it is feasible to study prior to marketing. Improved risk management, including post-approval surveillance, will help minimise the dangers, but cannot prevent them entirely.

The pharmaceutical industry has likewise undergone important changes. The costs of bringing a new drug to market keep rising at an accelerating pace, compounded by the fact that the 12–15 years that it takes on average from discovery to marketing increases the costs spent on compounds that fail along the way and so never return the research investment. Even if a drug reaches the market, there remains the substantial opportunity costs for the development capital that could have been invested elsewhere over that period. The latest estimate from the Tufts Center for the Study of Drug Development puts the average out-of-pocket cost, including failures, of developing a new chemical entity to the point of NDA approval at $403 million ($121m preclinical plus $282m clinical). When the cost of capital is included, this figure rises to $802 million ($336m preclinical plus $466m clinical).[2]

In recent years, also, the drug industry has been increasingly criticised for excessive profits and for the growing percentage of healthcare costs attributable to prescription drugs. Public sentiment on this issue has suffered both from unwillingness to recognise the high costs of new drug development and to meet, on a national basis, the challenge of paying for medical advances that improve the quality of life and the savings of healthcare money.

For a decade or more after the 1962 Amendments there existed in the agency (or at least in certain members of its reviewing staff) a hostile, adversarial attitude toward the drug industry, the latter often being characterised as unscrupulous seekers of profit from drug sales not justifiable in terms of patient wellbeing. Congressional hearings were typically preoccupied with adverse reactions from drugs, rather than with excessive delays in drug development time. However, when this situation and the accompanying drug lag was recognised and debated publicly, and even more so with the advent of AIDS, public and congressional pressures shifted toward impatience over delays in the marketing of effective remedies for serious diseases not treatable with older drugs. The picture

273

changed to one where new drug approval was no longer deemed to be a zero-sum game where benefit for some was possible only at the expense of harm to others. Instead, it became more acceptable to look upon drug development as a process wherein approval could be speeded by efficient and timely review of relevant animal and human data so that every sector could benefit – the sick, industry, the medical profession and the FDA.

9.4.2 Improvements for the 21st century

9.4.2.1 Further speeding drug development, and increasing success rates

9.4.2.1.1 Speed and success rates The drug development process now takes far too long and clearly needs to be further speeded up. Equally or more important is the success rate of the overall process, which needs to be increased. It has been estimated (J DiMasi, personal communication) that increasing the success rate by 10% across a portfolio of drugs at all stages of clinical development would have the same effect on development costs as reducing the development time by more than 20%.

9.4.2.1.2 Discovery and early development Having better new chemical entity (NCE) candidates and better ways of choosing which of them should enter into development would be an important step forward. Although the enormous increase in power of the biological and pharmaceutical sciences has increased the quality of development candidates over recent years, nevertheless prediction of consistently successful development candidates still eludes us, and the overall success rate of drugs in clinical development has changed little over the last few decades. Much hope is currently held out for the potential effects of genomics and biomarkers in improving the quality of targets, drug candidates, and their progression through early development, but at present these promises are still hypothetical.

9.4.2.1.3 FDA's skills Using the increased skills and talents of the greater number of qualified staff now at FDA (made possible in particular by the budget expansions of PDUFA) is another avenue; DiMasi and Manocchia[3] have shown that early and continuing discussions between the regulators and the regulated, in the form of FDA-sponsor conferences, facilitate drug approval. This is what one would expect if, at the time of filing an NDA, all the important questions had been asked and answered.

9.4.2.1.4 Animal data It may also be possible for time and money to be saved by eliminating requirements for animal toxicity data that are found to be no longer necessary. Excessive use of toxicity data has been criticised by some, reminiscent of the days when LD50 values in laboratory animals were routinely performed even when the precision sought in such studies was unnecessary for product development.

9.4.2.1.5 "Naturalistic" studies   The inclusion/exclusion criteria needed in formal clinical trials inevitably produce experimental populations that are not typical of patient populations in routine medical practice. More attention therefore needs to be paid to the "naturalistic" study of drugs in general clinical practice. Such studies could lead to an increased understanding of both effectiveness and risk in the intended patient population. Benefits will almost certainly accrue by identifying empiric relations between genetic make-up and drug response, with the possibility of increasing benefit or decreasing harm. Progress in this area is unfortunately predicted too optimistically at present by scientists who should be aware of the length of time that will be required to achieve these goals, but nevertheless ultimate progress will be made if we apply ourselves to the task.

9.4.2.1.6 Direct-to-consumer advertising   There needs to be continuing debate over the nature and effectiveness of direct-to-consumer advertising about pharmaceuticals. Whereas some patients do not wish to play an aggressive role in affecting physician prescribing, others do. The latter, understandably, do not consider themselves naïve innocents who are too ill informed to play a useful role. And many physicians (perhaps most?) do not feel that they will be inevitably forced to prescribe badly because of patient pressures. On the other hand, there is scope for abuse here, and a balance needs to be identified and sought.

9.4.2.1.7 Secondary indications   The current restrictions by the FDA on the advertising of secondary or tertiary indications (that is, unapproved by the FDA) for drugs need to re-evaluated. Experience has taught us that often not all the uses of a drug are known at the time of first marketing, and indeed it is not unusual for later approved uses to be more important medically than the original indication.

9.4.2.1.8 Incentives for obtaining new data   Because additional uses may first be demonstrated when a drug's patent has expired (or is close to expiration), a company may be reluctant to spend the time and money to obtain formal FDA approval of new uses primarily to benefit generic manufacturers. Optimal medical practice, however, calls for access to persuasive data on new indications.

Drug development and regulation promises to be an interesting ride through the 21st century.

References

1   Food and Drug Administration Modernization Act of 1997 (FDAMA).
2   Harris G. Cost of Developing Drugs Found to Rise. *Wall Street Journal* Dec/3/01, B14.
3   DiMasi JA, Manocchia M. Initiatives to speed new drug development and regulatory review: the impact of FDA-sponsor conferences. *Drug Info J* 1997;**31**:771–8.

10: Technical requirements for registration of pharmaceuticals for human use: the ICH process and the Common Technical Document

PATRICK F D'ARCY, DEAN WG HARRON

10.1 Introduction

The International Conference on Harmonisation of Technical Requirements for Registration of Pharmaceuticals for Human Use (ICH) is a unique project that brings together the regulatory authorities of Europe, Japan, and the United States with experts from the pharmaceutical industry in the three regions to discuss scientific and technical aspects of product registration. Its purpose is to make recommendations on ways to achieve greater harmonisation in the interpretation and application of technical guidelines and requirements for product registration in order to reduce or obviate the need to duplicate the testing carried out during the research and development of new medicines. The objective of such harmonisation is a more economical use of human, animal, and material resources, and the elimination of unnecessary delay in the global development and availability of new medicines while maintaining safeguards on quality, safety, and efficacy, and regulatory obligations to protect public health.

10.2 ICH organisation

10.2.1 Members

Under ICH, harmonisation involves the European Union, Japan, and the United States of America, with the assistance of observers from WHO, EFTA, and Canada. The six co-sponsors of the Conference are:

- European Commission – European Union (EU)
- European Federation of Pharmaceutical Industries' Association (EFPIA)
- Ministry of Health and Welfare, Japan (MHW)
- Japan Pharmaceutical Manufacturers Association (JPMA)
- US Food and Drug Administration (FDA)
- Pharmaceutical Research and Manufacturers of America (PhRMA).

In addition, the International Federation of Pharmaceutical Manufacturers Associations (IFPMA) participates as an "umbrella" organisation for the pharmaceutical industry, and provides the ICH secretariat.

10.2.2 The Steering Committee

The ICH Steering Committee (SC) oversees the preparations for ICH, and the harmonisation initiatives that are undertaken under the ICH Process. The Committee normally meets two or three times a year.

10.2.3 Expert working groups (EWGs)

The Steering Committee is advised, on technical issues concerned with harmonisation topics, by expert working groups. These are joint regulatory/industry groups for which experts are nominated from the six co-sponsors of the conference. The working groups deal with individual harmonisation topics under general headings: "Safety" (preclinical toxicity and related tests), "Quality" (pharmaceutical development and specifications), "Efficacy" (clinical testing programmes and safety monitoring) and "Multidisciplinary" (cross-cutting topics, including regulatory communications and timing of toxicity studies in relation to clinical studies).

In October 1994, the ICH Steering Committee announced a "new direction" in the harmonisation work coming within the remit of ICH. In response to developments in communications technology and the need to avoid divergence in the three regions, which could affect the efficiency of the regulatory process, it was agreed that two aspects on regulatory communications should be included in the ICH programme; these are the development of an international medical terminology and agreement on electronic standards for the transfer of information and data.

10.3 The ICH process

On the basis of experience to date, the Steering Committee has outlined a stepwise ICH process (Figure 10.1) for monitoring the progress of the harmonisation work and identifying the action needed in order to reach a defined endpoint.

277

10.3.1 ICH meetings and conferences

It was agreed from the start that the focus for discussions of tripartite harmonisation should be an international conference or series of conferences.[1-4] The Steering Committee recognised the importance of ensuring that the process of harmonisation is carried out in an open and transparent manner, and that ICH discussions and recommendations are presented in open fora.

- *The First International Conference on Harmonisation* (ICH 1) was held in Brussels in November 1991, hosted by the European Commission and EFPIA.
- *The Second International Conference on Harmonisation* (ICH 2) took place in Orlando, Florida, October 27–29, 1993.
- *The Third International Conference on Harmonisation* (ICH 3) took place in Yokohama, Japan, November 29 to December 1, 1995.
- *The Fourth International Conference on Harmonisation* (ICH 4) took place in Brussels, July 16–18, 1997.
- *The Fifth International Conference on Harmonisation* (ICH 5) took place in San Diego, USA, November 9–11, 2000.

10.3.2 Status of ICH harmonisation initiatives

At the close of ICH 4, the total number of finalised tripartite ICH guidelines had reached 33 (Table 10.1), with a further four at the Step 2 stage.

It is generally assumed that, following the ICH 4 meeting, international harmonisation had reached the end of phase 1 and would be brought together with a focus on developing a common technical document (CTD) to improve efficiency in documenting new medicines for regulatory purposes.

The adoption of the CTD may be the major event that will require a global conference (ICH 5/ICH 6?; see later), both to present the final document and to consider implementation issues.

The arguments in favour of a CTD have been forcefully presented. Having harmonised the technical requirements for the demonstration of quality, safety and efficacy of a new medicinal product under the first phase of the ICH process, it seemed reasonable that the three regions should now agree on the way in which this information should be presented for the purpose of obtaining authorisation to place the product on the therapeutic market. This would obviously save unnecessary duplication and reworking and reduce the time and resources required for submission of the regulatory documents, ultimately benefiting patients in the three regions and in the rest of the world.

The industrialists performed a feasibility study in record time in Europe and the USA to determine some of the resource requirements for producing

278

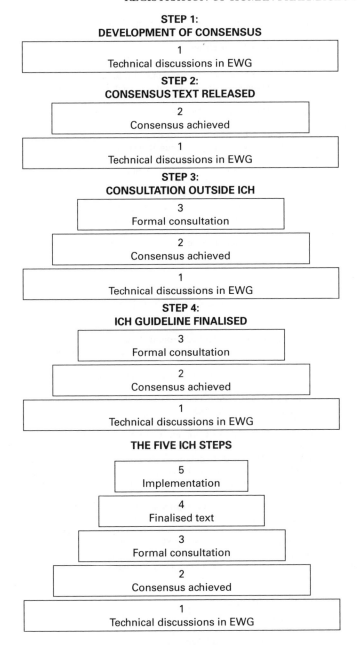

Figure 10.1 The ICH process.

Table 10.1 Step 4 tripartite harmonised and Step 2 draft consensus guidelines.

Step 4 Tripartite harmonised guidelines
1. The Extent of Population Exposure to Assess Clinical Safety for Drugs Intended for Long-term Treatment of Non-Life-Threatening Conditions
2. Clinical Safety Data Management: Definitions and Standards for Expedited Reporting
3. Data Elements for Transmission of Individual Case Safety Reports
4. Clinical Safety Data Management: Periodic Safety Update Reports for Marketed Drugs
5. Structure and Content of Clinical Study Reports
6. Dose-Response Information to Support Drug Registration
7. Guideline for Good Clinical Practice
8. Studies in Support of Special Populations: Geriatrics
9. General Considerations for Clinical Trials
10. Stability Testing of New Drug Substances and Products
11. Stability Testing: Photostability Testing of New Drug Substances and Products
12. Stability Testing for New Dosage Forms Annex to the ICH Harmonised Tripartite Guideline on Stability Testing for New Drugs and Products
13. Text on Validation of Analytical Procedures
14. Validation of Analytical Procedures: Methodology
15. Impurities in New Drug Substances
16. Impurities in New Drug Products
17. Impurities: Guideline for Residual Solvents
18. Viral Safety Evaluation of Biotechnology Products Derived from Cell Lines of Human or Animal Origin
19. Quality of Biotechnological Products: Analysis of the Expression Construct in Cells used for Production of R-DNA Derived Protein Products
20. Quality of Biotechnological Products: Stability Testing of Biotechnological/Biological Products
21. Derivation and Characterisation of Cell Substrates used for Production of Biotechnological/Biological Products
22. Guideline on the Need for Carcinogenicity Studies of Pharmaceuticals
23. Testing for Carcinogenicity of Pharmaceuticals
24. Dose Selection for Carcinogenicity Studies of Pharmaceuticals
25. Addendum to "Dose Selection for Carcinogenicity Studies of Pharmaceuticals" Addition of a Limit Dose and Related Notes
26. Guidance on Specific Aspects of Regulatory Genotoxicity Tests for Pharmaceuticals
27. Genotoxicity: A Standard Battery for Genotoxicity Testing of Pharmaceuticals
28. Note for Guidance on Toxicokinetics: The Assessment of Systemic Exposure in Toxicity Studies
29. Pharmacokinetics: Guidance for Repeated Dose Tissue Distribution Studies
30. Detection of Toxicity to Reproduction for Medicinal Products
31. Toxicity to Male Fertility: An Addendum to the ICH Tripartite Guideline on Detection of Toxicity to Reproduction for Medicinal Products
32. Preclinical Safety Evaluation of Biotechnology-Derived Pharmaceuticals
33. Non-Clinical Safety Studies for the Conduct of Human Clinical Trials for Pharmaceuticals

Step 2 Draft consensus guidelines
34. Ethnic Factors in the Acceptability of Foreign Clinical Data
35. Statistical Principles for Clinical Trials
36. Specifications: Test Procedures and Acceptance Criteria for New Drug Substances and New Drug Products: Chemical Substances
37. Duration of Chronic Toxicity Testing in Animals (Rodent and Non-rodent Toxicity Testing)

a CTD. They evaluated the time and resources required to convert a new drug application (NDA) to a European Union (EU) application and vice versa. For eight international companies, it took an average of three to four months to convert one submission to the other: obviously a costly operation in terms of time and resources, but the report showed the feasibility of developing the CTD and this was presented to regulators in advance of an ICH Steering Group meeting. The feasibility report revealed slight differences between the three regions in the proposed format of technical dossiers. Agreed harmonisation of format was considered to be relatively easy to achieve, but harmonising content was considered to be harder as differences were greatest between the three regions with regard to the detail required in reports submitted to the regulatory authorities.

Thus the CTD is feasible, but it is a formidable challenge. ICH has already demonstrated its ability to deliver and enforce consensus decisions based on good science and mutual trust. There is therefore an opportunity to develop in common a more logical, more efficient, more user-friendly way of compiling the technical requirements for registration purposes, taking into account the most recent advances of regulatory science and the extraordinary potentials of new information technologies. The ICH Steering Committee agreed to a two-year schedule to produce a document. It was also considered – and this is an important development – that the CTD would apply to generics and OTC products, and that their manufacturers should also be involved in discussions as to content. Up to this point, generic manufacturers and OTC producers had been largely ignored by ICH.

Against this background a Fifth International Conference on Harmonisation took place and a meeting report was prepared.[5]

10.4 ICH 5 Meeting Report: Fifth International Conference on Harmonisation[5] (reproduced with permission)

10.4.1 CTD finalised

Prior to the Conference, during which the ICH Expert Working Group and Steering Committee met, the ultimate objective of ICH 5 was achieved. The common technical document (CTD) was agreed, setting out a harmonised format for regulatory submissions.

- **Module 1 – Administrative Information and Prescribing Information**, which contains documents specific to each region including, for example, application forms or the proposed label for use in the region; the content and format of this module will be specified by the relevant regulatory authorities
- **Module 2 – Summaries:** in addition to a table of contents and a one-page introduction, this module contains the Quality Overall Summary,

the Non-clinical Overview, and the Clinical Overview; these are followed by the Non-clinical Written Summaries, the Non-clinical Tabulated Summaries, and the Clinical Summary; separate documents (M4Q, M4S, and M4E) give guidance on the format and content of the summaries

- **Module 3 – Quality** covers information on manufacture, specifications, quality control and stability, which must be presented in the structured format described in Guideline M4Q
- **Module 4 – Non-clinical Study Reports** covers reports on animal and *in vitro* tests, which must be presented in the order described in Guideline M4S
- **Module 5 – Clinical Study Reports** covers human study reports and related information presented in the order described in Guideline M4F.

10.4.2 Implementation of the CTD

All three of the ICH regulatory parties – the European Commission, FDA, and MHW – made firm commitments to implement the CTD, when their representatives spoke in a panel on "What the CTD will mean to Regulators" in the Closing Plenary.

By common agreement at the ICH Steering Committee meeting, all three parties will accept applications in the CTD format from 1 July 2001.

This will be on a so-called "voluntary" basis, as the time required before implementation can become mandatory will vary according to the formal steps needed in the three regions. It was apparent that a question in the minds of many in the audience was whether the new format would really replace current requirements. At several points in the CTD there is provision for authorities to ask for additional information according to "regional requirements".

Harmonisation of the requirements for summaries (Module 2) has been the most challenging task for the CTD working groups. A background note in the CTD text (see Box 10.1) identifies the current requirements that will be changed by the CTD, but there was concern, for example, that the FDA would still retain an additional "regional" requirement for the integrated safety summary (ISS) and integrated efficacy summary (IES).

Dr Janet Woodcock, Director of the FDA CDER, confirmed that implementation of the CTD would require changes in the CFR and hoped that it would be possible to "rewrite a more flexible and less specific CFR". She cautioned, however, that this would take time and that the full consultations required under the FDA's Good Guidance Practices must be followed. In response to questions about the ISS, she indicated that this was still regarded as a "crucial document" in the assessment of safety but that FDA recognised the need to address the subject further in order to achieve the goal of a single clinical summary.

> **Box 10.1 Extract from the "Organisation of the Common Technical Document" (M4)**
>
> **Background**
>
> "... Each region has its own requirements for the organisation of the technical reports in the submission and for the preparation of the summaries and tables. In Japan, the applicants must prepare the GAIYO, which organises and presents a summary of the technical information. In Europe, expert reports and tabulated summaries are required, and written summaries are recommended. The US FDA has guidance regarding the format and content of the new drug application. To avoid the need to generate and compile different registration dossiers, this guideline describes a format for the common technical document that will be acceptable in all three regions."

Ms Emer Cooke, Principal Administrator in the Pharmaceuticals and Cosmetics Unit of the European Commission Enterprise Directorate-General, presented a timetable under which the CTD could be fully implemented in the EU by July 2002:

- revision of *Notice to Applicants*, Vol IIB, first quarter of 2001
- acceptance of applications in the new format, July 2001
- proposal for revision to Directive 75/318/EEC (technical directive), mid- to end-2001
- date for CTD to become mandatory, provisionally July 2002.

Dr Yoshinobu Hirayama, Director, Evaluation Division 1, of the MHW Pharmaceuticals and Medical Devices Evaluation Centre, confirmed that "the current GAIYO will be replaced by CTD Module II documents". He cautioned, however, that although the CTD provides a common content and format, there will be cases where differences would necessarily occur in dossiers for the three regions (for example, there may be different dosage recommendations and different quality requirements). He sympathised with the impact on industry, which would feel "the burden of transition more than regulators", and indicated that the transition time before the CTD became mandatory might depend on how much preparatory work needs to be done by industry.

10.4.3 e-CTD

Progress on the electronic version of the CTD was discussed. It was anticipated that the e-CTD specification would reach draft consensus (or Step 2 of the ICH process) in May 2001 and be finalised (Step 4) by the end of 2001.

10.4.4 ICH 6 announced

The Sixth International Conference on Harmonisation will take place in Japan in the last quarter of 2003. In the meantime, the next ICH Steering Committee meeting was held in Tokyo, Japan, in May 2001. The priority before that was "continuing work on the implementation of the CTD along with the principles and work plan defined by the ICH Steering Committee".

The Steering Committee issued a statement on the future of ICH which emphasises the intentions of ICH to focus its activities on: implementing and maintaining existing guidelines, preventing disharmony, encouraging scientific dialogue and harmonisation in new areas (for example new technologies or therapies), and undertaking efforts towards global cooperation with non-ICH regions and countries. At its May 2001 meeting, the Steering Committee is expected to discuss practical aspects of the paper, including the possibility of harmonisation efforts in the area of post-marketing activities.

There were, however, no announcements of specific new harmonisation topics.

10.4.5 Globalisation of ICH

The Steering Committee has set up a subcommittee, the Global Cooperation Group (GCG). Its objective is "to facilitate making information available on ICH, ICH activities and ICH guidelines to any country or company that requests the information". The co-Chairpersons of the GCG are Dr Elaine Esber, Associate Director for Medical and International Affairs, CBER, FDA, and Dr Bert Spiker, Senior Vice President for Scientific and Medical Affairs, PhRMA.

10.4.6 Other ICH guidelines

A number of ICH guidelines, in addition to the CTD, reached a significant stage in the expert working group meetings held immediately prior to the Conference.

Quality topics

Q7A   Guideline on Good Manufacturing Practices for Active Pharmaceutical Ingredients was finalised at *Step 4* of the ICH process.
Q1A   Revisions to the Stability Testing Guideline were finalised.
Q1D   A Stability Guideline on Matrixing and Bracketing was released for consultation.

Safety topics

S7   Guideline on Safety Pharmacology Testing was finalised at *Step 4* of the ICH process.

284

S5/M3 Revisions to Toxicokinetics/Pharmacokinetics sections of the Reproductive Toxicology and Timing of Clinical Studies Guidelines were agreed.

10.4.7 Final texts made available

Before the Conference participants departed, they were given a copy of the harmonised guidelines (ICH Code "M4") on a CD-ROM. The text of the Safety Pharmacology Guideline (S7) was also on CD and Guideline Q7 was distributed in hard copy. The documents warned, however, that the texts may be "subject to editorial change", and the final version will be posted on the ICH website [http://www.ifpma.org/ich7.html] and those of the FDA, EU and MHW.

Post-ICH 5, Dr Manuel Zahn, Head of Regulatory Support at Knoll Ag, Ludwigshafen, Germany, provided an update on the common technical document (CTD).[6]

10.5 The Common Technical Document (CTD)

Manuel Zahn provided an update post-ICH 5 (reproduced with permission).

10.5.1 Organisation of the CTD

The common format of the CTD has been changed slightly compared to the Step 2 version agreed in July 2000 (for example, the "Overall Summary" is now called "Overview"). Once again, the CTD pyramid is presented here (Figure 10.2), and also the new version of the Organisation (Table 10.2).

10.5.2 Benefits for authorities and applicants

A common format is of value to both applicants and reviewers as the order of documents is logical, more user-friendly, shortens review time, saves resources and facilitates the exchange of information and discussions. Janet Woodcock, Director of FDA's CDER, speaking at ICH 5, expects more "reviewable" applications, more complete, well-organised submissions, a format which is more predictable, and, as a consequence, more consistent reviews.

10.5.3 Hurdles for harmonisation of the content of Module 3 (Quality)

Unfortunately, until now it was not possible to harmonise the content of the quality dossier in addition to the format. One of the major reasons for this is the fact that there are some areas where there has never been an ICH guideline (for example for the synthesis of drug substances, manufacturing of drug products, process validation and packaging material). This means that national guidelines apply. Also, it seems to be a high priority for the FDA to develop new national guidelines and regulations incorporating ICH guidelines where they exist. In consequence, applicants may be able

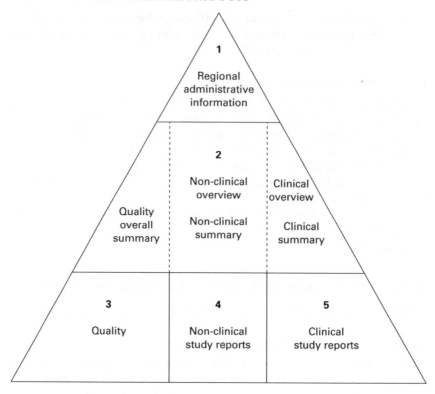

Figure 10.2 Diagrammatic representation of the ICH common technical document (CTD) (overview).

to submit common dossiers but should not expect identical query letters or common decisions issued by the various regulatory agencies concerned.

The other reasons for disharmony of the content is the fact that the three major pharmacopoeias are different in terms of monographs and methods required, with the consequence that industry is forced to duplicate testing and generate different specifications, analytical testing, validation of methods, stability testing, and summaries. In order to harmonise General Methods of Analysis and Excipient Monographs, in 1989 the *Pharmeuropa* (Ph Eur), the *Japanese Pharmacopoeia* (JP), and the *United States Pharmacopeia* (USP) formed a Pharmacopoeial Discussion Group (PDG) (for details of the PDG process see Table 10.3). However, progress is slow. At the time of ICH 5, only four of 11 General Chapters defined as essential in Q6A (Table 10.4) had reached Stage 6 of the PDG Procedure, six are still in Stage 4, and one in Stage 3. Only one Excipient Monograph out of 50 reached Stage 6, 31 are in Stage 5, and nine in Stage 4.

In addition to these regulatory issues there are some homemade limitations to common quality documentation (for example, in the USA,

Table 10.2   Organisation of the common technical document (CTD) for the registration of pharmaceuticals for human use (new table of contents).

Module 1:   Administrative Information and Prescribing Information

    A.   Module 1 Table of Contents
    B.   Documents Specific to Each Region (for example, application forms, prescribing information)

Module 2:   Common Technical Document Summaries

    A.   Overall Common Technical Document Table of Contents
    B.   Introduction
    C.   Quality Overall Summary
    D.   Non-clinical Overview
    E.   Clinical Overview
    F.   Non-clinical Summary

        1.   Pharmacology

            a.   Written Summary
            b.   Tabulated Summary

        2.   Pharmacokinetics

            a.   Written Summary
            b.   Tabulated Summary

        3.   Toxicology

            a.   Written Summary
            b.   Tabulated Summary

    G.   Clinical Summary

        1.   Summary of Biopharmaceutics and Associated Analytical Methods
        2.   Summary of Clinical Pharmacology Studies
        3.   Summary of Clinical Efficacy
        4.   Summary of Clinical Safety
        5.   Synopses of Individual Studies

Module 3:   Quality

    A.   Table of Contents
    B.   Body of Data
    C.   Key Literature References

Module 4:   Non-clinical Study Reports

    A.   Table of Contents
    B.   Study Reports
    C.   Literature References

Module 5:   Clinical Study Reports

    A.   Table of Contents of Clinical Study Reports and Related Information
    B.   Tabular Listing of All Clinical Studies
    C.   Clinical Study Reports
    D.   Literature References

pharmaceutical companies normally prefer to market tablets in polyethylene bottles, in contrast to blister packs for the European market, and different trade names, colours or pack sizes are also unavoidable in certain cases). The consequence of these differences is the fact that a

Table 10.3 The pharmacopoeial discussion group process.

PDG Stage No.	Status
Stage 1	Selection of subjects to be harmonised and nomination of a coordinating pharmacopoeia for each subject
Stage 2	Investigation on the existing specifications, on the grade of products marketed and on the potential analytical methods
	Preparation of a first draft text ("Stage 3 draft")
Stage 3	Publication of the draft text in the forum of each pharmacopoeia: *Pharmeuropa (Ph Eur)*, *Japanese Pharmacopoeial Forum (Japanese Pharmacopoeia)* and *Pharmacopeial Forum (United States Pharmacopeia)*
	Comments received and consolidated
	Preparation of a second draft text ("Stage 4 draft")
Stage 4	Publication of the Stage 4 draft
	Comments received and consolidated
	Preparation of a revised version ("Stage 5A draft")
Stage 5A	Stage 5A draft reviewed and commented on
	Revised provisional harmonised document prepared and reviewed until consensus is reached by all three pharmacopoeias ("Stage 5B draft")
Stage 5B	Consensus document is signed off by the three pharmacopoeias
Stage 6	Adoption of the signed-off document by the organisation responsible for each pharmacopoeia
	Publication of the adopted document by the three pharmacopoeias in supplements or new editions
Stage 7	Implementation of published document in each region

common Module 3 (Quality) and therefore a common Quality Summary in Module 2 cannot be compiled.

10.5.4 Implementation of the CTD format in ICH regions

As of 1 July 2001 all three authorities in the ICH regions are committed to accept CTD-formatted applications on a voluntary basis, and the CTD will become mandatory as of 1 July 2002.

In the meantime, national regulations and guidelines need to be changed in order to avoid any legal conflict within the regulatory framework of each nation involved. In the EU in particular, the *Notice to Applicants* Volume 2B, and Directive 75/318/EEC are affected. The Japanese MHW confirmed that the GAIYO (a 200-page summary in Japanese) will be

Table 10.4 Status of harmonisation of pharmacopoeial general chapters defined as essential in ICH guidelines Q6A.

General chapter	Coordination pharmacopoeia	Status in PDG process
Bacterial endotoxins	JP	Stage 6
Extractable volume of parenteral preparations	Ph Eur	Stage 6
Residue or ignition/sulphated ash	JP	Stage 6
Test for particulate contamination	Ph Eur	Stage 6
Sterility	Ph Eur	Stage 4
Dissociation test for solid dosage forms	USP	Stage 4
Disintegration test	USP	Stage 4
Uniformity of mass	USP	Stage 4
Uniformity of dosage units	USP	Stage 4
Microbial limits for non-sterile products	Ph Eur	Stage 4
Colour/clarity	Ph Eur	Stage 3

replaced by Module 2 of the CTD by changing the current PAB/NDD Notification No. 21 dated 31 March 1992.

In March 2001, the regulators communicated what actions were necessary and what kind of changes were to be made.

In May 2001 in Tokyo, Japan, the Implementation Working Group (IWG) met for the first time to discuss issues that might come to the surface, and to coordinate a smooth implementation of the ICH CTD guideline. Members of the IWG were more or less identical to those of the former CTD EWGs.

It goes without saying that in addition and in parallel to the legal changes to be made, several internal aspects have to be faced by the regulatory agencies concerned, for example:

- the impact of the new format on the current review process has to be checked
- current good review practices need to be adapted
- new templates and technical guidelines are to be set up
- internal training of reviewers and document staff will be required
- a feedback mechanism for applicants based on experience in the voluntary phase will have to be created.

Internationally operating pharmaceutical companies as well as CROs are busy these days with similar activities in order to gain first-hand experience with the new format, and to take part in the voluntary phase by filing applications simultaneously as soon as possible.

Sooner rather than later, CTD-formatted dossiers should also be made acceptable for other types of products (for example generics, line extensions, herbals, radiopharmaceuticals and blood products). Also, applications for clinical trials (for example CTX in the UK, IND in the

USA), as well as applications for variations, and Drug Master Files could be formatted according to the CTD guideline. However, before this becomes reality, national regulations and guidelines need to be adapted accordingly.

10.5.5 Impact on non-ICH countries

In addition to the ICH regions USA, EU and Japan, which agreed to accept a CTD-formatted dossier as of July 2001, other authorities in non-ICH countries announced that they will also accept this, in particular the ICH observers Canada and Switzerland.

The Swiss authorities intend to make the CTD format mandatory as of 1 July 2002 for new chemical entities (NCEs), as of 1 January 2003 for generics, and as of 1 July 2003 for OTC products and herbals. The same applies to the other EFTA countries (i.e. Iceland, Norway and Liechtenstein).

Mike Ward, representing the Canadian authorities' point of view in San Diego, supported a simultaneous filing of applications, and therefore expects an early acceptance of CTD-formatted dossiers. We should all be "singing from the same songbook". However, Mr Ward mentioned some challenges linked to the implementation of the CTD in Canada (for example, defining and adopting requirements, systems and procedure for CTD-based NDS is a complex task; also, the electronic submissions will need to be adjusted to the CTD format). All of this has to be done with limited resources.

On the other hand, an implementation master plan has been drafted and just needs to be completed. The Canadian authorities seem to be committed to ICH and the CTD. Health Canada will continue with its templates used since 1996 for the comprehensive summaries and evaluation reports, adapted according to the CTD guideline.

CEEC countries, South Africa, Australia, New Zealand, and countries in Latin America, the Middle East and southeast Asia are expected to adopt the CTD guideline sooner or later, or at least will hopefully not insist in any particular national format. This means, in consequence, that applicants would just need to compile one common dossier in a modular approach following the CTD format, and would be able to submit this to the authorities concerned in all their target countries at the same time.

10.5.6 Consequences

As the ICH and pharmacopoeia experts continue to develop harmonised guidelines, there is hope that in addition to the format, the content of a registration dossier will also be harmonised. One of the consequences of reaching this final goal, however, could be a mutual recognition of regulatory decisions, and may be even a common decision based on identical data submitted.

10.5.7 Recent developments: Brussels, February 2002

The ICH process is continuous, with the Steering Committee meeting in Brussels on February 2002 reporting on the CTD, eCTD, and MedDRA, the setting up of the Global Cooperation Group, and the status of the technical guidelines. This information can be obtained from the website: www.ifpma.org/lchl.htm. As has been stated the sucess of the ICH process and full implementation of the CTD is fraught with difficulties, not only from current regional reporting differences but also from the impact of local factors such as disease prevalence, ethnicity, and local medical practice. It will require "goodwill" and the "Wisdom of Solomon" to bring together the many disparate views. This of course will be encouraged with the eCTD, which will provide a medium to transfer data through the world instantaneously. These changes will require companies to develop their own technical and human resources to meet the "e" demand.[7]

With the adoption of the ICH CTD from July 2002 and mandatory use in the EU and Japan from July 2003 (and its use strongly encouraged by the USFDA), "aids" to finding our way round the CTD are beginning to appear. One of these is produced by Quintiles Regulatory Affairs Europe as a teaching aid and is reproduced in the *Regulatory Affairs Journal*.[8]

Originally the ICH process, which had its first conference in 1991, was supposed to terminate at ICH3 in 1995. The importance of this issue has superseded any time limitations and preparations are well under way for ICH6 in Osaka 2003.

10.5.8 Recent developments: Washington, September 2002[9]

- Electronic version of Common Technical Document (eCTD) has been adopted and would move forward for adoption in the three ICH Regions
- Paper version of CTD Upgraded/Clarification on Quoting References in the Scientific Literature
- ICH has published a list of frequently asked questions (FAQs) on its website.
- ICH guidelines on Pharmacovigilance have been further developed
- Open workshop on Gene Therapy convened and recommended amongst other topics; the need to review the safety issue relating to Germ-Line integration following administration of either viral or non-viral based vectors
- The steering committee agreed to establish an EWG to develop harmonised Guidelines on Bioequivalence of Biotech Products (Q5)
- Implementation Working Group (IWG) set up to develop recommendations and clarifications for the E5 Guideline on Ethnic Factors in Acceptability of Foreign Clinical Data
- Other guidelines being further developed include

- Residual Solvents (Q3C(M))
- Impurities in new drug products (Q3B)
- Safety Pharmacology Studies for assessing the potential for delayed ventricular repolarisation (QT interval prolongation) by human pharmaceuticals (S7B)

- MeddRA Version 5.1 released
- ICH6, 12–15 November 2003, Osaka

  - To include a special symposium on co-operation with NON-ICH countries
  - Next Steering Committee meetings: February 2003 Tokyo; September 2003 Brussels.

References

1 Cone M, D'Arcy PF, Harron DWG. ICH international conference on harmonisation of technical requirements for registration of pharmaceuticals for human use. *Int Pharm J* 1996;**10**:104–6.
2 D'Arcy PF. ICH 3: a report and background. *Adverse Drug React Toxicol Rev* 1996;**15**:125–7.
3 D'Arcy PF. ICH 4: a report and background. *Adverse Drug React Toxicol Rev* 1997;**16**: 199–206.
4 D'Arcy PF, Harron DWG. Proceedings of the Fourth International Conference on Harmonisation, Brussels 1997. Belfast: Queen's University, 1998.
5 Cone M. Meeting Report: Fifth International Conference on Harmonisation. *Regulatory Affairs J* 2000;**11**:954–5.
6 Zahn M. The Common Technical Document (CTD) Post-ICH 5. *Regulatory Affairs J* 2001;**12**:113–17.
7 Nick C. The CTD and beyond: surviving the impact. *Regulatory Affairs J* 2002;**13**:373–4.
8 Winzenrieth A. CTD roadmap. *Regulatory Affairs J* 2002;**13**:463–8.
9 Cone M. ICH Update. *The Regulatory Affairs Journal* 2002;**13**:814–16.

References (5) and (6) were reproduced with the kind permission of the *Regulatory Affairs Journal* (e-mail: *editors@raj.co.uk*, website: *http://www.raj.co.uk*).

Appendix 1: European guidelines relevant for pharmaceutical physicians

A1.1 Clinical Guidelines (General)

286/95   Note for guidance on non-clinical safety studies for the conduct of human clinical trials for pharmaceuticals (ICH)

289/95   Note for guidance on ethnic factors in the acceptability of foreign clinical data (ICH)

291/95   Note for guidance on general considerations for clinical trials (ICH)

462/95   Note for guidance on clinical investigation of medicinal products in children (EWP)

560/95   Note for guidance on the investigation of drug interactions (EWP)

5608/95   *Concept paper on a directive on the implementation of Good Clinical Practice and clinical trials (EC Consultative Paper)*

280/96   Note for guidance on modified release oral and transdermal dosage forms: Section II (pharmacokinetic and clinical evaluation) (Draft 15) (EWP)

363/96   Note for guidance on statistical principles for clinical trials (ICH)

364/96   Note for guidance on choice of control group in clinical trials (ICH)

197/99   Points to consider concerning endpoints in clinical studies with haematopoietic growth factors for mobilisation of autologous stem cells (EWP)

482/99   Points to consider on switching between superiority and non-inferiority (EWP)

908/99   *Points to consider on multiplicity issues in clinical trials (EWP)*

1776/99   Points to consider on missing data (EWP)

2158/99   Concept paper on the development of a CPMP points to consider on biostatistical/methodological issues arising from recent CPMP discussions on licensing applications: choice of delta (EWP) (Free)

2330/99   Points to consider with applications: 1. Meta-analyses 2. One pivotal study (EWP)

2711/99   Note for guidance on clinical investigation of medicinal products in paediatric population (ICH) (EWP)

2863/99   Concept paper on the development of a CPMP points to consider on biostatistical/methodological issues arising from recent CPMP discussions on licensing applications: adjustment for baseline covariates (EWP) (Free)

2747/00   Note for guidance on coordinating investigator signature of clinical study reports (EWP) (Free)

287/95   *See* **Pharmacovigilance Guidelines**

288/95   *See* **Pharmacovigilance Guidelines**

A1.2   Clinical Guidelines (Therapeutic Class)

205/95   Note for guidance on evaluation of anticancer medicinal products in man (Rev. 1) (EWP)

235/95   Note for guidance on clinical investigation of medicinal products for the treatment of cardiac failure (EWP)

238/95   Note for guidance on clinical investigation of medicinal products in the treatment of hypertension, Revision 1, incorporating an addendum (Rev. 1) (previously numbered EWP/5931/94) (EWP)

552/95   Note for guidance on postmenopausal osteoporosis in women (Rev. 1) (EWP)

553/95   Note for guidance on medicinal products in the treatment of Alzheimer's disease (EWP)

556/95   Points to consider on clinical investigation of slow-acting anti-rheumatic medicinal products in rheumatoid arthritis (EWP)

558/95   Note for guidance on evaluation of new anti-bacterial medicinal products (EWP)

559/95 Note for guidance on the clinical investigation of medicinal products in the treatment of schizophrenia (EWP)

563/95 Note for guidance on clinical investigation of medicinal products in the treatment of Parkinson's disease (EWP)

602/95 Points to consider on the assessment of anti-HIV medicinal product (Rev. 3)

281/96 Note for guidance on clinical investigation of drugs used in weight control (EWP)

986/96 Points to consider: the assessment of the potential for QT interval prolongation by non-cardiovascular medicinal products

021/97 Points to consider on hormone replacement therapy (EWP)

504/97 Points to consider on clinical investigation of medicinal products in the treatment of patients with acute respiratory distress syndrome (EWP) (Free)

518/97 Note for guidance on clinical investigation of medicinal products in the treatment of depression (Rev. 1) (EWP)

784/97 Points to consider on clinical investigation of medicinal products used in the treatment of osteoarthritis (EWP)

785/97 Concept paper on the development of a CPMP points to consider on the evaluation of drugs for the treatment of the irritable bowel syndrome (EWP) (Free)

519/98 Note for guidance on clinical investigation of steroid contraceptives in women (BWP)

559/98 Concept paper on the development of a CPMP note for guidance on clinical investigation of medicinal products for the treatment of osteoporosis in men (EWP) (Free)

560/98 Points to consider on clinical investigation of medicinal products for the treatment of acute stroke (EWP)

561/98 Note for guidance on clinical investigation of medicinal products for the treatment of multiple sclerosis (EWP)

562/98 Points to consider on clinical investigation of medicinal products in the treatment of patients with chronic obstructive pulmonary disease (COPD) (EWP)

563/98 Note for guidance on clinical investigation of medicinal products for the treatment of venous thromboembolic disease (EWP)

565/98 Points to consider on clinical investigation of medicinal products for treatment of Amyotrophic Lateral Sclerosis (ALS) (EWP)

566/98   Note for guidance on clinical investigation of medicinal products in the treatment of epileptic disorders (EWP)

567/98   Note for guidance on clinical investigation of medicinal products for the treatment and prevention of bipolar disorder (Rev. 1) (EWP)

570/98   Points to consider on the clinical investigation of new medicinal products for the treatment of Acute Coronary System (ACS) without persistent ST-segment elevation (EWP)

571/98   Concept paper on the revision of a CPMP note for guidance on clinical investigation of medicinal products for the treatment of cardiac failure (EWP) (Free)

707/98   Points to consider on clinical investigation of medicinal products for prophylaxis of intra- and post-operative venous thromboembolic risk (EWP)

714/98   Note for guidance on clinical investigation of medicinal products for the treatment of peripheral arterial occlusive disease (EWP)

1119/98   Points to consider on the evaluation of diagnostic agents (EWP)

2284/99   Points to consider on clinical investigation of medicinal products for the management of Crohn's disease (EWP)

2655/99   Points to consider on pharmacokinetics and pharmacodynamics in the development of antibacterial medicinal products (EWP)

541/00   ICH principles document for the clinical evaluation of new antihypertensive drugs (ICH)

612/00   *Note for guidance on the clinical investigation of medicinal products for treatment of pain (EWP)*

1080/00   *Note for guidance on clinical investigation of medicinal products on treatment of diabetes mellitus (EWP)*

2922/00   *Note for guidance on the clinical investigation of medicinal products in the treatment of asthma (EWP)*

18/01   *Note for guidance on the clinical investigation of medicinal products for the treatment of urinary incontinence in women (EWP)*

49/01   Concept paper on the development of an appendix to the CPMP note for guidance on the clinical investigation of medicinal products in the treatment of schizophrenia, on methodology of clinical trial concerning the development of depot preparations of approved medicinal products in schizophrenia (EWP) (Free)

512/01   Concept paper on the development of a CPMP note for guidance on the evaluation of medicinal products for the treatment of dyslipoproteinaemia (EWP) (Free)

788/01   Concept paper on the development of a CPMP note for guidance on the evaluation of medicinal products for the treatment of migraine (EWP) (Free)

967/01   Concept paper on the development of a CPMP note for guidance on the evaluation of medicinal products indicated for thrombolysis in acute myocardial infarction (AMI) (Free)

1343/01 Concept paper on the development of a CPMP points to consider document on the evaluation of new anti-fungal agents for invasive fungal infections (EWP) (Free)

1533/01 Concept paper on the development of an addendum on acute cardiac failure to the CPMP note for guidance on clinical investigation of medicinal products in the treatment of acute cardiac failure (CPMP) (Free)

A1.3   Pharmacovigilance

175/95   Note for guidance on the procedure for competent authorities on the undertaking of pharmacovigilance (PhVWP) (Rev. 1)

180/95   Guideline for PMS studies for metered dose inhalers with new propellants

285/95   Note for guidance on recommendations on electronic transmission of individual case safety reports message specification (ICH)

287/95   Note for guidance on clinical safety data management: data elements for transmission of individual case safety reports (ICH) (previously numbered 144/95)

005/96   Revised note for guidance on the Rapid Alert System (RAS) and Non-Urgent Information System (NUIS) in human pharmacovigilance (Rev. 1) (PhVWP)

183/97   Conduct of pharmacovigilance for centrally authorised products

053/98   Principles of providing the World Health Organisation with pharmacovigilance information (PhVWP) (Free)

108/99   Notice to marketing authorisation holders: Pharmacovigilance guidelines (PhVWP)

2056/99 Note for guidance on electronic exchange of pharmacovigilance information for human and veterinary medicinal products in the European Union

2058/99 Joint pharmacovigilance plan for the implementation of the ICH E2B, M1 and M2 requirements related to the electronic transmission on individual case safety reports in the community (EMEA)

2278/00 CPMP position paper on possible pre-clinical studies to investigate addiction and dependence withdrawal related to the use of Selective Serotonin Uptake Inhibitors (SSRIS) (CPMP)

1417/01 Concept paper on the development of a CPMP note for guidance on the use of medicinal products during pregnancy: need for post-marketing data (PhVWP/EWP) (Free)

1618/01 European concept paper on compliance with pharmacovigilance regulatory obligations (PhVWP)

560/95 *See* **Clinical Guidelines (General)**

Reproduced with permission from the Medicines Control Agency from *The MCA European Guideline Service, Retrospective Catalogue and Order Form 1993–2001.* Published by the MCA Euro Direct Publication Service, Room 10–238 Market Towers, Medicines Control Agency, 1 Nine Elms Lane, London SW8 5NQ, T: + 44(0)20 7273 0352, F: + 44(0)20 7273 0353, e-mail: info@mca.gov.uk.

Index

Page numbers in **bold** type refer to figures: those in *italics* refer to tables or boxed materials *v* indicates a comparison
To save space in the index, the following abbreviations have been used
CSD: Committee on Safety of Drugs (UK)
EU: European Union
FDA: Food and Drug Administration (USA)
GMP: good manufacturing practice
ICH: International Conference on Harmonisation
IND: investigational new drug (USA)
NDAs: New Drug Applications (USA)
OTC: over-the-counter drugs
SPC: summary of product characteristics

299

© BMJ Publishing Group 2003
BMJ Books is an imprint of the BMJ Publishing Group

First published by BMJ Books in 2003
BMJ Books, BMA House, Tavistock Square,
London WC1H 9JR

www.bmjbooks.com

British Library Cataloguing in Publication Data
A catalogue record for this book is available from the British Library

ISBN 0 7279 1780 3

Typeset by SIVA Math Setters, Chennai, India
Printed and bound in Spain by GraphyCems, Navarra

The WITHDRAWN Regulation of Medical Products

Edited by

JP Griffin BSc, PhD, MBBS, FRCP, FRCPath, FFPM

Chairman, John Griffin Associates Ltd
Visiting Professor, University of Surrey Postgraduate Medical School
Former Director, Association of the British Pharmaceutical Industry, London
Formerly Professorial Head of the Medicines Division, DHSS, London

and

J O'Grady MD, FRCP, FFPM, MRCPath, FBIRA

Medical Director for Europe, Daiichi Pharmaceutical Co. Ltd, London
Visiting Professor of Clinical Pharmacology, University of London
Member of British Pharmacopoeia Commission

BMJ Books